Child and Adolescent Psychiatry and the Media

Child and Adolescent Psychiatry and the Media

EUGENE V. BERESIN, MD
Professor of Psychiatry
Harvard Medical School
Executive Director, Clay Center for Young Healthy Minds
Department of Psychiatry
Massassachusetts General Hospital/Harvard Medical School
Boston, MA, United States

CHERYL K. OLSON, MPH, ScD
Principal
Cheryl K. Olson, ScD, LLC
San Carlos, CA
United States

ELSEVIER

ELSEVIER

3251 Riverport Lane
St. Louis, Missouri 63043

CHILD AND ADOLESCENT PSYCHIATRY AND THE MEDIA   ISBN: 978-0-323-54854-0

Notices

Content Strategist: Lauren Boyle
Content Development Manager: Kathy Padilla
Content Development Specialist: Karen Miller
Publishing Services Manager: Jameel Shereen
Project Manager: Nadhiya Sekar
Designer: Gopalakrishnan Venkatraman

Printed in United States of America

Last digit is the print number: 9 8 7 6 5 4 3 2 1

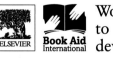

Working together
to grow libraries in
developing countries

www.elsevier.com • www.bookaid.org

List of Contributors

Eliza Abdu-Glass, BA
Research Assistant
Psychiatry
Massachusetts General Hospital
Boston, MA, United States

Robert R. Althoff, MD, PhD
Associate Professor
Psychiatry
University of Vermont
Burlington, VT, United States

Jessica E. Becker, MD
Resident Physician
MGH/McLean Psychiatry Residency
    Program
Massachusetts General Hospital
Boston, MA, United States

Eugene V. Beresin, MD
Executive Director
Clay Center for Young Healthy Minds
Professor of Psychiatry
Massachusetts General Hospital/Harvard Medical
    School
Boston, MA, United States

Jeff Q. Bostic, MD, EdD
Psychiatry Faculty
Medstar Georgetown University
    Hospital
Washington, DC, United States

Patricia A. Cavazos-Rehg, PhD
Associate Professor
Psychiatry
Washington University
St. Louis, MO, United States

Neha P. Chaudhary, MD
Fellow Physician
Child and Adolescent Psychiatry
Massachusetts General Hospital/Harvard Medical
    School
Boston, MA, United States

Ruben Echevarria, MA
Northwestern University
Evanston, IL, United States

Jabari Evans, MSW
Center on Media and Human Development
Northwestern University
Evanston, IL, United States

Michael Feldmeier, MD
Second-Year Fellow
UCLA West LA VA Child Fellowship Program
San Fernando Mental Health Clinic
Granada Hills, CA, United States

Christopher J. Ferguson, PhD
Professor
Psychology
Stetson University
DeLand, FL, United States

Lisa Fortuna, MD
Medical Director of Medicine and Adolescent Psychiatry
Boston University School of Medicine
Boston, MA, United States

Wanda P. Fremont, MD
Professor
Director
Division of Child and Adolescent Psychiatry
SUNY Upstate Medical University
Syracuse, NY, United States

Brianna Hightower, MA
Center on Media and Human Development
Northwestern University
Evanston, IL, United States

James J. Hudziak, MD
Director
Vermont Center for Children, Youth, and Families
Professor
Psychiatry, Medicine, Pediatrics, and Communication
    Sciences
Director
Wellness Environment
University of Vermont
Burlington, VT, United States

Abigail M. Judge, PhD
Assistant in Psychology
Department of Psychiatry
Massachusetts General Hospital
Clinical Instructor in Psychology
Harvard Medical School
Boston, MA, United States

Sylvia J. Krinsky, MD
Assistant Professor of Psychiatry
Child Psychiatry
Tufts University School of Medicine
Boston, MA, United States

Lawrence A. Kutner, PhD
President
Lawrence Kutner, Ph.D., LLC
San Carlos, CA, United States

Alexis R. Lauricella, PhD, MPP
Associate Director
Center on Media and Human Development
Northwestern University
Evanston, IL, United States

Maria Jose Lisotto, MD
Child and Adolescent Psychiatry Fellow
Psychiatry
Massachusetts General Hospital/McLean Hospital
Boston, MA, United States

Silvia B. Lovato, MA
Center on Media and Human Development
Northwestern University
Evanston, IL, United States

Ardis C. Martin, MD
Child, Adolescent, and Adult Psychiatrist
Pacific Coast Psychiatric Associates
Walnut Creek, CA, United States

Cheryl K. Olson, MPH, ScD
Principal
Cheryl K. Olson, Sc.D., LLC
San Carlos, CA, United States

Allison Optican, MD
Resident Physician
Department of Psychiatry
Washington University School of Medicine in St. Louis
St. Louis, MO, United States

Ranna Parekh, MD, MPH
Director
Diversity and Health Equity
American Psychiatric Association
Washington, DC, United States

Caroly Pataki, MD
Health Sciences Clinical Professor
Psychiatry & Biobehavioral Sciences
Geffen School of Medicine at UCLA
Los Angeles, CA, United States

Holly S. Peek, MD, MPH
Instructor
Psychiatry
Harvard Medical School
Boston, MA, United States
Associate Medical Director
McLean Klarman Eating Disorders Center
McLean Hospital
Belmont, MA, United States

Eric Piacentini, BS
Graduate Student in Computer Engineering
Santa Clara University
Santa Clara, CA, United States

Sarah Pila, MA
Center on Media and Human
   Development
Northwestern University
Evanston, IL, United States

Paulina Powell
Student
Candidate for a Bachelor of Science Degree in
   Psychology
Northeastern University
Boston, MA, United States

David C. Rettew, MD
Director
Child & Adolescent Psychiatry Residency Program
University of Vermont Medical
   Center
Burlington, VT, United States

David H. Rubin, MD
Director
Child and Adolescent Psychiatry Residency Training
Massachusetts General Hospital and McLean
   Hospital
Boston, MA, United States

John Sargent, MD
Professor
Psychiatry and Pediatrics
Tufts University School of Medicine

Director
Division of Child and Adolescent
   Psychiatry
Tufts Medical Center
Boston, MA, United States

Steven C. Schlozman, MD
Assistant Professor
Psychiatry
Harvard Medical School/Massachusetts General
   Hospital
Boston, MA, United States

Sven Smith, PhD, JD
Professor
Sociology
Stetson University
DeLand, FL, United States

Anthony D. Sossong, MD, MS
Medical Director
McLean-Franciscan Community-Based Acute Treatment
   Program
McLean Hospital
Belmont, MA, United States

Roxy Szeftel, MD
Clinical Professor of Psychiatry
UCLA Department of Psychiatry and Biomedical
   Sciences
Program Director
UCLA West LA VA Child Fellowship Program
San Fernando Mental Health Clinic
Granada Hills, CA, United States

Kara Sydelle Tabor-Furmark, MD
Psychiatrist
UCLA Child and Adolescent Mood Disorders Clinic
Adelpha Psychiatric Group
Encino, CA, United States

Elvira Perez Vallejos, PhD
Associate Professor of Digital Technology for Mental
   Health
Division of Psychiatry and Applied Psychology
The University of Nottingham
Nottingham, United Kingdom

Ellen A. Wartella, PhD
Director
Center on Media and Human Development
Northwestern University
Evanston, IL, United States

Liora Zhrebker, BA
Clinical Research Coordinator
Psychiatry
Massachusetts General Hospital
Boston, MA, United States

Preface

In 2005, The Child and Adolescent Psychiatric Clinics of North America published the first edition of Child Psychiatry and the Media. Since then, the reach of media and knowledge of media effects on youth, families, clinicians, and society at large have expanded tremendously. Much of this has been due to the development and proliferation of new technologies, and digital media in particular.

When we put together our first book, most homes had an average of three TVs, and many had at least one desktop computer. Since then, most households, children, and parents have laptops, tablets, and—most notably—smartphones. The family-room television has transformed into a smart TV that comes with apps and immediate access to WiFi or mirroring from cell phones. In short, media have become embedded in the fabric of our daily lives in ways we would never have predicted. Perhaps the best example is the ubiquity of social media and its immediacy in connecting people, promoting real and "fake" news, and, at times, escalating drama in our lives.

Media not only influences our children, for better or worse, but becomes a means by which clinicians can draw from it to further conversation or even use it for diagnostic and therapeutic purposes. Beyond its influence on our patients, it has a profound influence on our own perceptions of society. In short, none of us can escape its power. But we can hope to understand its influence and provide guidance for youth, parents, and clinicians.

In this issue, we wish to provide an update on the state of the art of media in our daily lives and clinical practice.

Children and adolescents cannot escape the consequences of media in many areas. In this book, we will examine the effects of violent media on youth, including the use of video games, the effects of reality TV on female body image, the consequences of viewing terrorist acts, how sex and substances in the media impact youth, media portrayals of family life, and how social media may be used by children in cyberbullying and sexting.

Several chapters provide insights and tips for parents and caregivers about how children of different ages and stages perceive, relate to and create with media, how families can responsibly use and sensibly limit digital media, and where to go for help.

Beyond guiding parents and youth, we want to provide guidance for clinicians. Above all, child and adolescent psychiatrists, psychologists, and clinicians of all allied health professions who work with youth and families need to be media literate. They need to know what content children are accessing and its possible effects. They also need to be proactive in helping assess the influence of media on kids. And they need to be able to provide parents and youth reasonable assurance on what media use and observation is developmentally appropriate and safe.

We also hope to help clinicians appreciate the important role that media can play in understanding ethnic and racial stereotypes and to become culturally competent by examining how culturally diverse groups of people are portrayed by others and tell their own stories. Further, we will show the potential for media to be important vehicles for destigmatizing mental illness, and examples of the opposite—how even children's media promote misinformation and inaccurate, if not dangerously misguided, views about mental illness and treatments.

Finally, this volume aims to help clinicians harness media for promoting mental health. This may be done through outreach to the news media, by sharing or discussing media content in our work with children and families, and increasingly via telepsychiatry to increase our clinical reach, given the incredible shortage of child and adolescent psychiatric clinicians worldwide.

We hope that this book will be a useful resource for clinicians and clinical educators. Media in its many forms is part of the fabric of our society and therefore must be part of our practice. With greater understanding of media effects comes greater ability to use media to promote the health and well-being of our children, adolescents, and families.

Gene Beresin and Cheryl Olson

Contents

CHAPTER 1

The Effects of Violent Media on Children

SVEN SMITH, PHD, JD • CHRISTOPHER J. FERGUSON, PHD

In the United States and elsewhere, each mass homicide involving a young male starts a familiar cycle of debate over the influence of popular culture on violence. Such discussions go back as far as the ancient Greeks, who worried over the effects of plays such as *Antigone* on youth. Public officials raise concerns about war play and toy guns on conduct.[1,2] Each new form of entertainment media arouses fears among parents and policy makers about potential harms. For more than a half-century, people have studied the effect of television and movie viewing on children,[3] extending the debate into video games as well. Some say violent media is harmful and others argue that the effects are inconsequential or unclear.

Three different questions are ever-present in this field of study. First, is there a psychological effect of violent media on behavior? Second, are there lasting effects of video game exposure on children? Finally, is there any relationship between violent media, including video games, and acts of physical assault or mass violence? The support for the arguments within these areas is developed from laboratory experiments and large, social science studies, and many of the findings in both of these arenas are very contentious. As of yet, no consensus has emerged among scholars about how to interpret this pool of research. Researchers argue about their substantive findings as well as the methods through which they gained these findings. Some have even suggested that the research methodology itself has been influenced by social narratives linking violent media to sensationalistic examples of societal violence.[4,5] We cover each of these three subtopics below.

MEDIA AND TELEVISION/MOVIE VIOLENCE

Studies involving the effects of violence in television programs and movies are comprised mostly of laboratory-based experiments and correlation-based surveys of convenience samples.

Experiments

Experiments designed to investigate the effect of media violence on youth have been mixed in regard to outcome. Despite these mixed results, some scholars continue to suggest short-term effects of violent media on aggression.[6] As an example of a typical media violence study, Thomas and colleagues[7] showed clips of either action-filled police dramas or volleyball games to small groups of youth (n = 28) or college students (n = 59) before showing them scenes of real-life aggression. The authors argued that participants who watched the crime drama were less physically aroused following the scene of real-life aggression than those watching the volleyball game.[8] However, there have been controversies regarding the degree that such studies inform us about "real-world" aggression.[9] In the case of the Thomas et al. study, the samples were tiny, and it's not clear whether a volleyball game is a good contrast to a police drama or the presence or absence of physical arousal is particularly meaningful. (Presumably, had the respondents been more aroused after the crime drama, this would have been interpreted as them being more interested in and approving of real-world aggression.) In other studies, researchers will commonly attempt to get participants to engage in behaviors that don't much resemble the kinds of aggressive behavior of concern to parents and society, involving attempts to harm another person psychologically or physically. Typical laboratory behavioral measures include punishing opponents with harmless bursts of white noise or filling in the missing letters of words (such that "kill" is more aggressive than "kiss").[10] Oftentimes, these measures are unstandardized, meaning that researchers can pick and choose from among various outcomes those which best fit their hypotheses.[11] Some researchers assert that these laboratory proxy measures of aggression are directly comparable to behaviors outside the laboratory.[12]

Other researchers consider using such outcomes as indicators of aggression to be controversial because the validity of the measures remains unclear.[13] These critics see a distinction between laboratory aggression and real-life actions. In other words, they express concern that, whatever the outcome, supposedly aggressive behaviors measured in laboratories and other controlled experimental environments do not predict violent behavior in real life.

These criticisms can be illustrated using a 2011 study by Krahé et al., which found evidence for small associations between exposure to media violence in the laboratory and mild aggression tasks (e.g., bursts of irritating white noise rendered to an opponent in a reaction time game), but that everyday-life exposure to movie violence did not predict aggression in the laboratory.[14] One reason for this apparent discrepancy may be that experiments provide exposure to only brief clips of media where violent content lacks any narrative context, unlike real-world experience of a movie or television show. Another concern is that the resultant aggressive behaviors also lack context, with apparent endorsement by the researchers themselves, rather than the disapproval that would follow in most real-world settings. One other issue is that closely pairing media violence clips with experimental behaviors that look like aggression could set up demand characteristics (i.e., hypothesis guessing by participants that causes them to change their behavior to what they think they *should* do to benefit the experiment[15]), producing artificial rather than realistic behaviors.

In sum, there is a great disparity between the laboratory measures of aggression utilized in much of the research on media violence and the real-world aggression discussed day-to-day as a true concern. Methodological problems, such as unstandardized aggression measures, the poor matching of conditions (such as police dramas compared to volleyball games), or obvious demand characteristics lead some to question the usefulness and generalizability of such experiments.[4,16] Another point of contention revolves around the brief media clips used in the experiments. The violence exposure is raw, without the possibility for motivation (such as knocking out a violent bully or resolving hostile conflicts with restrained violence) or the calming influence of reason. It lacks the dialogue, plot line, or other context found in the entirety of a movie or television show.

Whatever their worth, it is important to note that these experiments have not provided consistent results. Some studies find small aggression effects; others do not. Thus, deriving conclusions from these studies is difficult. Unfortunately, there are concerns that some scholars have misrepresented the data as more consistent than it actually is, in attempts to advocate for social change.[17]

Societal Data

Researchers have also looked beyond the laboratory in studying factors related to aggression in youth. Such scholars instead work within the framework of correlative studies that involve questions regarding media consumption and indicators of aggression or violence in real-life relationships. The ongoing debate regarding the effects of watching violence on television, the movie screen, or computer screen continues here as well. Some of this research has suggested that, for youth and young adults, there is a correlation between greater amounts of violent media consumption and greater amounts of aggression.[18] (Of course, there may be other reasonable explanations for this observation. For instance, individuals from lower-income neighborhoods with a poverty of extracurricular options may watch more TV and, due to their socially disadvantaged status, be at higher risk for aggression.)

Other studies have failed to support this correlation. In particular, longitudinal studies suggest that one's peer associations, family, mental health, and personal traits are likely to predict criminal behavior, but media exposure does not.[19,20] (Some older longitudinal studies may also be compromised by changing social perceptions. For example, one[21] classified relatively mild action-oriented television shows such as Road Runner cartoons or *The Six Million Dollar Man* as "violent content" when few people would do so today.) These findings are supported by evidence that youth violence has greatly decreased, while media violence has demonstrably increased.[4,22,23] Likewise, reviews of preventative efforts for youth violence rarely mention reducing media violence as a useful avenue.[24]

As with experimental studies, there have been numerous critiques of this research's ability to support violent media consumption as a risk factor for violent or aggressive behavior. First, many studies do not control for the effects of important third variables which may explain any small relationship between violent media and aggressiveness. Correlations often disappear once these variables, related to personality, family environment, genetics, or mental health, are controlled.[4] For example, gender is an important factor to control given that boys both consume more violent media and act more aggressively. Likewise, genetic traits may predict both a person's natural aggressiveness and proclivity toward viewing violent media.[25] Failure to control for such variables can result in spurious correlations.

Correlational studies of media violence frequently invent ad hoc aggression measures rather than using those that have been standardized, validated, and tested (see Savage, 2004 for discussion[26]). Scholars commonly misrepresent both the magnitude of effect as well as the consistency of findings in correlational research. One example is a study by Coyne[27] following 467 adolescents over 3 years to examine the impacts of physical and relational aggression on television to similar behavioral outcomes. Physical aggression on TV was interpreted as predicting physical aggression in boys (using a relaxed $P = .10$ standard for statistical significance) although the effect size was near zero ($r = 0.02$). Similarly, although TV relational aggression was statistically significant in predicting relational aggression among teens, the effect size was merely $r = 0.06$. Thus, the relationship between TV aggression exposure and teen aggression was a very weak support for any practical association. Given that no documented effort was made to control for other theoretically important variables (which could possibly render the original relationship insignificant), communicating this as meaningful evidence linking TV aggression to real-world aggression is deeply misleading. Put simply, correlational research has failed to consistently find that media violence exposure is a risk factor for aggressive behaviors, whether mild or serious.

VIDEO GAMES AND ADOLESCENTS

Many of the same arguments regarding generalized media also pertain to video games and the effect of the violence contained therein.

Video Games and Youth Aggression

As with other media, much of the discussion regarding children and video games has centered around aggression. Public fear of the effects of video game violence has only increased as the games have grown more graphic in their display of violence. Some researchers have implied that their studies may be generalized to mass shooting events, such as the Virginia Tech massacre,[28] and put forth the notion that video games predispose adolescents toward a lifetime of aggressive behavior. Social scientists remain divided over whether there is a true connection between video games and the aggression levels of the youth who play them. Even if it were true that video games promote some minor acts of aggression (e.g., giving people hot sauce to eat when you know they don't like spicy foods), it does not tell us much about the violent criminal acts most of society is concerned with.

Experimental studies of video game effects randomly assign individuals to violent or nonviolent games and then compare their outcomes on aggression measures similar to those seen in other media violence research. However, serious validity issues have emerged for many of these studies. To begin, most studies fail to adequately match these different styles of games (violent and nonviolent) with regard to other characteristics (e.g., difficulty and intensity).[29] As with other experiments involving media violence, serious concerns remain regarding the validity of aggression measures in experimental studies and whether these measures truly measure "aggression" or other variables such as competitiveness.

A classic example is the Taylor Competitive Reaction Time Test, often used in studies of media violence. Respondents in a reaction-time game give supposed opposing players (who do not, in fact, exist) bursts of annoying white noise as punishment for losing in the game. As respondents can set louder and longer bursts, it was thought this measure may tap into aggression. However, given that respondents have explicit permission from the experimenter to set loud noise blasts, and the other player is apparently consenting to receiving them as part of the game, it is not clear that this measure meets definitions of aggression as opposed to friendly competition. Further, the measure is unstandardized with, at last count, over 150 different ways of "extracting" aggression from it. These different methods of extracting aggression don't correlate well with each other, making it possible for a researcher, using the same sample, to make it appear as if video games increase, decrease, or have no influence on aggression.[11]

Similar to other forms of media violence, results from studies of violent video games have been mixed. Many recent experiments have not found evidence for violent game effects on aggressive behaviors or hostile emotion.[9,30,31] Although some research has produced support for minor aggression increases due to violent game play,[32] other studies have found little or no effect for violent games on aggression.[4,31] Some empirical research suggests that violent video games *decrease* aggression,[33−35] particularly when played cooperatively. Further, longer periods of gameplay appear to be associated with reduced aggression in some players.[31] Thus, conclusive statements of effects are difficult to support.

Correlational studies of violent video game effects have likewise been mixed. Weak correlations found in some studies could very possibly be explained by additional variables such as depression, social associations, other personal struggles such as personality disorders, or domestic violence.[36] As with general media violence viewing, being male may correlate with video game usage and also predict greater levels of aggressive behavior. Therefore gender and other third variables should be taken into account when attempting to determine how great a relationship violent video games may have with aggressive behavior.[37]

The landscape of violent video game research resembles that of violent media more generally. Overall, research evidence is weak, inconsistent, and marred by serious methodological limitations. As we'll discuss in a later section, this has not prevented some scholars and groups such as the American Psychological Association (APA) from claiming that research conclusively links violent video games to aggression.[38]

Sexist Games

Another area of video game effects research focuses on players' views of gender and appropriate treatment of women. In the past decade, concerns that some games promoted sexual objectification of women have received greater attention.[39] Some scholars express concern that these video games are teaching sexism to youth as part of a larger narrative perpetuated by mainstream media. They further argue that sexism in video games correlates with negative views of women in real life and that girls and young women are encouraged to see females as submissive and sexually objectified when playing such games.[40]

Our critique of this material is nearly identical to the critiques of the research that claims that media causes aggression. Results of studies on sexist content in media have not been consistent.[41] In fact, research has found support for the notion that certain combinations of sex and violence in media (such as crime dramas) can have little effect or even positive effects on viewer/player attitudes toward women.[42]

Results of studies regarding sexism in video games have been mixed, with some finding evidence for effects on negative outcomes such as benevolent (but not hostile) sexism toward women.[43] Benevolent sexism refers to overly positive and protective attitudes toward women, such as viewing women as more morally pure or needing the protection of men. Other studies have not found evidence that playing games with sexist content influences sexist attitudes.[44] One experimental study of 86 women found that using sexualized avatars may decrease female players' rape myth acceptance (score on a scale of false beliefs, e.g., that women invite or deserve rape), unless the avatar has the player's own face (raising the possibility that playing a character representing a sexualized version of oneself might be psychologically harmful).[45]

Several other critiques have been made of studies purporting to show that games promote sexist beliefs in their players. First, there is no standard accepted definition of what may be considered a sexist game or sexist sequence within a game. For instance, if the absence or minimal role of female characters would be considered sexist, this opens up numerous games to such a charge, including *Pac Man*. But it may be difficult to imagine such games having a strong influence on player attitudes. Other games, such as the *Grand Theft Auto* series, have potentially sexist content. However, "sandbox" games such as these often leave it to player choice whether such content is even accessed, making real-world effects difficult to assess. Second, there is a dearth of theory to support why games labeled as sexist by researchers would discourage empathy regarding women or increase sexist attitudes. Empathy development appears to be driven mainly by a mixture of genetics and early childhood experiences with family and culture. Most empathy development is completed by the time children are likely to access more controversial games. Third, in many studies examining the impact of sexist games, methodological concerns and even data mismanagement have been critical problems (see Ref. 46 for discussion).

An example of the problems in this area involve an experimental study of Italian adolescents by Gabbiadini et al.,[47] which claimed a link between "sexist" video games and a reduction in empathy toward women among male players who identified with the game avatar. Ferguson and Donnellan sought to replicate this study and evaluate the strength of its claims; they found a number of issues with procedures and measures. For example, random assignment of subjects, while claimed, had not in fact been done. Age had become hopelessly conflated with game condition, such that most of the younger adolescents played sexist games and the older adolescents nonsexist ones. When reanalyzed, the evidence was not sufficient to make claims of either direct or indirect effects for sexist games on player empathy toward girls and women.[47] This is a useful reminder of the need to check the methodology of studies before blindly accepting claims made in abstracts or press releases.

Positive Effects of Video Game Use

There has also been a lively, though smaller, debate in the literature regarding the positive ramifications of video games on young users. Young adults and adolescents agree that there are many benefits in video games.[48,49] Jackson and colleagues reported findings that 12-year-olds demonstrated greater creativity when they played video games.[50] Lenhart and colleagues similarly found that video game play is a largely positive activity for much of youth, particularly in relation to social interaction, reduced loneliness, and stress reduction.[51] Granic et al.[52] conclude that gaming is a way for modern youth to take part in activity that is viewed as socially positive.

Other research has extended the breadth of discovery for the positive ramifications of video game play in youth. Research that examined whether video games are useful for inclusion in education has generally returned affirmative results.[53] For example, Adachi and Willoughby concluded that video games which required some strategizing promoted problem-solving skill confidence and also contributed to better academic performance.[29] Ventura, Shute, and Zhao[54] suggest that the gaming environments teach players that persistence beyond failure provides reward. Although there are reasonable concerns that research on positive effects, just as with negative effects, could be ripe for overstatement (such as claims that games can boost IQ or prevent dementia), there are indicators that there are some benefits to playing games, including for stress relief and socialization opportunities among gamers.[53] It is also worth noting that it may be beneficial for the field to focus on specific games or game genres rather than considering games (or violent games) as a universal sweeping category. This may help add sophistication to a debate that has often failed to establish clear conceptual boundaries for what effects it hopes to test.

MEDIA VIOLENCE AND THE POLICY REALM

The American Psychological Association 2015 Policy Statement and Resultant Debate

In 2005, the APA released a policy statement wherein it institutionally supported the notion of a link between media and aggression (2005).[38] In 2013, the APA decided to update its policy statement regarding video game violence. A task force of APA members was appointed by a process which was not made transparent. The majority of members had previously taken strong public stances against video games, which led to questions about the objectivity of the task force and its stated purpose. Hearing about this process, over 230 scholars in criminology, psychology, and media signed a letter to the APA requesting they refrain from releasing policy statements conclusively linking video games to aggression or violence.[55]

The 2015 APA task force's report concluded that violent video game use does affect aggression and that this effect is manifested both as an increase in negative outcomes (such as aggressive behavior, cognitions, and affect) and as a decrease in positive outcomes (such as prosocial behavior, empathy, and sensitivity to aggression).[56] This report was not received positively among many scholars or in news media coverage,[57] and claims of bias persisted. Concerns also emerged that the task force had only considered a small number of empirical articles in their meta-analysis and had largely excluded null studies. In 2017, the APA's Division 46 (Media Psychology and Technology) released a public education statement noting that conclusive statements about aggression effects were not possible to make based on the data and that journalists and policy makers should refrain from linking video games to violence.[58]

The argument between the scholars who believe the effects of video games are real and properly evidenced and those who believe them to be minor or wholly lacking in proper empirical support continues. This argument deals much with methodology as much as it does with the results and generalizability of those results. Elson and Ferguson,[59] in their overview of video game research, found that much of the research relied upon by those who promote the idea that video games encourage an increase in aggression is limited by significant methodological issues (as detailed earlier in this chapter). Publication bias also remains a significant problem for the field. At present, the research base is not of a quality or consistency necessary to support claims of a clear link between video game violence and aggression or violence in society.

MASS HOMICIDES AND MEDIA

The 1990s saw the creation of video game rating boards, such as the British Board of Film Classification and Pan European Game Information and the Entertainment Software Ratings Board in the United States, in response to political outcry of a need to militate against alleged dangers of video games and violent media. Some states attempted to regulate the sale of games indicated as violent to minors.[60] Political influence, often hastily misplaced, encouraged the trend wherein certain homicides were attributed to video games or another media influence.[61] Public officials claimed that one cause of the violent behavior by some young shooters could be violent video game play. For example, the perpetrator in the Sandy Hook shooting was initially alleged to have been an obsessed violent video game player in news media and by some politicians and scholars. An official report later indicated that the perpetrator had played primarily nonviolent games, particularly *Dance Dance Revolution*.[62] Similar false claims were made about Seung Hui Cho, the shooter in the Virginia Tech massacre in 2007. The official report[63] of that state's review panel stated that as a child, Cho "played video games like *Sonic the Hedgehog*. None of the video games were war games or had violent themes" (p. 32). In college, "Cho's roommate never saw him play video games" (p. 42).

Despite the fact that most academic research involved minor measures of aggression that had little to do with violent shootings, it became increasingly common during the 2000s for scholars to draw causal implications between mass violence and violent media.[28] The behavior of such scholars may have done much to promote cultural beliefs linking violent games and media to mass shooting events and other acts of societal violence.[22]

NATIONAL STUDIES OF SCHOOL SHOOTINGS

Considering the uncertainty in this area and the political push for investigation of the causal effects of video games on children, there have been two attempts by the federal government to analyze mass killers: one by the US Secret Service and Department of Education performed in 2002 ("SSDE Report") and another by the Congressional Research Service ("CRS"). The SSDE report was based on the research performed on the descriptive analysis of 41 school shooters performing 37 school shootings between 1974 and 2000. In addition, the Secret Service interviewed the 10 surviving perpetrators and individually investigated the court, mental health, and school records of these attackers. Their most interesting finding was that the attackers' video game usage was *below* that of persons of similar age. Specifically, only 15% of the shooters admitted or were known by witnesses or records to display interest in violent media. The report details that the most common violent media to which the shooters were exposed were the shooters' own journals and log entries. Thirty-seven percent of the shooters created hate-filled prose.[64]

The CRS, in an attempt to develop a profile of mass murderers, enlarged the focus from school shootings to mass killings in general. However, its findings were even more supportive of a notion that video games do not encourage aggression in youth. The report explained that most mass killings are not performed by youth but by middle-aged white males with histories of mental illness. Most notable in the report is the absence of any claims of media effects. In other words, the CRS did not find video games or mass media of any kind as a constant theme in its research. The report's only mention of media is that mass media exacerbates the public's fear of mass killings. As such, no confirmatory evidence has emerged to suggest that mass killings are induced or even mildly encouraged by video game playing or violent media.

CONCLUSION

There are indications that researchers are becoming more aware of the possibility that mass fear, political movement, or research agendas may be encouraging the questionable conclusion that adolescents are effected by media to become overly aggressive, delinquent, or even violent. Media violence can unfortunately serve to distract attention and funding from well-supported risk factors for harmful aggression and violence. Regarding societal violence, what should society be focusing on, if not video games? The SSDE's report provides some guidance on this matter. The SSDE reports that 81% of all perpetrators of the school shootings informed others before they committed the acts; similarly, 93% demonstrated behaviors that caused alarm to some people in the perpetrator's social sphere. This suggests that society should focus away from video games and movies, and rather on improving communication with law enforcement, and on improving mental health services. This fits with the recent recommendations of the APA's division for Media Psychology and Technology, which specifically suggest that politicians and news media avoid linking violent media to societal violence. Focusing on media can distract society from more pressing issues that cause violence, including income and educational disparities, poor mental healthcare, and gun control issues.

There are signs that both scholars and the general public have become more skeptical of claims linking violent media to societal violence. Many scholars,[65] clinicians,[66] and the public challenge the claims linking violent video games to adolescent acts of aggression.[67] It is clear that this research field is in need of revitalization. Scholars need to be more cautious in linking violent media to aggression or societal violence as there is no solid research base on which to make sweeping claims of effects. Adoption of open science principles, such as preregistration (scholars publishing their data collection and analysis plan in advance of data collection so that results cannot be easily tinkered with to produce a desired outcome), may help provide greater understanding of effects, as may purposeful efforts to avoid publication bias. Until the field reforms, it is likely to remain part of social science's replication crisis, in which many previous findings thought to be true are proving false when tested under more rigorous methods of open science.[68]

REFERENCES

1. Levin DE. Beyond banning war and superhero play. *Young Child.* 2003;61.
2. Watson M, Peng Y. The relation between toy gun play and children's aggressive behavior. *Early Educ Dev.* 1992;3(4): 370–389.
3. Anderson J. The production of media violence and aggression research: a cultural analysis. *Am Behav Sci.* 2008;51(8):1260–1279. Available from: PsycINFO, Ipswich, MA.
4. Ferguson C. Do angry birds make for angry children? A meta-analysis of video game influences on children's and adolescents' aggression, mental health, prosocial behavior, and academic performance. *Perspect Psychol Sci.* 2015; 10(5):646–666.
5. Anderson C, Gentile D. *Media Violence, Aggression, and Public Policy. Beyond Common Sense: Psychological Science in the Courtroom.* Malden: Blackwell Publishing; 2008: 281–300.
6. Bushman B, Huesmann L. Twenty-five years of research on violence in digital games and aggression revisited: a reply to Elson and Ferguson (2013). *Eur Psychol.* 2014;19(1): 47–55.
7. Thomas MH, Horton RW, Lippincott EC, Drabman RS. Desensitization to portrayals of real-life aggression as a function of exposure to television violence. *J Personal Soc Psychol.* 1977;35(6):450–458.
8. Homas M, Horton R, Lippincott E, Drabman R. Desensitization to portrayals of real-life aggression as a function of television violence. *J Personal Soc Psychol.* 1977;35(6): 450–458.
9. Ferguson C, Rueda S, Cruz A, Ferguson D, Fritz S, Smith S. Violent video games and aggression: causal relationship or byproduct of family violence and intrinsic violence motivation? *Crim Justice Behav.* 2008;35(3):311–332.
10. Anderson C, Dill K. Video games and aggressive thoughts, feelings, and behavior in the laboratory and in life. *J Personal Soc Psychol.* 2000;78(4):772–790.
11. Elson M, Mohseni M, Breuer J, Scharkow M, Quandt T. Press CRTT to measure aggressive behavior: the unstandardized use of the competitive reaction time task in aggression research. *Psychol Assess.* 2014;26(2):419–432.
12. Bushman B. Moderating role of trait aggressiveness in the effects of violent media on aggression. *J Personal Soc Psychol.* 1995;69(5):950–960.
13. Kutner L, Olson C. *Grand Theft Childhood: The Surprising Truth about Violent Video Games and What Parents Can Do.* New York, NY, US: Simon & Schuster; 2008.
14. Krahé B, Möller I, Huesmann L, Kirwil L, Felber J, Berger A. Desensitization to media violence: links with habitual media violence exposure, aggressive cognitions, and aggressive behavior. *J Personal Soc Psychol.* 2011;100(4): 630–646.
15. Orne M. On the social psychology of the psychological experiment: with particular reference to demand characteristics and their implications. *Am Psychol.* 1962;17(11): 776–783.
16. Savage J, Yancey C. The effects of media violence exposure on criminal aggression: a meta-analysis. *Crim Justice Behav.* 2008;35(6):772–791. Available from: PsycINFO, Ipswich, MA.
17. Markey P, Males M, French J, Markey C. Lessons from Markey et al. (2015) and Bushman, et al. (2015): sensationalism and integrity in media research. *Hum Commun Res.* 2015;41(2):184–203.
18. Anderson C, Shibuya A, Saleem M, et al. Violent video game effects on aggression, empathy, and prosocial behavior in Eastern and Western countries: a meta-analytic review. *Psychol Bull.* 2010;136(2):151–173.
19. Ferguson C. Video games and youth violence: a prospective analysis in adolescents. *J Youth Adolesc.* 2011;40(4): 377–391.
20. Breuer J, Vogelgesang J, Quandt T, Festl R. Violent video games and physical aggression: evidence for a selection effect among adolescents. *Psychol Popul Media Cult.* 2015; 4(4):305–328.
21. Huesmann L, Moise-Titus J, Podolski C, Eron L. Longitudinal relations between children's exposure to TV violence and their aggressive and violent behavior in young adulthood: 1977–1992. *Dev Psychol.* 2003;39(2):201–221.
22. Markey P, French J, Markey C. Violent movies and severe acts of violence: sensationalism versus science. *Hum Commun Res.* 2015;41(2):155–173.
23. Centers for Disease Control. *Nonfatal Assaults among Persons Aged 10–24 Years — United States, 2001–2015*; 2018. Retrieved from: https://www.cdc.gov/mmwr/ volumes/67/wr/mm6705a1.htm?s_cid=mm6705a1_w.
24. Lösel F, Farrington D. Direct protective and buffering protective factors in the development of youth violence. *Am J Prev Med.* 2012;43(2, suppl 1):S8–S23.
25. Schwartz J, Beaver K. Revisiting the association between television viewing in adolescence and contact with the criminal justice system in adulthood. *J Interpers Violence.* 2016;31(14):2387–2411.
26. Savage J. Does viewing violent media really cause criminal violence? A methodological review. *Aggress Violent Behav.* 2004;10(1):99–128. https://doi.org/10.10 16/j.avb.2003.10.001.
27. Coyne S. Effects of viewing relational aggression on television on aggressive behavior in adolescents: a three-year longitudinal study. *Dev Psychol.* 2016;52(2):284–295.
28. Anderson C. An update on the effects of playing violent video games. *J Adolesc.* 2004;27(1):113–122.
29. Adachi P, Willoughby T. The effect of violent video games on aggression: is it more than just the violence? *Aggress Violent Behav.* 2011;16(1):55–62.
30. Przybylski A, Deci E, Rigby C, Ryan R. Competence-impeding electronic games and players' aggressive feelings, thoughts, and behaviors. *J Personal Soc Psychol.* 2014; 106(3):441–457.
31. Unsworth G, Devilly G, Ward T. The effect of playing violent video games on adolescents: should parents be quaking in their boots? *Psychol Crime L.* 2007;13(4): 383–394.

32. Sestir M, Bartholow B. Violent and nonviolent video games produce opposing effects on aggressive and prosocial outcomes. *J Exp Soc Psychol.* 2010;46(6):934−942.

33. Charles E, Baker C, Hartman K, Easton B, Kreuzberger C. Motion capture controls negate the violent video-game effect. *Comput Hum Behav.* 2013;29(6):2519−2523.

34. Velez J, Mahood C, Ewoldsen D, Moyer-Gusé E. Ingroup versus outgroup conflict in the context of violent video game play: the effect of cooperation on increased helping and decreased aggression. *Commun Res.* 2014;41(5): 607−626.

35. Jerabeck J, Ferguson C. The influence of solitary and cooperative violent video game play on aggressive and prosocial behavior. *Comput Hum Behav.* 2013;29(6): 2573−2578.

36. Ferguson C, Cruz A, Martinez D, Rueda S, Ferguson D, Negy C. Personality, parental, and media influences on aggressive personality and violent crime in young adults. *J Aggress Maltreat Trauma.* 2008;17(4):395−414.

37. Ferguson C, Miguel C, Hartley R. A multivariate analysis of youth violence and aggression: the influence of family, peers, depression, and media violence. *J Pediatr.* 2009; 155(6):904−908.

38. American Psychological Association. Resolution on Violence in Video Games and Interactive Media. http://www.apa.org/about/policy/interactive-media.pdf.

39. Beck V, Boys S, Rose C, Beck E. Violence against women in video games: a prequel or sequel to rape myth acceptance? *J Interpers Violence.* 2012;27(15):3016−3031.

40. Dill K, Thill K. Video game characters and the socialization of gender roles: young people's perceptions mirror sexist media depictions. *Sex Roles.* 2007;57(11−12):851−864.

41. Garos S, Beggan J, Kluck A, Easton A. Sexism and pornography use: toward explaining past (null) results. *J Psychol Hum Sex.* 2004;16(1):69−96.

42. Lee M, Hust S, Zhang L, Zhang Y. Effects of violence against women in popular crime dramas on viewers' attitudes related to sexual violence. *Mass Commun Soc.* 2011;14(1): 25−44.

43. Stermer S, Burkley M. SeX-Box: exposure to sexist video games predicts benevolent sexism. *Psychol Popul Media Cult.* 2015;4(1):47−55.

44. Breuer J, Kowert R, Festl R, Quandt T. Sexist games=Sexist gamers? A longitudinal study on the relationship between video game use and sexist attitudes. *Cyberpsychol Behav Soc Netw.* 2015;18(4):197−202.

45. Fox J, Bailenson J, Tricase L. The embodiment of sexualized virtual selves: the Proteus effect and experiences of self-objectification via avatars. *Comput Hum Behav.* 2013; 29(3):930−938.

46. Ferguson Christopher J, Donnellan M Brent. The association between sexist games and diminished empathy remains tenuous: lessons from Gabbiadini et al.(2017) and Gabbiadini et al.(2016) regarding sensationalism and accuracy in media research. *Journal of Youth and Adolescence.* 2017:2467−2474.

47. Gabbiadini A, Riva P, Andrighetto L, Volpato C, Bushman BJ. Acting like a tough guy: violent-sexist video games, identification with game characters, masculine beliefs, & empathy for female violence victims. *PLoS One.* 2016;11(4):e0152121.

48. Olson CK. Children's motivations for video game play in the context of normal development. *Rev Gen Psychol.* 2010;14(2):180−187.

49. Whitbourne S, Krauss S, Akimoto K. Reasons for playing casual video games and perceived benefits among adults 18 to 80 years old. *Cyberpsychol Behav Soc Netw.* 2013; 16(12):892−897.

50. Jackson L, Zhao Y, Kolenic A, Fitzgerald H, Harold R, Von Eye A. Race, gender, and information technology use: the new digital divide. *Cyberpsychol Behav.* 2008;11(4):437−442.

51. Lenhart A, Kahne J, Middaugh E, et al. *Teens, Video Games, and Civics: Teens' Gaming Experiences Are Diverse and Include Significant Social Interaction and Civic Engagement.* Pew Internet & American Life Project; 2008.

52. Granic I, Lobel A, Engels R. The benefits of playing video games. *Am Psychol.* 2014;69(1):66−78.

53. Annetta L, Lamb R, Minogue J, et al. Safe science classrooms: teacher training through serious educational games. *Inf Sci.* 2014;264:61−74.

54. Ventura M, Shute V, Zhao W. The relationship between video game use and a performance-based measure of persistence. *Comput Educ.* 2013;60(1):52−58.

55. Consortium of Scholars. *Scholars' Open Statement to the APA Task Force on Violent Media* (Delivered to the APA Task Force, 9/26/13). http://christopherjferguson.com/APA%20Task%20Force%20Comment1.pdf.

56. American Psychological Association. *Resolution on Violence in Video Games and Interactive Media.* http://www.apa.org/pi/families/review-video-games.pdf.

57. Wofford T. *APA Says Video Games Make You Violent, but Critics Cry Bias;* August 2015. Retrieved from: http://www.newsweek.com/apa-video-games-violence-364394.

58. American Psychological Association. *APA's Division 46 (Media Psychology and Technology).* https://div46amplifier.com/2017/06/12/news-media-public-education-and-public-policy-committee/.

59. Elson M, Ferguson C. Twenty-five years of research on violence in digital games and aggression: empirical evidence, perspectives, and a debate gone astray. *Eur Psychol.* 2014;19(1):33−46.

60. Ferguson CJ, Coulson M, Barnett J. Psychological profiles of school shooters: positive directions and one big wrong turn. *J Police Crisis Negot.* 2011;11(2):141−158.

61. Copenhaver A. Violent video game legislation as pseudo-agenda. *Crim Justice Stud.* 2015;28(2):170−185.

62. State's Attorney for the Judicial District of Dansbury. *Report of the State's Attorney for the Judicial District of Danbury on the Shootings at Sandy Hook Elementary School and 36 Yogananda Street, Newtown, Connecticut on December 14, 2012.* Danbury, CT: Office of the State's Attorney Judicial District of Danbury; 2013.

63. Virginia Tech Review Panel. *Report of the Virginia Tech Review Panel*; 2007. Retrieved from: http://www.governor.virginia.gov/TempContent/techPanelReport.cfm.

64. Ferguson C. The school shooting/violent video game link: casual relationship or moral panic? *J Investig Psychol Offender Profil.* 2008;5(1–2):25–37.

65. Quandt T, Van Looy J, Vogelgesang J, et al. Digital games research: a survey study on an emerging field and its prevalent debates. *J Commun.* 2015;65(6):975–996.

66. Ferguson C. Clinicians' attitudes toward video games vary as a function of age, gender and negative beliefs about youth: a sociology of media research approach. *Comput Hum Behav.* 2015;52:379–386.

67. Przybylski A. Who believes electronic games cause real world aggression? *Cyberpsychol Behav Soc Netw.* 2014; 17(4):228–234.

68. Open Science Collaboration. Estimating the reproducibility of psychological science. *Science.* 2015;349(6251):1–8.

FURTHER READING

1. Media Psychology and Technology Division. *Societal Violence and Video Games*; 2017. Retrieved from: https://div46 amplifier.com/2017/06/12/news-media-public-education-and-public-policy-committee/.

CHAPTER 2

Distorted Reality: Reality Television and the Effects on Female Body Image

HOLLY S. PEEK, MD, MPH

INTRODUCTION

Reality television programming is a huge part of our television-viewing culture. From the birth of reality TV's popularity with MTV's *The Real World* in the 1990s and ABC's *Survivor* in 2000, reality TV has blossomed to include a wide variety of content. This programming ranges from shows featuring the drama-filled lives of the rich and famous to shows featuring "regular people" as they compete in dating competitions or undergo major transformations through plastic surgery and weight loss. A Nielsen report from 2011 demonstrated that since 2002–03, reality TV has consistently captured the largest percentage of audience watching the top 10 broadcast programming.[1] Preteens and adolescents seem to be particularly drawn to this genre of television programming, with reality programs ranking as some of the most-viewed television programming by this demographic.[2]

But not all is real in the reality world of television. While this may be clearer to mature audiences, the line between reality and television can be blurred for children and adolescents. Unlike sitcoms, animated films, and fashion magazines, reality TV inherently gives the indication that what is being portrayed on the screen is in fact *reality*. What exactly are our youth learning from reality TV, if anything?

The Girl Scouts of America conducted a survey of 1100 girls aged 11–17 years across the United States to discover their thoughts on reality television.[3] Of those surveyed, 47% identified themselves as "regular" viewers of reality television, 30% watched the programming "sometimes," and 23% "rarely" watched. Regardless of the frequency of viewership, a majority of the girls believed the reality shows reflected real life, stating they were "mainly real and unscripted."

This becomes particularly problematic when many reality shows depict women idealizing beauty, thinness, and material wealth, as well as giving poor examples of appropriate behavior among peer groups by promoting drama and interpersonal aggression. Additionally, many have argued that mass media are one of the principal factors behind body dissatisfaction, concerns about weight, and disordered eating.[4] When reality television blurs the line between entertainment and reality, the potential for this form of media to impact perceptions of viewers, particularly more-vulnerable youth, seems to be high.

In this chapter, we will look at how female body image has been portrayed in mass media, especially television, and how this has played a role in the development of body dissatisfaction and its clinical implications for child and adolescent mental health. We will then explore the theoretical underpinnings of the mass media effects on body image dissatisfaction. Although reality television is a relatively new player in the world of media research, we will discuss some of the research specific to reality television programming that has been published in the past decade in terms of body image portrayals and the effects on adolescent females. We will conclude with a discussion of the potential role of media literacy programs.

FEMALE BODY IMAGE PORTRAYALS IN MASS MEDIA

In present-day entertainment, television, magazines, and movies often depict thin or underweight female body types that drastically differ from the body type of the average American woman. This has not always been the case, as the body image of women in entertainment has been evolving into more tall and slender body types over the past several decades. In the 1950s, the average American model was within 5% of the size of the average American woman. Currently, the average female model is 15%–20% below what would be considered a healthy weight for her height,[5] and 98%

of the American female population is not as thin as fashion models.[6] Given that 70.7% of the US adult population is classified as overweight or obese and that 20.6% of adolescents are classified as obese,[7] there is a large disparity between body types presented in the media and body types that represent the reality of the US population.

In fact, underweight female characters have been shown to be overrepresented in television sitcoms in both North America and other western countries, while overweight characters are underrepresented.[8–10] Female characters in G-rated animated films are even created with a thin-idealized body image and are more likely to have thin waists and large chests.[11] There are also major differences in the way characters of varying body types are portrayed in some television shows. For instance, when overweight characters are presented in sitcoms, they are often the subjects of humor or are unpopular.[8,10] In a content analysis of prime-time television sitcoms, the below-average-weight female characters received significantly more positive comments from male characters in regard to their weight and shape when compared to heavier female characters. Alarmingly, 12% of female characters dieted or restricted food intake, as indicated by their behaviors and conversations on the show. Those who were dieting gave themselves more verbal punishment for their weight and shape when compared with those not dieting and also made more negative comments about other women's weight and bodies.[10]

Given the evolution toward overwhelming representation of thin-ideal messages in the media over the decades, it is important to understand the associations between these portrayals and the potential impact on adolescent females in terms of their body image and related issues.

THE EFFECTS OF TELEVISION ON FEMALE BODY IMAGE

Self-report measures have shown that a majority of female adolescents and young adults in Western society experience body dissatisfaction.[6,12,13] A longitudinal study of US adolescent girls found that, in contrast to boys, female body dissatisfaction is amplified from middle school into high school.[13] The consideration of body image dissatisfaction is important when evaluating the mental health of adolescents and young adults, as poor body image is associated with the development of a host of concerning issues, including low self-esteem, obesity, depression, social anxiety, and the development of eating disorders.[14]

The media are pervasive shapers of our culture in the United States. From television and movies, to magazines and advertisements, to the multitude of social media platforms that are readily available, we are bombarded with messages containing information that we often unquestionably, and unfortunately, hold to be true. Adolescents and young adults are particularly vulnerable to these messages and have been shown to use media for a source of information about attractiveness and ideal body shapes and sizes.[12] The thin-idealized body types that are often portrayed in the media are both unhealthy and generally unobtainable, yet continue to be idealized and culturally valued.[15]

The body images portrayed in the media do not go unnoticed by young girls, as media research has indicated that media images can affect girls' perceptions of the culturally "ideal" body image and that of their own. Research has shown associations between media exposure and body image dissatisfaction, a preference for the thin-ideal, a heightened estimation of the importance of physical appearance, as well as symptoms of eating disorders.[16] A meta-analysis of 25 studies showed that a majority of females aged 8–18 years compare themselves to models appearing in advertisements and fashion layouts in magazines. Additionally, girls' body image was significantly more negative after viewing thin media images, which was particularly true for teenage girls.[17] Concerns are also raised for younger girls, with studies indicating elementary school girls who read fashion magazines report greater body dissatisfaction and disordered eating.[17] In a cross-sectional survey of females from the 5th–12th grade in the United States, 69% reported that fashion magazine images influenced their concept of their ideal body shape, and 47% reported the images made them want to lose weight. Additionally, the frequency of reading these magazines was correlated with higher levels of body dissatisfaction.[6] A major limitation is the correlational nature of the association between body dissatisfaction and viewing thin-idealized images in this study, as it does not necessarily indicate a causal effect.

A Dutch study focusing on girls from grades 4–6 showed that 11- to 12-year-old girls who watched a thin-idealized program showed greater body dissatisfaction.[18] In this study, 60 girls were tested on 3 different days. In each session, they were shown a 20-min television clip in a random order: a television clip explicitly focused on the thin ideal, a soap opera featuring thin actresses but not explicitly focused on the thin ideal, and a neutral clip. After each session, their body dissatisfaction was assessed using the Children Figure Rating Scale, which has been shown to be valid for use in children across many studies. Only the older preadolescent girls (the sixth graders) showed greater body dissatisfaction after watching the thin-idealized television clip versus the neutral clip. Interestingly, the greater degree of body dissatisfaction with age is similar to the findings of a study based on adolescents in the United States, which demonstrates that for girls, increases in age are associated with increases in body dissatisfaction.[13] Perhaps this is due to the physical developments of puberty leading to a physical change away from the thin ideal, leading to more body dissatisfaction.

Self-comparisons with television characters have also been shown to lead to body dissatisfaction. In a study of 1003 Israeli adolescent girls in grades 7−8 and 10−11, their favorite female television characters were mostly identified as thin or average in body size. The thinner the character, the more the girls compared the character's body to their own. The larger the gap between a girl's self-perceived body size and the body size of her favorite characters, the more negative was her body image.[9]

A critique can be made that a majority of media-related body image research is based on that of females in North America and other Westernized countries. Perhaps one of the best-known studies, by Becker,[19] looked at the impact of television 3 years after it was introduced to a rural community in Fiji that had previously not been exposed to the widespread media images in Western society. The indigenous culture in Fiji valued larger appetites and body shapes. Thirty school girls were interviewed and narrative data were collected relating to television and body image after they were exposed to Westernized media. Results suggest that television did redefine cultural ideals for body appearance. Girls reported modeling the behavior and appearance of television characters and made admiring comments about their thinness and apparel choices. The girls also commonly expressed an ability and desire to reshape their bodies, specifically by modifying their diet and increasing physical activity for weight control. Some expressed disparagement of their own bodies and the beginnings of disordered eating behaviors, such as restrictive eating, purging, and the use of diet pills. They seemed driven to obtain this new Western esthetic for more competitive social positioning, such as economic opportunities and peer approval, associating the thin-idealized body image portrayed on television with success: an association

not found in the indigenous society before the introduction of television.[19]

The causal direction of associations between media use and body dissatisfaction is often debated in media research. However, it appears that media use is at the very least a risk factor in development of maladaptive beauty ideals, which may lead to further body dissatisfaction and other harms to health.[12,20]

MEDIA AND BODY IMAGE EFFECTS: THEORETICAL APPROACHES

The associations between media content and its deleterious effects on the body image of young girls and adolescents have been shown in numerous studies. These associations are complex, however, and (as is often the case with media effects research) it can be difficult to demonstrate causal relationships. Given this complexity of the potential effects of thin-idealized media portrayals on the body image of young females, it is interesting to consider the theoretical underpinnings. Multiple disciplines offer different viewpoints on how these effects may take place. Ultimately, a combination of these theoretical approaches may best explain how media exert their influence on body image.

Social Comparison Theory

The social comparison theory, first outlined by Festinger in 1954, states that people are constantly evaluating themselves and comparing themselves to others, specifically others whom they perceive as representing realistic goals to attain. This process is automatic, meaning people often make these comparisons without conscious realization.[21,22] "Downward comparisons" occur when a person compares herself to someone else and finds the other to be lacking. "Upward comparisons," by contrast, leave the person feeling that she herself is lacking.[23] Furthermore, the social comparison theory suggests that people are motivated to meet their goals after making such comparisons.[21,22] In terms of body image, upward comparisons, in particular, predict higher body dissatisfaction and disordered eating behaviors.[14]

In terms of body image and the media, people may compare themselves to thin-idealized media images in a form of upward comparison. Researchers have suggested social comparisons as a mechanism by which exposure to media images may induce negative effects on body image. In fact, a number of studies have indicated that women who frequently compare themselves to thin idealized images are at greater risk for body dissatisfaction and disordered eating behaviors.[14,20,24] In one study, a group of 84 young adult college women from Australia were exposed to either a series of music video clips that emphasized the appearance of thin and attractive females or music video clips that did not emphasize this esthetic. Each group was given a set of statements to rate, with some women in each group receiving a set of statements that would encourage comparisons between themselves and the women in the music videos. For instance, they were asked to agree or disagree on a Likert scale statements such as "The people in this video clip are physically attractive" and "I would like my body to look like the bodies of the women in this video clip." It was found that viewers of the thin-idealized music videos showed increased social comparisons and body dissatisfaction compared to women watching neutral music videos. The effects of body dissatisfaction were mediated by the level of comparisons, meaning that women primed to compare themselves to the video had higher dissatisfaction.[25]

Given the overrepresentation of thin-idealized women portrayed in the media, women who are heavier viewers of television are presented with numerous images with a potential for upward comparison. Additionally, those who are primed to compare themselves to media images are more likely to experience higher body dissatisfaction. In terms of the social comparison theory, self-comparison to these idealized images and motivation to attain these goals may lead to dissatisfaction in body image.

Cultivation Theory

The cultivation theory suggests that exposure to television media messages can influence the thoughts and behaviors of its viewers.[26,27] The basis of this is the "cultivation hypothesis," which states that those who spend more time watching television are more likely to perceive the world in ways that reflect recurrent messages or themes presented in fictional television.[28]

The theory was first developed in the 1960s by George Gerbner, with the idea of "cultivation analysis," when researchers looked at the contribution of television viewing to audiences' concept of social reality in many different contexts.[28] For instance, Gerbner and colleagues found that compared to light viewers of crime television, heavier viewers had an exaggeration of perception of victimization, mistrust, and danger and were more likely to state "people cannot be trusted" and others are "just looking out for themselves.".[28-30] The theory posits that heavier viewers are more likely

to view the world in a way that is more consistent with the messages and lessons portrayed on television.

In terms of body image messages in television media, cultivation theorists find that heavier consumers of unrealistic and thin-idealized media may internalize those images as sociocultural norms, potentially resulting in body dissatisfaction. Given that television programs and commercials do portray a much higher-than-average proportion of thin, underweight female images, frequent viewers may internalize this unrealistic concept of appearance and believe that the thin-idealized images are standard.[31] When comparing to self, this may lead to body dissatisfaction. There is mixed evidence supporting this theory, with some research indicating that heavier television viewership leads to body dissatisfaction, and other research finding no meaningful link.[32]

Central to the cultivation theory is the concept of "heuristic processing." This processing occurs when a person accesses readily available information from their memories when making quick judgments, rather than systematically searching their memories for perhaps more accurate accounts. Ideas and constructs that are more frequently activated are more likely to be quickly accessed over time.[23] Using the concept of cultivation theory in the media, the more that a person is exposed to thin-idealized messages on television, the more likely they are to incorporate these ideals into their own social schemas. Subsequently, the more likely they are to access this standard from their memory when making evaluations on their own body image, leading to the potential for body dissatisfaction.

It has been noted that heavy cumulative exposure to media messages may shape viewers' concepts of reality, attitudes, and behavior, particularly when a person has little direct personal experience.[33,34] When considering the child and adolescent population specifically, the increased impact on those with "little direct personal experience" perhaps makes this population more susceptible to media effects. For instance, if a child has little direct knowledge of what constitutes a healthy body type, she may be more likely to be influenced by thin idealized images in the media than an adult with greater exposure to the topic. This also resonates with the concept of heuristic processing, when a child with little knowledge on a subject accesses these readily available memories to make her judgments.

It's important to consider that cultivation of attitudes and ideas through television media messages may not serve to create new beliefs in viewers, but may rather reinforce their already existing beliefs.[23] Furthermore, people often seek out programming that reflects and reinforces their existing attitudes; per the cultivation theory, the heavier viewership can further strengthen these attitudes.[28]

Uses and Gratification Theory

The uses and gratification theory offers yet another framework to view the effects of media on body image. Both the social comparison and cultivation theories place the media viewer in a more passive role, as if the media being viewed is having a direct one-way effect on the consumer, even without conscious viewer awareness. Per these theories, when viewers are repeatedly exposed to certain images, values, and themes in the media, such as thin-idealized body images, they may make upward comparisons to themselves or adopt these into their own social schemas which may be cultivated or strengthened over a period of time.

The uses and gratification theory, on the other hand, puts the viewer in a more active role. This theory sees the viewer as an active media consumer who deliberately selects and uses media for her own gratifications or rewards, which may include relaxation, escape, information, and personal identity, or as a resource for behavioral or appearance standards.[35,36] In the instance of fashion magazines, a person may look at this form of media to learn information about the latest fashion trends. Someone also may watch a particular sitcom on television for the entertainment value. In these two examples of media consumption for separate gratifications (information/appearance standards vs. entertainment), there is a difference in information processing involved for the consumer, leading to a difference in attitudinal and behavioral effects based on the motives for consumption of the media.[35] In other words, in the uses and gratification theory, the consumer is actively choosing a form of media for a specific reason or need and therefore would be affected in different ways based on the purpose for the media chosen.

The uses and gratification and cultivation theories can also be integrated. For example, someone may choose a sitcom to watch for the entertainment value rather than standards of appearance; however, they may also be influenced by messages and images contained in the sitcom that idealizes thinness.

To further demonstrate this, in a cross-sectional study by Tiggeman,[35] television-viewing habits in a sample of 1452 male and female adolescents from a South Australian high school was analyzed by total time of television exposure, exposure to different program types (sitcoms, soap operas, news, sports, etc.), and motivations for viewing these programs in relation to the adolescents' body image and disordered eating behaviors. The study found that total television-

viewing time was not related to body image, but the time spent watching the genre of soap operas specifically was related to a drive for thinness and internalization of cultural beauty ideals. Tiggeman theorized that the association with the soap opera genre specifically is related to the sense of "realness" of the drama, as compared to other forms of dramas or sitcoms. When we consider reality television in this chapter, this is an important consideration. Adolescents motivated to watch soap operas for social learning or as an escape from their negative affect were more strongly predicted to have body image disturbances, whereas those watching for the motive of entertainment did not.

Personality Traits

When looking at the uses and gratification, cultivation, and social comparison theories, it is clear that the pathway of media effects on adolescent body image may be multifactorial, and perhaps we could more accurately view this complex relationship using a combination of all three of these theories. In addition, there are personal traits of individuals which also make them more susceptible to media effects and can be mediators when considering these theoretical perspectives.

When considering the uses and gratification theory particularly, individual personality types may drive the use of media and lessons learned from it.[37] Histrionic personality traits, including features such as attention-seeking drives and emotional shallowness, have been shown to be predictive of negative outcomes, including excessive focus on one's appearance, relational aggression, and willingness to compromise values for fame. In fact, in an analysis of the Girl Scouts of America Study, histrionic traits were a stronger predictor for these negative outcomes than reality television viewing itself, although individuals with a higher degree of histrionic traits were more likely to seek out reality television programming.[37]

Neuroticism is another personality trait that has been linked to negative effects when presented with idealized body images in the media. Individuals with neurotic traits are more emotionally reactive, more likely to experience a negative affect, easily upset, and prone to overreacting to unpleasant experiences.[38] They are also more sensitive to evaluations of others and have a strong desire for social approval, making them at greater risk for negative body image.[39] When considering the social comparison theory, neurotic individuals are more likely than those with low levels of neuroticism to make upward comparisons.[38] Upward comparisons can predict higher body dissatisfaction and disordered eating behaviors.[14] It thus makes sense that those with eating disorders are more likely to have high levels of neuroticism and also engage in upward comparisons.[38,40,41] Research on college women has indicated that when presented with an idealized body image, those with high neuroticism have greater shifts in body self-esteem and indicate more body dissatisfaction, when compared to less neurotic women.[38]

Attachment style is another personal characteristic to consider as a vulnerability for poor body image. Bartholomew and Horowitz describe four attachment styles for adults, including secure, preoccupied, fearful, and dismissing.[42] Preoccupied attachment style presents as those who are anxious in relationships and wanting emotional intimacy with others but worrying that others do not want to become as close to them.[39] In a study of college students, those with this preoccupied attachment styles reported poorer body image than those with other forms of attachment.[43] To our knowledge, there is no direct research on attachment style and media body image effects; however, one could hypothesize that those with a more anxious attachment style would be more susceptible to negative effects of idealized body image presented in the media.

So in addition to considering the theoretical ways in which thin-idealized media may have an impact on adolescent body image, it's important to remember that individual temperamental and personality characteristics may also make some adolescents more susceptible to these effects.

REALITY TELEVISION AND BODY IMAGE

The popularity of reality television has blossomed since the early 2000s, with the development of hundreds of diverse programs that have dominated the American television markets. Reality TV contains several sub-genres, including dating shows (*The Bachelor, The Bachelorette*), talent and competition shows (*America's Got Talent, American Idol, American Ninja Warrior*), "real-life" or "docusoap" shows (*Keeping Up with the Kardashians, The Real World, Jersey Shore*), weight loss shows (*The Biggest Loser*), and makeover or cosmetic surgery shows (*The Swan, Extreme Makeover, Dr. 90210*).

Reality TV has traditionally been popular among preteen and teenaged audiences. Surveys from a 2009 Nielsen report showed that a high percentage of this age group has watched these shows.[44] Research from CommonSense.org shows a vast diversity of ways in which teens and tweens spend their screen time, including social media, music, computer games, mobile games, video games, and television. Using a nationally representative sample, the study found that the average American teen uses 9 h of media daily, not including use for schoolwork or homework. (This time includes "multitasking," such as perusing social media while on the school bus.) Television screen time can be further broken down into watching a TV broadcast or watching in a "time shifted" manner, as with On Demand or Netflix. TV shows can also be watched online, streamed through a computer, tablet, or smart phone. Despite the plethora of media options to choose, the media activities that teens and tweens most enjoy and dedicate the most time to are television and music, with 62% of tweens and 58% of teens watching TV every day.[45] Given that the number of reality TV programs is continuously growing, there is a high likelihood that this age group will continually be exposed to the media messages that reality TV delivers.[2,44]

With the popularity of these shows, research over the past decade has began to focus on the effects that reality TV has on influencing viewers' values and behaviors. For example, studies have found that adolescents purchase products that reality stars use or display.[2,46] A study of 334 male and female undergraduate students aged 18−24 years used self-report questionnaires to examine the effects that reality dating shows have on young adults' views on dating. The results indicate that watching reality dating shows is correlated with the endorsement of a sexual double standard, the belief that dating is a game, and a focus on personal appearance. Similarly, viewers were more likely to see men and women in heterosexual relationships as inherently in opposition to one another (what the researchers referred to as "adversarial sexual beliefs") as measured by agreement with statements such as "a lot of women seem to get pleasure out of putting men down" or "men are out for only one thing." These effects were significant whether the viewers were watching for entertainment or with the goal of learning about dating.[46]

The introduction of this chapter mentioned The Girl Scouts of America's *Real to Me* survey of 1100 girls aged 11−17 years. In that survey, 47% of the girls identified themselves as "regular" viewers of reality TV, and a majority of the girls believed that reality shows were "mainly real and unscripted" and reflected real life. The regular viewers were more focused on the value of their physical appearance than girls who were not regular viewers. The former indicated that they "spent a lot of time on their appearance," "think that a girl's value is based on how she looks," and "would rather be recognized for their outer beauty than their inner beauty."[3,34] A major limitation of one-time surveys such as this is that they cannot show causality.

However, the Girl Scouts survey does indicate that regular reality TV viewership is correlated with girls placing more value on their appearance. Perhaps this may be explained by the uses and gratifications theory, with appearance-focused girls seeking out this programming and being more actively involved in the viewership.

Like traditional television programming, reality TV has also been shown to focus on thin-idealized female body types. This is illustrated by a study on MTV's reality TV shows of the "docusoap" subgenre, which has historically been distinctively popular with adolescents and young adults. Docusoaps blur the line between documentary and soap opera formats, giving the viewers a "fly on the wall" perspective of the lives of the cast members while also presenting a "constructed reality" delivered by careful editing meant for a dramatic effect.[47] Examples of some of these docusoaps include *Jersey Shore, The Real World, Laguna Beach, Newport Beach,* and *The Hills.* Because the documentary-style presentation of these shows implies that viewers are actually watching reality, it has been speculated that adolescents may be more susceptible to the negative effects of modeling cast members' problematic behaviors.[47–49] Given that adolescents are also the most susceptible to develop body image disturbances,[47,50] it is interesting to consider the depiction of body ideals portrayed in this docusoap subgenre.

Flynn et al.[47] examined the body ideals in the five MTV docusoaps mentioned above. They found that close to half the bodies of women cast members were classed as "curvaceously thin," meaning thin with large breasts. Over two-thirds of the women's bodies were considered "low fat," demonstrating that thinness was the most common female body characteristic seen. Women, compared to men, exhibited a higher level of body exposure, with widespread partial nudity and some full nudity in the shows. The cast members with the idealized body type had higher levels of body exposure when compared to others. It is clear from this study that the presentation of body image in this reality show subgenre is far from real, given the percentage of lean bodies in the docusoaps when compared to overweight or obese body types is inverse that of US statistics, with 20.9% of adolescents qualifying as obese and over two-thirds of adults as either overweight or obese.[7] In fact, there were no characters classified as obese in any of these shows.[47]

Cosmetic Surgery Reality Television and Body Image

When considering the relationship between reality TV and body image, it makes sense to carefully consider the genre of makeover and cosmetic surgery reality programming. Most of the research surrounding the relationship between body image and reality TV does focus on this subgenre because of its inherent media message of placing high value on idealized beauty.

As evidenced by the multitude of thin-idealized media messages, the Westernized culture of the United States also reflects this high value on idealized beauty. This is apparent in plastic surgery trends over the past 2 decades. The number of cosmetic surgical and non surgical procedures performed in the United States increased by 1600% between 1992 and 2002.[51] In 2003, 8.3 million people underwent these surgeries, and in 2008, 12.1 million.[15,52] Between the years of 2000 and 2016, cosmetic procedures have increased further by 132%.[53] There is a large gender differential in these numbers, with 92% of procedures being performed on females, although cosmetic surgery patients are increasingly gender diverse.[15,53] Additionally, these procedures are becoming more widely accepted, particularly among college-aged women.[51,52,54]

Beginning with the airing of *Extreme Makeover* in 2002, a variety of cosmetic surgery and makeover shows have followed, including *Dr. 90210, The Swan, Botched,* and *I Want a Famous Face.* Although each show has its own unique twist, the primary theme is that of an individual dissatisfied with aspects of his or her life having the ability to transform through the use of surgical cosmetic procedures.[55] Some of these transformations are so extreme that postsurgery patients are hardly recognizable to friends and family. There is often a follow-up, purporting to demonstrate how these individuals have improved their lives by transforming their appearance, including changes in their romantic relationships, employment opportunities, and overall happiness. The idea that these dramatic physical changes lead to complete psychological and social change has been referred to as the "myth of transformation" and is a questionable motive for individuals to want to pursue plastic surgery.[15] It should also be noted that the risks and sometimes-difficult postoperative recoveries are rarely a focus of the programming; instead, they depict the postsurgical individual as fully recovered and happy.[55]

Correlational research has shown that cosmetic surgery media exposure is associated both with body dissatisfaction and a desire for these procedures.[55] As has been discussed in this chapter, there are certain individual traits that may make females more susceptible to responding negatively to this type of idealized body imagery than others, including those who have a higher internalization of the thin ideal, place a high importance on appearance in their sense of self-worth, and have more materialistic values.[55]

In an experimental study by Ashikali, Ditmar, and Ayers, these factors were examined in terms of the impact of a cosmetic surgery reality show on adolescent girls' body image and their attitudes toward plastic surgery. In this experimental study, 99 girls aged 11—18 years were exposed to the reality TV show *Dr. 90210* or a control exposure of a home makeover show. The results indicated that exposure to the cosmetic surgery show led to increased weight and appearance dissatisfaction.[55]

In another experimental design, researchers looked at the effects of a reality TV cosmetic surgery program on eating disordered attitudes, behaviors, and self-esteem. Participants consisted of 147 college women assigned to watch a cosmetic surgery show, *The Swan*, or a reality TV home improvement program. *The Swan* presents women undergoing extensive plastic surgery and an intense diet and exercise routine in order to transform themselves from an "ugly duckling," to a "beautiful swan." Consistent with other reality television research, women in the cosmetic makeover viewing group who reported a higher baseline internalization of the thin-ideal reported lowered self-esteem at posttesting, which persisted over a 2-week follow-up period.[52]

This study also investigated how disordered eating behaviors, such as restrictive eating, may be a mediator in the effects of exposure to cosmetic surgery reality shows. Previous media research has shown that those with restricted eating patterns actually may have an increase in social self-esteem following exposure to thin-ideal media, perhaps because restrictive eaters are more invested in their appearance and believe that achieving the thin ideal is attainable based on what they see in the media.[52,56] In the context of reality television, it is possible that these ideals may appear to be even more attainable, given that the media is inherently presented as "reality."

Markey and Markey conducted two studies to examine the influence of cosmetic surgery reality television on young adults' interest in altering their appearance using these surgical methods.[15] This study was unusual in that it included both male and female university students. In the first part of the study, 170 participants were initially given a survey assessing factors such as their impression of reality shows featuring cosmetic surgery, their appearance satisfaction, and their interest in cosmetic surgery. In this survey, women had a greater body dissatisfaction and greater desire to alter their appearance using plastic surgery when compared to men, which is consistent with national trends of women compromising the majority of plastic surgery patients. Additionally, those who had a positive impression of reality shows featuring cosmetic surgery also desired to obtain these procedures for themselves. In the second part of the study, 189 participants were randomly assigned to watch 20-min clips of *Extreme Makeover* or assigned to a control group viewing a reality home improvement show. Participants who watched *Extreme Makeover* wanted to alter their own appearance using cosmetic surgery more than participants who watched the home makeover show. This indicated a possible causal influence on viewing these shows on the desire to pursue cosmetic surgery, at least in the short term.[15] There was no attempt to measure whether this interest in pursuing plastic surgery lasted over time, so perhaps the expressed interest in plastic surgery in the postexposure assessments is a reflection of priming. Given that this experimental exposure lasted approximately 20 min and "real-world" exposure to reality television could potentially be on a daily basis, it would be interesting to see exposures long term and an assessment of the longevity of these effects.

Markey and Markey followed up with a study examining young adults' qualitative responses after watching *Extreme Makeover*.[12] The analysis showed that both men and women tended to view the show's message of a female pursuing beauty ideals as important, focusing on the physical and psychological benefits of cosmetic surgery as a tool to enhance appearance. Women in the study who viewed the show more positively were more likely to desire cosmetic surgery than those who viewed it more negatively.[12] This of course does not prove causality; however, based on the previous experimental studies, there is some evidence that exposure to this media increases an individual's desire to pursue surgery at least in the short term.

There was no gender difference when looking at how young adult men and women viewed the idealization of female beauty in the reality TV programming, with men being as impressed by the potential benefits of cosmetic surgeries as women. As suggested by some researchers and as supported by the cultivation theory, men may be internalizing female beauty ideals from the media just as women do.[12]

It is clear that cosmetic surgery reality shows do not inherently *cause* individuals to have decreased body satisfaction, low self-esteem, and eating disordered behaviors and attitudes or to pursue plastic surgery. However, repeat exposure to this reality programming for individuals who are susceptible to the negative effects of this beauty-idealizing media (i.e., those with highly internalized thin ideals), may contribute to increased body dissatisfaction and pressures to engage in appearance-altering behaviors, as well as the development of mental health pathology such as eating disorders, depression, and anxiety.

MEDIA LITERACY

There is an association between the thin-idealized body images presented in the media and the effects on body image of young women. Body dissatisfaction, in turn, is associated with a number of negative consequences such as depressive symptoms, low self-esteem, obesity, disordered eating, and the development of eating disorders.[57] Although we can recognize that the images presented in the media do not reflect that of the average female in the United States, the trend toward this presentation has remained a part of our culture for several decades and has been slow to change. Ultimately, we are faced with the question of how we counteract these messages and prevent the development of negative consequences for children and adolescents.

Censorship is certainly an option to decrease any negative effects of media on children and adolescents; however, this may not be desirable or even practical given the pervasiveness of thin-idealized media messages.[34,58,59] Teaching media literacy has been widely supported, including by the American Academy of Pediatrics, whose 2010 policy statement endorsed media literacy education as potentially reducing negative media effects.[60]

Media literacy is defined as the ability to understand, analyze, evaluate, and challenge media messages.[34,61] Teaching the critical thinking skills required for media literacy differs from taking an informational approach. This has been seen in other public health research; when students are trained to critically examine and resist pressures toward alcohol, tobacco, and drug use, it is more effective in preventing these behaviors than informational sessions.[61] Various media literacy programs have been linked to less aggressive attitudes and behaviors, decreased substance abuse behaviors, and overall decreased television viewing.[34,58,60]

Teaching adolescent and school-aged children media literacy in regard to body image has shown some positive results, although more research in this area is needed. In general, those who have high levels of media literacy are more skeptical about the realism of media messages and have the ability to assess how realistic or unrealistic an image may be. Self-reported engagement in media literacy strategies is associated with having a more positive body image.[57] Additionally, media literacy has been shown to mitigate negative effects for adolescents particularly vulnerable to media messages, such as those having a high thin-ideal internalization and a tendency to upwardly compare themselves to images in the media.[57] An example of a media literacy intervention was created by The Dove Self-Esteem Fund, featuring a short video of a real-life demonstration of how media images of women are manipulated. In a study of 127 British preteen girls, those who were shown this intervention video were less likely to make negative comparisons between themselves and the media models.[62]

A 2016 systematic review examined the relationships between the level of media literacy and the level of body image dissatisfaction and disordered eating outcomes. The 16 studies included in the review were from the United States, Australia, and Israel, with a majority of participants from preadolescent through college age. In interventional studies, media literacy was shown to increase from baseline in postintervention, and even at a 3-month follow-up. Body-image-related outcomes were also improved, including positive outcomes for body satisfaction in boys, improvements in internalization of the thin-ideal in girls, body size acceptance in girls, and drive for thinness in both boys and girls. Media literacy interventions did not show improvements in eating disorder-related outcomes; however, only one intervention in the review focused on eating-related content while other interventions focused on appearance or general media literacy. Limitations of the studies include a general lack of experimental design in a majority of the intervention studies and an inability to determine if the reductions in body image concerns were truly mediated by changes in media literacy.[63]

Although more research is needed to optimize how media literacy interventions may most effectively be used, this sort of intervention has shown promise in many areas. By teaching youth to be media literate and cultivating the idea of becoming critical viewers of the media, subsequent negative exposure effects may be disrupted.

CONCLUSION

Negative body image and body image dissatisfaction is associated with a number of serious and concerning mental health affects, including obesity, depression, social anxiety, and eating disorders. Although there are number of factors that may contribute to body image dissatisfaction among children and adolescents, exposure to media images has been associated with the development of this dissatisfaction. Although direct long-term causal effects between the exposure to thin-idealized media and body dissatisfaction have been difficult to demonstrate in research studies, a theoretical understanding of these effects can be understood through the social comparison, cultivation, and uses and gratification theories. Additionally, there are factors that make young people more susceptible to potential negative affects, including personality types and attachment styles.

Television media research has shown that there is an overabundance of thin-idealized images in American media. With the development and popularity of reality television, this trend has continued. Given the popularity of reality television among children and adolescents, coupled with reality television inherently giving the impression that the media portrayals are *real*, it is important to consider what children may be learning from this programming.

This chapter does not focus on the body image of child and adolescent males and does not imply that this research is any less important. Historically, men have not been granted the same consideration regarding their body dissatisfaction and negative clinical outcomes.[64,65] However, more research is beginning to show that body dissatisfaction in men is quite prevalent and can lead to many of the same clinical issues. Although this research is not discussed in this particular chapter, it would be a necessary topic of discussion in future editions.

Additionally, social media, including Snapchat, Instagram, and other visual communication platforms, are hugely popular among the teenage population. Similar to reality television, social media are often inherently presumed to be representative of real life. These media also may have an effect on the development of thin-idealizations and body dissatisfaction and many of the theoretical approaches mentioned in this chapter may also apply. As these forms of media gain even more popularity, it will be important to continue media and body image research.[66]

REFERENCES

1. Nielsen. *10 Years of Primetime: The Rise of Reality and Sports Programming*. Media and Entertainment; 2011. Available at: http://www.nielsen.com/us/en/insights/news/2011/10-years-of-primetime-the-rise-of-reality-and-sports-programming.html.
2. Patino A, Kaltcheva VD, Smith MF. The appeal of reality television for teen and pre-teen audiences. *J Advert Res*. 2011;51(1):288−297.
3. Girl Scout Research Institute. *Real to Me: Girls and Reality TV*; 2011. Available at: https://www.girlscouts.org/content/dam/girlscouts-gsusa/forms-and-documents/about-girl-scouts/research/real_to_me_factsheet.pdf.
4. Lopez-Guimera G, Levine MP, Sanchez-Carracedo D, Fauquet J. Influence of mass media on body image and eating disordered attitudes and behaviors in females: a review of effects and processes. *Media Psychol*. 2010;13(4):387−416.
5. Wiseman CV, Sunday SR, Becker AE. Impact of the media on adolescent body image. *Child Adolesc Psychiatr Clin N Am*. 2005;14:453−471.
6. Field AE, Cheung L, Wolf AM, Herzog DB, Gormaker SL, Colditz GA. Exposure to the mass media and weight concerns among girls. *Pediatrics*. 1999;103(3):e36.
7. Centers for Disease Control and Prevention, 2016. Available at: http://www.cdc.gov/nchs/fastats/obesity-overweight.htm.
8. Fouts G, Vaughan K. Television situation comedies: male weight, negative references, and audience relations. *Sex Roles*. 2002;46(11−12):439−442.
9. Te'eni-Harari T, Eyal K. Liking them thin: adolescents' favorite television characters and body image. *J Health Commun*. 2015;20:607−615.
10. Fouts G, Burggraf K. Television situation comedies: female body images and verbal reinforcements. *Sex Roles*. 1999; 40(5−6):473−481.
11. Smith SL, Cook CA. *Gender Stereotypes: An Analysis of Popular Films and TV*. Los Angeles: Geena Davis Institute for Gender and Media; 2008. Available at: https://seejane.org/wp-content/uploads/GDIGM_Gender_Stereotypes.pdf.
12. Markey C, Markey P. Emerging adults' responses to a media presentation of idealized female beauty: an examination of cosmetic surgery in reality television. *Psychol Pop Media Cult*. 2012;1:209−219.
13. Bearman SK, Presnell K, Martines E, Stice E. The skinny on body dissatisfaction: a longitudinal study of adolescent girls and boys. *J Youth Adolesc*. 2006;35:229−241.
14. Bailey SD, Ricciardella LA. Social comparisons, appearance related comments, contingent self-esteem and their relationships with body dissatisfaction and eating disturbance among women. *Eat Behav*. 2010;11:107−112.
15. Markey C, Markey P. A correlational and experimental examination of reality television viewing and interest in cosmetic surgery. *Body Image*. 2010;7:165−171.
16. Holstrom AJ. The effects of the media on body image: a meta-analysis. *J Broadcast Electron Media*. 2004;48:196−217.
17. Groesz LM, Levine MP, Murnen SK. The effect of experimental presentation of thin media images on body satisfaction: a meta-analytic review. *Int J Eat Disord*. 2002;31:1−16.
18. Anschutz DJ, Spruijt-Metz D, Van Strien T, Engels R. The direct effect of thin ideal focused adult television on young girls' ideal body figure. *Body Image*. 2011;8:26−33.
19. Becker AE. Television, disordered eating, and young women in Fiji: negotiating body image and identity during rapid social change. *Cult Med Psychiatry*. 2004;28:533−559.
20. Tiggemann M, Polivy J, Hargreaves D. The processing of thin ideals in fashion magazines: a source of social comparison or fantasy? *J Soc Clin Psychol*. 2009;28:73−93.

21. Festinger L. A theory of social comparison processes. *Hum Relat.* 1954;7:117−140.
22. Botta R. Television images and adolescent girls' body image disturbance. *J Commun.* 1999;49(2):22−41.
23. Van Vanoderen KE, Kinnally W. Media effects on body image: examining media exposure in the broader context of internal and other social factors. *Am Commun J.* 2012; 14(2):41−57.
24. Dittmar H, Howard S. Ideal-body internalization and social comparison tendency as moderators of thin media models' impact on women's body-focused anxiety. *J Soc Clin Psychol.* 2014;23:747−770.
25. Tiggeman M, Slater A. Thin ideals in music television: a source of social comparison and body dissatisfaction. *Int J Eat Disord.* 2003;35(1):48−58.
26. Hammermeister J, Brock B, Winterstein D, Page R. Life without TV? Cultivation theory and psychosocial health characteristics of television-free individuals and their television-viewing counterparts. *Health Commun.* 2005; 17(3):253−264.
27. Shanahan J, Morgan M. *Television and Its Viewers: Cultivation Theory & Research.* Cambridge, England: Cambridge University Press; 1999.
28. Morgan M, Shanahan J. The state of cultivation. *J Broadcast Electron Media.* 2010;54(2):337−355.
29. Gerbner G, Gross L. Living with television: the violence profile. *J Commun.* 1976;26(2):173−199.
30. Gerbner G, Gross L, Morgan M, Signorielli N. The "mainstreaming" of America: violence profile no. 11. *J Commun.* 1980;30(3):10−29.
31. Eisend M, Moller J. The influence of TV viewing on consumers' body image and related consumption behavior. *Mark Lett.* 2007;18:101−116.
32. Nabi RL. Cosmetic surgery makeover programs and intentions to undergo cosmetic enhancements: a consideration of three models of media effects. *Hum Commun Res.* 2009; 35:1−27.
33. Russell CA, Russell DW, Boland WA, Grube JW. Television's cultivation of American adolescents' beliefs about alcohol and the moderating role of trait reactance. *J Child Media.* 2014;8(1):5−22.
34. Peek H, Beresin E. Reality check: how reality television can affect youth and how a media literacy curriculum can help. *Acad Psychiatry.* 2016;40(1):177−181.
35. Tiggeman M. Television and adolescent body image: the role of program content and viewing motivation. *J Soc Clin Psychol.* 2005;24(3):361−381.
36. Nabi R, Stiff CR, Halford J, Finnerty KL. Emotional and cognitive predictors of the enjoyment of reality-based and fictional television programming: an elaboration of the uses and gratifications perspective. *Media Psychol.* 2006;8(4):421−447.
37. Ferguson CJ, Salmond K, Modi K. Reality television predicts both positive and negative outcomes for adolescent girls. *J Pediatr.* 2013;162:1175−1180.
38. Roberts A, Good E. Media images and female body dissatisfaction: the moderating effects of the five-factor traits. *Eat Behav.* 2010;11:211−216.
39. Frederick DA, Sandhu F, Morse PJ, Swami V. Correlates of appearance and weight satisfaction in a U.S. National sample: personality, attachment style, television viewing, self-esteem, and life satisfaction. *Body Image.* 2016;17: 191−203.
40. Cassin S, Ranson K. Personality and eating disorders: a decade in review. *Clin Psychol Rev.* 2005;25:895−916.
41. Corning A, Krumm AJ, Smitham DA. Differential social comparison processes in women with and without eating disorder symptoms. *J Couns Psychol.* 2006;53(3): 338−349.
42. Bartholomew K, Horowitz LM. Attachment styles among young adults: a test of a four-category model. *J Personal Soc Psychol.* 1991;61:226−244.
43. Cash TF, Theriault J, Annis NM. Body image in an interpersonal context: adult attachment, fear of intimacy and social anxiety. *J Soc Clin Psychol.* 2004;23:89−103.
44. Nielsen. *Nielsen 2009 Report on Television.* New York: Nielsen Media Research; 2009.
45. Watson ST. The line between reality and reality shows blurs. *McClatchy-Tribune Bus News.* 2008.
46. Zurbriggen E, Morgan E. Who wants to marry a millionaire? Reality dating television programs, attitudes toward sex, and sexual behaviors. *Sex Roles.* 2006;54:1−17.
47. Flynn MA, Park SY, Morin DT. Anything but real: body idealization and objectification of MTV docusoap characters. *Sex Roles.* 2015;72:173−182.
48. Baruh L. Publicized intimacies on reality television: an analysis of voyeuristic content and its contribution to the appeal of reality programming. *J Broadcast Electron Media.* 2009;53:190−210.
49. Stefanone MA, Lackaff D, Rosen D. The relationship between traditional mass media and Bsocial media: reality television as a model for social network site behavior. *J Broadcast Electron Media.* 2010;54:508−525.
50. American Psychiatric Association. *Diagnostic and Statistical Manual of Mental Disorders.* 4th ed. Washington, DC: American Psychiatric Association; 1994.
51. Sarwer D, Crerand C. Body image and cosmetic medical treatments. *Body Image.* 2004;1:99−111.
52. Mazzeo S, Trace S, Mitchell K, Gow R. Effects of a reality TV cosmetic surgery makeover program on eating disordered attitudes and behaviors. *Eat Behav.* 2007;8: 390−407.
53. American Society of Plastic Surgeons. 2016 Cosmetic Plastic Surgery Statistics. Available at: https://www.plasticsurgery.org/documents/News/Statistics/2016/cosmetic-procedure-trends-2016.pdf.
54. Sarwer DB, Cash TF, Magee L, et al. Female college students and cosmetic surgery: an investigation of experiences, attitudes, and body image. *Plast Reconstr Surg.* 2005; 113(3):931−938.
55. Ashikali EM, Dittmar H, Ayers S. The effect of cosmetic surgery reality tv shows on adolescent girls' body image. *Psychol Pop Media Cult.* 2014;3(3):141−153.
56. Joshi R, Herman CP, Polivy J. Self-enhancing effects of exposure to thin-body images. *Int J Eat Disord.* 2004; 35(3):333−341.

57. McLean SA, Paxton SJ, Wertheim EH. Does media literacy mitigate risk for reduced body satisfaction following exposure to thin-ideal media? *J Youth Adolesc.* 2016;45: 1678−1695.

58. Geraee N, Kaveh MH, Shojaeizadeh D, Tabatabaee HR. Impact of media literacy education on knowledge and behavioral intention of adolescents in dealing with media messages according to stages of change. *J Adv Med Educ Prof.* 2015;3(1):9−14.

59. Brown JD, Witherspoon EM. The mass media and American adolescents' health. *J Adolesc Health.* 2002; 31(suppl 6):153−170.

60. Council on Communications and the Media. Media education. *Pediatrics.* 2010;126:1012−1017.

61. Wade TD, Davidson S, O'Dea JA. A preliminary controlled evaluation of a school based media literacy program and self-esteem program for reducing eating disorder risk factors. *Int J Eat Disord.* 2003;33(4):371−383.

62. Halliwell E, Easun A, Harcourt D. Body dissatisfaction: can a short media literacy message reduce negative media exposure effects amongst adolescent girls? *Br J Health Psychol.* 2011;16(Pt. 2):396−403.

63. McLean SA, Paxton SJ, Wertheim EH. The role of media literacy in body dissatisfaction and disordered eating: a systematic review. *Body Image.* 2016;19:9−23.

64. McCabe M, Ricciardelli L. Body image dissatisfaction among males across the lifespan: a review of past literature. *J Psychosom Res.* 2004;56(6):675−685.

65. Dallesasse SL, Kluck AS. Reality television and the muscular male ideal. *Body Image.* 2013;10:309−315.

66. Fardouly J, Diedrichs P, Vartanian L, Halliwell E. Social comparisons on social media: the impact of Facebook on young women's body image concerns and mood. *Body Image.* 2015;13:38−45.

CHAPTER 3

Sexting and Cyberbullying in the Developmental Context: Use and Misuse of Digital Media and Implications for Parenting

ABIGAIL M. JUDGE, PHD • ANTHONY D. SOSSONG, MD, MS

INTRODUCTION

Mobile phones, the Internet, and social media are linchpins of social behavior among US adolescents.[a] In particular, smartphones are the mobile communications hub that teens use to access the Internet, text messaging apps, and online social networking sites. Survey data from Pew Internet Research (2015) reports that nearly three-quarters (73%) of US teens aged 13–17 years have smartphones; only 12% of teens report having no cell phone of any kind.[1] The majority of teens access the Internet from mobile devices daily or more often (94%), and almost a quarter (24%) of surveyed youth aged 13–17 years report going online "almost constantly."[1] Many adolescents report that phones are essential to their social life and that they "can't live without their phones."[2]

The implications of smartphone use on adolescents' well-being remains a source of debate. Concerns about the "always on" nature of mobile phones have existed since their invention,[3] including questions about how constant accessibility may reorganize our most important relationships: among peers, between parent and child, between device and self.[4] Ever since, empirical research on smartphone use and psychosocial well-being has evolved, with the popular media emphasizing a dystopian narrative about smartphones and teens.[5,6] For example, recent articles in major media venues have likened smartphones to "portable dopamine pumps,"[7] and implicated teen smartphone use in an impending mental health crisis among a cohort dubbed *iGen* (i.e., individuals born between 1995 and 2012).[8]

It is important to maintain a historical perspective in the face of such alarm. The emergence of new technology is typically associated with narratives that alternate between danger, misuse, and harm on the one hand and untold possibility and innovation on the other.[9] When young people are the earliest adopters of a technology, there are typically even greater concerns about a technology's potential to corrupt youth, create new risk, and upset family hierarchies.[10,11] The invention of home telephones, for example, raised concern about new and troubling "opportunities to stray from the family circle without detection."[11] Of course, there are significant differences between a home-based landline and the smart phones of today. With smartphones, youth may "stray from the family circle" while in the presence of family, raising some legitimate questions about autonomy, safety, and monitoring. The fact remains, however, that a primarily alarmist perspective on youth and digital media leaves stakeholders such as child psychiatrists and psychologists, educators, and parents uncertain about how much concern is appropriate. Digital media *has* transformed life, for children and adults alike, but the nature of these changes is far more nuanced than most popular depictions allow.

In addition to the historical perspective, we put forth the importance of a developmental framework when considering adolescents' use and misuse of digital media. A developmental psychopathology perspective assumes the possibility of adaptive and maladaptive development within a context of ongoing maturation.[12]

---

[a]In this chapter, we define *digital media* as the collective of mobile communications technologies, social networking platforms, and the Internet.

This perspective also includes the influence of family, social, and cultural factors on developmental changes. Such a framework can help direct clinical attention to youth whose use is more problematic and inform areas for intervention. In this chapter, we focus on the use and potential misuse of digital technology and social media among US adolescents grounded in such a developmental framework. We begin with the epidemiology of digital media use among "tweens" (aged 8–12 years) and US teens, including associations between technology use and online and offline vulnerability and risk. This perspective helps define normative and more problematic forms of use within a young person's development.

We then critically review the literature on two behaviors at the interface of adolescence and digital media which have attracted significant attention in the popular press and more recently the scientific literature: cyberbullying and "sexting"/youth-produced sexual images. We consider available evidence through the lens of developmental psychopathology[12] and the co-construction model of digital media use, which holds that children's use of digital media is highly connected to the developmental processes of their lives.[13] These theoretical perspectives help avoid the polarizing claims that digital media is inherently destructive or inherently transformative.[9] On balance, we suggest that teens' use of digital media carries both potential benefits and risks, and a developmental analysis helps identify moderators of these outcomes. Although it is premature to use the language of best practices, we conclude with suggestions for psychiatric practice with an emphasis on the implications for working with parents given the importance of family context on child adjustment—even in the digital age.

NORMATIVE CONTEXT OF DIGITAL MEDIA USE

Children's use of digital media to interact with peers increases between childhood and adolescence, which corresponds with the increasing salience of peer relationships from early to mid and late adolescence.[14] It is challenging to obtain valid estimates of how "tweens" (youth aged 8–12 years) use social networking, which may be due to the Childhood Online Privacy Protection Act.[b] This act prevents children younger than 13 years from registering on social media sites, although many parents help their

children bypass this restriction.[2,15] In the Common Sense Census (2015) survey of media use among a nationally representative sample of teens and tweens ($n = 2600$), 15% of youth aged 8–12 years used social media, as compared with 58% of youth aged 13–17 years.[16] Although most surveyed tweens do not use social media, those who do so are quite devoted to this and to screen media in general (e.g., use of devices to access TV, music). Surveyed boys overwhelmingly spend more time video gaming than girls. Survey data indicate these tweens average 1 h and 43 min per day on social media, and 57% report that they enjoy social networking "a lot," which is more than any online activity other than listening to music. This cohort of tweens are predominantly female and more likely to be from families earning less than $35,000 a year. These tweens are the heaviest screen users of all the tweens studied, with estimates of almost 8 h/day with screen media.[16]

In general, survey data suggest that black youth and children from lower socioeconomic groups tend to spend more time with screen media (e.g., watching TV, videos, video gaming, social media) than Hispanic, white, or higher-socioeconomic status (SES) youth do.[16] Although each of these groups reportedly enjoy screen media, the black and low-SES youth spend more time doing so. Study authors note that it is not the case that lower-income youth are more likely to engage in media-related activities such as watching TV, listening to music, or using social media than their peers. Rather, it's that those who do use media spend more time doing so.[16]

There are more extensive data on how adolescents interact with digital media. Smartphone ownership is more common among teens than tweens, with nearly three-quarters of teens aged 13–17 years owning smartphones.[16] Teens are diversifying their use of social networking platforms, with 71% of surveyed youth using more than one site, usually some combination of Facebook, Instagram, and Snapchat.[1] The Associated Press and NORC Center for Public Affairs Research (2017) reported Instagram and Snapchat as the most popular social networks for teens aged 13–17 years.[17] Social networking site preferences vary by socioeconomic status, with teens from less-affluent families (i.e., households earning less than $50,000) preferring Facebook and more-affluent teens preferring Snapchat and Twitter.[1] These data are consistent with previous ethnographic research on how socioeconomic differences can pattern the popularity of social networking sites.[9]

The majority of teen cell phone owners (91%) use text messaging, either directly through their mobile

---

[b]Personal communication, Michael Rich, MD, MPH, Center on Media and Child Health, Boston Children's Hospital, October 4, 2017.

phones or through an app (e.g., WhatsApp, Kik). Research and clinical experience suggest that teens' primary motivation for texting is communication with friends.[1,2] Texting apps are more common among African-American and Hispanic youth.[1] These data converge with another national survey reporting that black teens are the most active of any group on social media and messaging apps and are more likely than white teens to use platforms like Snapchat or Instagram and messaging apps like Kik, and to use them more frequently.[17]

The use of anonymous sharing apps or sites where individuals can ask questions or anonymously self-disclose via text or images appears rare, with only 11% of teens with cell phones reporting use.[1] Girls are somewhat more likely to use anonymous sharing apps, as are youth from more affluent families. These data may have particular relevance to the topic of cyberbullying, to be discussed later.

Correspondence Between Online and Offline Risk

Previous research posited a *co-construction model* of Internet use, which assumed that teens' digital worlds are highly connected to the developmental processes of their lives.[13] This means, for example, that the nearly constant digital chatter of a "group-chat" among 13-year-old girls can be understood to reflect the increased salience of social bonds and conformity associated with social development in early adolescence.[18] As the developers of the co-construction model have opined:

> We expect that youth will bring people and issues from their offline worlds into their online worlds. Thus, we anticipate that core adolescent issues such as sexuality, identity intimacy, and interpersonal connection will figure prominently in their online contexts.[19]

This correspondence holds for problematic behavior as well. A teen who has experienced sexual abuse offline is, as a possible response to victimization, more likely to interact sexually with an adult online.[20]

A preponderance of research supports the co-construction model, indicating that technology-related risk is very often intertwined with preexisting, offline risk.[19–23] A 2014 critical review summarized evidence about the factors associated with increased risk of online harm among adolescents: personality factors (e.g., low self-esteem, high sensation-seeking, moral disengagement), psychological difficulties, and lack of parental and peer support.[23] The authors note that

this is consistent with the literature on childhood vulnerability where it is well known that risk factors tend to compound one another, and teens who take risks in one domain are more likely to take risks in another.[23,24]

Another consideration in estimating risk is that the majority of research on digital media is cross-sectional, a design that prevents causal inferences. For example, a recent critical review examined the available evidence on associations between standardized measures of problematic smartphone use and the severity of psychopathology.[25] The majority of studies used college student samples, and we should be cautious about generalizing these findings to adolescents and young teens due to developmental differences. Across all reviewed studies, depression severity was consistently related to problematic smartphone use, demonstrating at least medium effect sizes, but correlational study design prevented causal explanations.[25] Although the authors discussed potential causal explanations, these models await empirical study. From a developmental perspective, it is most likely that bidirectional effects exist, with smartphone use driving certain kinds of psychopathology and psychopathology, in turn, further motivating problematic use.[26,27]

Despite the strong associations between online and offline risk, certain features of online environments and mobile communications (e.g., accessibility, potential anonymity, and rapid, text-based communication) may increase the likelihood of impulsive action[19] and amplify the emotional impact of online victimization.[28] These technical features, coupled with teens' neurodevelopmental immaturity, can increase the likelihood of isolated poor choices that may not be representative of an individual's overall well-being.[29,30] Adolescents' developmental tasks interact with certain aspects of the Internet (e.g., social networking as a site for exploration of self-presentation and psychosocial identity; self-disclosure online compared to face-to-face encounters).[31] Such interactions may be positive, such as an adolescent who identifies as gay and lacks a supportive community at his school but finds such a community online via Twitter which helps him consolidate his sexual identity. Other interactions may be more problematic, for example, an adopted adolescent with significant attachment problems who is drawn to conversing with adults via online chat applications where she is vulnerable to inappropriate relationships. Assessment must therefore focus on the extent to which the misuse of technology indicates a developmental "glitch" remediable with support and psychoeducation or is a harbinger of underlying difficulties with self-regulation, self-esteem, attachment, etc.[32–34]

We next review two behaviors at the intersection of adolescent development and digital media: cyberbullying and adolescent "sexting." These behaviors may be used in the service of healthy development (e.g., consensual adolescent sexting), as well as the expression of more troubling dynamics and risk (e.g., cyberbullying; nonconsensual sexting).

CYBERBULLYING

Cyberbullying is defined as a form of interpersonal aggression that is intentionally and repeatedly carried out in a digital/electronic context (e.g., instant messages, e-mail, text messages, social media sites, Web pages, online games, or digital images).[35] The term cyberbullying therefore encompasses many behaviors: flaming (i.e., an online fight), harassment (i.e., repetitive, offensive messages), outing/trickery (i.e., soliciting personal information from someone and then electronically sharing that information without the individual's consent), exclusion (e.g., blocking someone), impersonation (e.g., posing as the victim and electronically communicating inappropriate or negative information with others as if it were coming from the victim), cyberstalking (i.e., using electronic communication to stalk and harass another person through repetitive, threatening messages), and the nonconsensual distribution of youth-produced sexual images.[36] There remains some dispute about what the key features of cyberbullying are (e.g., intent to cause harm, repetition, and an imbalance of power), which has resulted in definitional and measurement issues within the broader literature.[23]

Cyberbullying: Prevalence and Correlates

In light of the unresolved questions about how cyberbullying should be defined and thus measured, it is not surprising that research has produced varying prevalence rates depending on the definition used. Prevalence estimates generally range between approximately 10% and 40%.[15,37,38] The majority of research has examined cyberbullying among middle-school and high-school samples, with most studies based in North America, Europe, and Australia (with fewer studies in Asian countries).[39] A meta-analysis of 131 studies on bullying in the digital age reported that prevalence estimates are higher when self-report study measures use behavioral checklists rather than provide a bullying definition or use the word "bully," likely due to social desirability.[39]

There is substantial cross-sectional overlap between online and offline bullying both in terms of victimization and perpetration.[39–43] Because the majority of available literature is correlational, future research is required to determine how exactly traditional bullying and cyberbullying are related. Importantly, a meta-analysis of youth cyberbullying research noted that traditional bullying explained only 20% of the variance in reports of cyberbullying, suggesting that not all youth who report being bullied in traditional ways also report being cyberbullied.[39] Other variables must also be assessed.

Spending more time online is a risk factor for cyberbullying, as is older age for cyberbullying but not victimization (i.e., older vs. younger adolescents are more likely to engage in cyberbullying).[28,39,44] Engagement in cyberbullying has also been correlated with a number of negative psychological variables (e.g., higher levels of anxiety, loneliness, depression, and lower self-esteem and life satisfaction).[39] A lack of affective empathy, or an individual's ability to share the emotions of others, has been associated with more frequent cyberbullying perpetration.[39] Like other dimensions of teens' digital life and consistent with the co-construction model,[19] cyberbullying is likely to be an extension of social interactions "in real life." For example, qualitative research on gang-involved ethnic minority adolescents described the use of social media to grieve, express trauma, and make and respond to threats (i.e., cyberbanging).[45]

Youth who engage in bullying as both victims and perpetrators are referred to as "bully-victims." Within the research on "bully-victims" who are involved in traditional bullying, this category of youth is small in terms of prevalence but is the most psychiatrically troubled and vulnerable.[46] It is not clear whether this same pattern holds for the "bully-victims" involved in cyberbullying. Some research on "bully-victims" involved in cyberbullying report higher rates of abuse/neglect and experiences of maladaptive parenting,[47] as well as greater psychiatric and psychosomatic problems (e.g., emotional and peer problems, sleep difficulties, conduct problems, hyperactivity, substance use).[48] Other studies have reported that rates of "bully-victims" are higher among youth who engage in cyberbullying than the published rates on traditional bullying.[41] The authors propose it may be "easier" to act as both bully-victims in a digital context given the lack of face-to-face social cues in digital interactions.

Despite the correlations between online and offline bullying, certain features of digital contexts may amplify the emotional experience and psychological consequences of cyberbullying. These include the potential reproducibility of cyberbullying (e.g., the ability to copy others on a message or forward material to others), the perception of uncontrollability of online communications, lack of verbal cues that potentially de-escalate or mitigate emotional reactions, and 24/7 accessibility.[23,28,39] These unique technical features of cyberbullying and their potential to cause greater harm are often emphasized in reports of individual teens where serious outcomes such as suicide have occurred.[49] Indeed, perhaps the most serious potential harm of cyberbullying is its association with suicidal ideation, suicide attempts, and completed suicide among adolescents, which we will discuss next.

Associations Between Cyberbullying and Suicidality

The emergence of cyberbullying and media coverage that linked this form of bullying with the suicides of individual teens during the late 1990s and early 2000s caused renewed social concern about bullying in general.[50] This, in turn, spurred increased popular attention and novel legal responses to cyberbullying, even though longitudinal research on the topic is limited.[50] Research suggests that the media continue to influence how bullying and suicidality are popularly represented, and the effects are not always positive. For example, a recent content analysis of US news stories ($n = 184$) on cyberbullying and suicide showed that few articles adhered to expert guidelines on reporting (i.e., Center for Disease Control, American Foundation for Suicide Prevention) shown to help protect against the contagion of suicidal behavior.[49]

Meta-analytic research has shown moderately strong relationships between cyberbullying and suicidal ideation, indicating that individuals reporting higher levels of cyberbullying also report having thought about committing suicide more often.[39] Youth who have experienced traditional bullying or cyberbullying, as an offender, victim, or both, had more suicidal thoughts and were more likely to attempt suicide than those who had not experienced this form of peer aggression.[39] Victimization by cyberbullying has been more strongly related to suicidal thoughts and behaviors than perpetrating cyberbullying.[51] A meta-analysis found that cyberbullying has been more strongly related to suicidal ideation when compared with traditional bullying.[52] Suicidality should therefore be assessed when any form of bullying is present: traditional or cyber, and whether the youth is a victim, perpetrator, or both.

It is also important to put findings about cyberbullying and suicidal ideation in developmental context and to consider cyberbullying alongside the multitude of other risk factors associated with adolescent suicide in order not to direct prevention and intervention efforts solely on digital technology.[50] For example, lesbian, gay, and bisexual adolescents have higher odds of reporting suicidal thoughts, plans, and attempts than their heterosexual peers.[53–55] A large investigation ($n = 75,344$) of US adolescents assessed variation in bullying and suicidal ideation based on race/ethnicity and sexual orientation. Sexual minorities from all race/ethnicity and gender categories were more likely to report suicidal ideation even with bullying held constant.[56] Such results emphasize the importance of considering how risk factors interact, and the effects of moderating factors such as stigma and social support in addition to the role of digital media.[56]

Contextual Factors and Cyberbullying

Research has identified contextual factors that influence development and maintenance or cyberbullying behavior, including the quality of parent-child relationships. Just as developmental adversity may be associated with cyberbullying and possibly "bully-victim" status, a positive social and family context can be protective. Parental involvement as well as a school climate characterized by safety, respect, fairness, and kindness of staff has been associated with less frequent cyberbullying as either a victim or perpetrator.[28,39] Perpetration of cyberbullying includes beliefs that aggression is an acceptable way to solve problems, high levels of family conflict, and low parental supervision.[39,44] Parental monitoring has been negatively associated with cyberbullying,[39] but not all parental monitoring is equally effective. Limited research exists on the kinds of parental monitoring that is most protective of youth and also supportive of teens' abilities to make self-protective choices as they mature.

A recent review considered the available evidence on the association between specific parenting strategies and cyberbullying.[57] Parental monitoring of adolescent activities online is also referred to as parental mediation of technology.[58] Mediation strategies include (1) *restrictive mediation* (e.g., limiting adolescents' online activities), (2) *evaluative mediation* (i.e., discussion and joint creation of Internet rules), and/or (3) *co-using* (e.g., parents' active participation in teens' online activities).[58] Research suggests that evaluative mediation is more highly associated with reduced cyberbullying victimization than restrictive mediation, where parents make decisions unilaterally.[59,60]

Evaluative mediation is consistent with an authoritative parenting style, which combines high levels of warmth and control, and is associated with children's lower cyberbullying perpetration.[57] These findings are consistent with the broader literature on parental monitoring and adolescents, a point we return to later in our discussion of practice recommendations. Although the research on parenting in the digital age is limited, surveillance is unlikely to be the most effective way to reduce risky online behaviors.[61] Rather, identifying factors that promote youth disclosure is a more promising approach.[57]

It is clear that prevention and intervention strategies for reducing cyberbullying must be multisystemic, and consider parent-child dynamics and how these relate to community, school, and society.[57,62] It is not certain from the literature what parenting strategies best prevent cyberbullying, let alone how these may be tailored to diverse families. We return to this topic and implications for parent guidance later.

One form of cyberbullying involves the misuse or nonconsensual distribution of youth-produced sexually explicit images.[63,64] Sharing of such images, commonly referred to as "sexting," is a topic in itself, which we discuss next.

"SEXTING" AND YOUTH-PRODUCED SEXUAL IMAGES

One of the most controversial forms of adolescents' technology use is "sexting," a phenomenon that emerged from the intersection of several volatile social topics: adolescent sexual behavior, new technology, and criminal law. The popular press coined the term sexting around 2008, and early popular coverage on the topic was tilted toward a presumption of danger due to inflated but widely publicized prevalence estimates, and several high-profile cases involving a disproportionate legal response.[6,33]

Since these reactionary beginnings, a peer-reviewed literature on the topic has developed. Research has recommended the more specific language of *youth-produced sexual images* when referring to the most legally problematic form of "sexting": pictures created by minors that depict minors, which could be child pornography under applicable criminal statutes.[64,65] Unlike bullying, where all forms are harmful, not all forms of consensual minor sexting are problematic— although most of the time when sexting occurs, some conversation about sex, sexuality, and relationships is required, including concerns about legal and reputational risks. We will review the literature in this area to aid psychiatrists in their assessment of adolescent sexting behaviors.

Research on teens' motivations to engage in sexting suggests that most episodes of sexting are best understood as romantic or sexual interest during a time that heightened sexual interest, drive, and activity is developmentally typical.[66,67] Prevalence estimates of sexting vary based on the definition used. When sexting is defined as images that are sexually explicit and more likely to meet the statutory definition of child pornography, estimates are quite low (1%).[65] When the definition of sexting includes ever appearing in, creating, or receiving sexually suggestive rather than explicit images, estimates are higher (9.6%) based on a nationally representative sample of youth aged 10–17 years.[65]

A critical review of sexting research concluded that the majority of youth who participate in research on sexting cite romantic and/or sexual motivations (e.g., "to be sexy or initiate sexual activity") for self-producing sexual images.[68] Empirically derived typologies distinguish between sexting with "experimental" motivations (e.g., romantic in nature; sexually attention-seeking) and so-called "aggravating" factors, whether intended or not (e.g., adult involvement, coercion, unwanted distribution to a third party).[64] Another research-based motivational continuum of sexting describes situations of mutual trust (i.e., exclusive closed, trusting relationships), self-interest (i.e., attention seeking, bragging rights, subtle coercion, joking around), and intent to harm (i.e., adults involved, explicit peer-based aggression).[63] Of course, the boundaries among these categories may shift unexpectedly due to the vicissitudes of adolescent relationships,[33] and the individuals involved may have different perspectives on how best to define what has transpired. It is nevertheless important to consider teens' motivations in producing a sexted image, their intended use of such images, and the implications of this behavior for psychosexual well-being.

The available literature on sexting consistently associates the behavior with a greater likelihood of sexual activity "in real life." A review cited 11 studies have investigated the relationship between sexting and sexual risk behaviors, 8 of which measured sexual activity.[68] All eight studies found that youth who had reported previous "sexting" were significantly more likely to be sexually active than nonsexters.[69–74] Research is mixed, however, on whether sexting is associated with higher-risk sexual activity (e.g., higher number of partners).[70–72,74,75] Data are also equivocal on whether sexting is associated with mental health or well-being, with mixed data on associations between sexting and self-reported depression, anxiety, or self-esteem problems,[68] and some evidence for an association between sexting and higher rates of substance use and impulsivity.[76]

One longitudinal study of sexting followed an ethically diverse sample of adolescents ($n = 964$; mean age 16 years) and reported that the odds of being sexually active at 1-year follow-up were 1.32 times larger for youth who sent a sext at baseline.[77] Although sexting was not temporally associated with other risky behaviors, results suggest that sexting can be understood as marker of sexual behavior and/or a predictor of initiating offline sexual behavior.

Possible Misuses of Adolescent Sexting

Perhaps the greatest possible misuse of adolescent sexting is the unwanted forwarding and dissemination of images by one member of the sexting dyad. Research on nonconsensual or "third-party" distribution of sexts suggests that this behavior is rare. A national study of Internet users aged 10–17 years reported only a small proportion of youth had forwarded youth-produced sexual images. Images were distributed in 10% of incidents when a youth appeared in or created the image and 3% when the youth received it.[64,65] While reassuring, unwanted dissemination is associated with very high levels of distress when it does occur, including shame, guilt, and helplessness.[78] These situations are also challenging for parents, schools, and law enforcement in terms of knowing which system should hold youth accountable,[63,79] and how best to support youth whose images are nonconsensually circulated since such images that can never be fully retrieved or expunged.

A related behavior is the extortion of sexual images, referred to as "sextortion," which is much less studied. A 2016 study surveyed a self-selected sample of youth aged 18–25 years who had been the targets of threats to expose sexual images.[78] Respondents were primarily female, with almost half (45%) reporting incidents of sextortion when they were younger than 18 year. Perpetrators carried out threats in 45% of cases. Scenarios involving sextortion were diverse. One common scenario included an aggrieved former partner threatening to distribute images that were consensually exchanged during the relationship, either to force reconciliation or humiliate the respondent. A second common sextortion scenario involved someone met online requesting a sexual image from respondents or another source used to demand more images or sexual interactions. Respondents described systemic factors that worsened their distress, including a lack of criminal laws addressing this phenomenon, perceived blame by law enforcement, and jurisdictional issues related to the Internet.[78]

Another potential harm of sexting is the perpetuation of sexual double standards among teens. Sexual socialization theory posits that frequent exposure to consistent themes about gender and sexual behavior can affect a young person's developing sense of what is expected for males and females, including subsequent behavior.[80] Research suggests gender differences in the *experience* of sexting may perpetuate sexual double standards. A qualitative study of males and females aged 12–18 years reported that females felt judged harshly whether they sent sexts or not (e.g., judged as a "slut" or "prude," respectively), with males not endorsing this same experience.[81] Another qualitative investigation in the U.K. of youth aged 12–15 years found that being asked for "nudes" is a new form of female desirability, albeit one rooted in gender-related contradictions.[82] For example, males in this study curried respect from peers through collected and rated images of females, while females were blamed for being photographed in the first place. Female respondents describe the practice as risky and potentially shaming of sexual reputation (i.e., "slut shaming").[82] Other qualitative research in the United States reported similar results, with females describing how males who engage in sexting are lauded whereas females are shamed.[63]

Although early media reports about sexting emphasized the possible legal risks for teens, arrests and prosecution stemming from adolescent sexting are rare. One study described 3477 cases of sexting handled by law enforcement in 2006–09.[83] Two-thirds of sexting cases handled by law enforcement involved aggravating circumstances that went beyond the creation and dissemination of sexually explicit images (e.g., adult involvement, 46%, or a minor engaged in nonconsensual or malicious behavior, 13%).[83] Research also suggests the role of aggravating factors in cases where adolescents are prosecuted for sexting. A convenience sample of state prosecutors who handled such cases identified variables associated with prosecutors bringing charges against juveniles.[84] Prosecutors who filed charges against a minor involved in sexting reflected four themes: (1) malicious intent/bullying/coercion of harassment (36%), (2) distribution, including of one's own image or forwarding of someone else's (25%), (3) the existence of a large age difference between the involved parties (22%), and (4) graphic nature of the images (9%).[84] Thus, the presence of aggravating factors is typically required for teens to be arrested and prosecuted for sexting. This category of sexting should therefore be considered statistically and also developmentally anomalous, and a reason for more concern and specialized intervention, whether psychoeducational, clinical, or some combination.

In sum, motivations for and the emotional impact of sexting will vary for the individual involved and should be assessed rather than assumed. Differences in the emotional experience of sexting may range depending on the young person's age, gender, perception of choice or pressure to send or receive images, and also his/her motivations.[63,64] Distress can also be present even when the sexting is consensual[65] and feelings about the experience may change following the initial encounter.[33] Psychiatrists should therefore consider each of these possible dynamics as part of assessment.

Educational Responses to Adolescent Sexting

In light of these findings, a combination of educational, legislative, and diversion strategies should replace a primarily law enforcement or prosecutorial response for the majority of situations where minors engage in consensual sexting.[6,79,85] Although educating youth about legal consequences may be part of effective education,[86] this is unlikely to be sufficient. Research on the most effective components of Internet-related educational programming recommends instructing skills related to the problem of interest (e.g., emotion regulation, healthy relationships and boundaries, curbing impulsivity), providing opportunities for role-play and skills practice, and multiple "doses" of education rather than one-time assemblies.[87,88]

With respect to sexting, we suggest that education target components of sexuality development related to adolescent sexting: sexual decision-making (e.g., consent), privacy violations, relational sexuality, reciprocity, and trust.[6,33] Clinicians should understand adolescent sexting as an expression of sexual behavior[77] and talk about it accordingly, including frank discussions of risk and pleasure, the importance of trust and communication with one's partner, and questioning the necessity of an image as compared to verbal, in-person communication. In light of adolescents' nascent prefrontal cortex development, it is important for education about sexting to account for the major differences in teens' decision making under conditions of relative calm versus emotional arousal. Adolescents can easily identify the risks of sexting during a school assembly, but this is much harder to do in situations of strong affect or "hot" cognition. Indeed, most situations where youth encounter "trouble" related to sexting is due to an impulsive response to emotional arousal (e.g., a break-up, a perceived slight).[79] Thus, education should include skills for regulating emotions at such times, and helping youth understand that their decision making is more likely to go "off-line" under conditions of high arousal due to adolescent brain development.

Education should also emphasize research-based estimates of sexting to counter the misperception that all teens engage in this behavior. Popular media has promoted the narrative of adolescent sexting as highly prevalent,[5,6] which research does not support.[64,68] Providing research-derived estimates is important since adolescents are likely to evaluate the risks associated with specific sexual behaviors through social comparisons with their best friends.[89] Teens are often surprised to learn that published prevalence rates of sexting are quite low (i.e., 1% for sexually explicit images that meet the statutory definition of child pornography and 9.6% for sexually suggestive images), in contrast with the perception that "everyone sends nudes." Youth perceptions of peer norms around sexual standards can affect sexual behavior even when the perceived norms are erroneous.[90–92] Simply educating teens about the tendency to misperceive the behavior of peers (i.e., pluralistic ignorance) can be an effective strategy to reduce risk behaviors[93] and can inform educational approaches to sexting.

CONCLUSION AND RECOMMENDATIONS: THE 4MS OF PARENT GUIDANCE

We have highlighted several themes in the evolving literature about the use and misuse of digital media among teens. First, the risk of technology misuse is not evenly distributed among teens, with problematic use of digital media most often associated with psychosocial difficulties "in real life."[20] Clinical attention to related offline challenges (e.g., social isolation, parent-child conflict, or risk-taking behavior) may indirectly address problems with digital media. At the same time, however, the unique dynamics of digital technology (e.g., potential anonymity, text-based communication, and disembodied communication) increase the likelihood of impulsive missteps, particularly given teens' neurodevelopmental immaturity.[30,33] Clinicians should therefore assess teens' digital media use as part of routine psychiatric assessment, and published recommendations can help inform this process.[32]

Consistent with our emphasis on developmental theory, parental influence on digital media use also matters, and we will emphasize this in our practice recommendations. The evidence base on parents' roles in preventing teens' online harm and victimization is provisional, since the majority of research is correlational and limits conclusions about causality. Nonetheless, we suggest that family remains the most central and enduring context for child development[94]—even in our digital age. The quality of parent-child relationships can protect youth as well as help foster their resilience when missteps occur. In our experience, however, parents are uncertain about how best to engage adolescents in conversations about mobile communications, digital technology, and social media. Our clinical experience has shown us ways in which parents feel intimidated, avoidant, or "deskilled" when it comes to talking about and setting limits on teens' technology use.[95,96] By "deskilled," we refer to our observations of many parents who are able to set limits effectively in other aspects of an adolescent's life but struggle to apply these same strategies (e.g., authoritative parenting) to digital life.

This section provides recommendations for how clinicians can advise parents about starting and maintaining conversations on these topics and on forms of parental monitoring associated with safer digital media use. We refer to these principles as the "4Ms of parent guidance," which are a distillation of available research on digital media as well as related constructs from the child development literature. The 4Ms apply to all of the behaviors we have reviewed in this chapter, and they include: *manner*, *modeling*, *monitoring*, and *meaning*.

Manner

The *manner* in which parents approach conversations and communicate with adolescents about complex topics impacts their children's behavior. For example, the manner and approach that parents take when talking with adolescents about topics such as sex provide important insights. Parents' responsiveness during conversations about sex is associated with teens' more protective sexual behavior (e.g., delayed age of intercourse and increased use of contraception).[97] A systematic review of interventions designed to improve parental communication about sex identified qualities associated with effective communication: parents who talk less and listen more, are less directive, ask more questions, and maintain a nonjudgmental, receptive stance.[98] Parents who dominate such conversations by talking more rather than listening and engaging the teen tend to have adolescents who are less knowledgeable about sexual health topics.[99,100]

Whatever monitoring strategies parents use, it is paramount that parents couch limits within a relationship of emotional warmth and support. In the absence of warmth, youth are more likely to experience monitoring as controlling and punitive, which may reduce compliance and increase reactivity/mistrust.[57] In contrast, authoritative parenting, which combines developmentally appropriate limits with high levels of warmth and collaboration, is most likely to foster disclosure and thus create opportunity for the kinds of parent-child conversations we are recommending.

Adolescents whose parents practice this warm, authoritative manner of communication report greater comfort discussing sex with their parents and discussion of more topics.[101] We recommend applying these findings to conversations about digital media, with future research to evaluate the effects on teen behavior. Clinicians can provide psychoeducation to parents about the impact of conversations on adolescent behavior and coach this manner of communication. While clinicians must be sensitive to the role of parents' values, including cultural and religious factors that inform how they wish to communicate about sex, they should also inform parents about the risk of no conversation. For example, children raised in families where sex is taboo are more susceptible to sexually explicit media influence than those raised in homes where sex is a permissible topic.[102,103] In the absence of effective sex education by parents, youth may rely on media for information, which may condone more sexually permissive norms and affect teen's sexual behavior.[104]

Modeling

In our experience, parents tend to underestimate the impact of their own use of digital media on their children. This is, in part, because teens can *appear* more sophisticated with new devices, and adolescents have been socially framed—largely by adults—as "digital natives."[105] Neglected in most discourse about youth and digital media is the continued presence and influence of adults on this landscape.[10] With respect to child psychiatry, we can remind parents that their use of digital technology does impact their children and that modeling still matters in a digital age.

Prior longitudinal research on the effects of parent-modeled media use on children's TV watching[106] provides a basis for speculating about similar effects with respect to digital media. Likewise, social cognitive theory[107] holds that youth observe the behavior of social referents around them and are likely to learn and emulate behaviors that result in favorable outcomes (e.g., enjoyment, extrinsic rewards). In fact, over half of the surveyed teens (58%) name their parents as the most influential in what they believe to be appropriate in terms of digital media use.[58] A study of adolescents (aged 12–17 years) and parents reported that parents' level of engagement in seven Internet activities predicted teen engagement in each activity.[108] Thus, there is some evidence that teens are following their parents' cues, with teens' being influenced by their parents' use of digital media.

Research suggests that parental use of mobile technology around young children is associated with fewer parent-child interactions,[109] and lower responsivity to children's bids for attention.[110] Thus, in addition to modeling effects, parents' restraint around digital technology may also impact relationship quality. Technology-based interruptions in parent-child interactions has been termed "technoference." A recent cross-sectional study of US parents ($n = 170$; mean child age 3 years) found that maternal and paternal problematic technology use predicted greater technoference in both parents' interactions with children. Maternal technoference also predicted both parents' reports of child internalizing and externalizing behaviors.[111] The directionality of these effects awaits longitudinal study, but results highlight the influence of digital media on family interactions, and the potential impact of modeling on child behavior as well as the quality of parent-child relationships.

We recommend educating parents about the possible effects of their own digital media use on their children, and their role as leaders in establishing the family culture. As teens mature, they are increasingly attuned to hypocrisy and are quick to point out times that parents do not abide by their own rules, which is extremely important in matters relating to digital media.[96] Whatever youth assert about their parents' lack of influence, or their own superior knowledge of all things digital, parents must also be reassured that their influence extends to digital spaces. Parents need not be experts with the latest app to have an impact, and parents knowing the effects of their own digital media use on their children is an important first step.

Monitoring

Parents often ask how much they should monitor their teen's texts, online presence, and social networking. There is a relative dearth of research, especially longitudinal studies, to help psychiatrists answer these questions. In general, we recommend monitoring strategies tailored to characteristics of the child and their behavior (e.g., age, psychosocial well-being, and any risk factors). Risk factors may include an untreated psychiatric diagnosis which affects social behavior, or other indications of vulnerability (e.g., suicidality, self-harm, poor boundaries).[32] It is first important to define what monitoring even means in the digital age.

The developmental concept of parental monitoring predates digital media and is conceptualized as "a set of correlated parenting behaviors involving attention to and tracking of the child's whereabouts, activities, and adaptations."[112] Subsequent research has reinterpreted parental monitoring as a form of parental knowledge based on child disclosure as much as parental solicitation and parental control.[61] Studies suggest that parent-child communication is much more important than control and surveillance with respect to adolescents' school performance, substance use, and norm-breaking.[61,113,114] Parents get most of their information about a child's activities from his/her willing disclosure rather than from their active surveillance and control.[61]

Seen in this way, "good monitoring" is best understood as a relationship property in which both child and parent participate.[61] Monitoring teens' digital media use therefore includes ways that parents can facilitate adolescent disclosure rather than rely exclusively, or even primarily, on surveillance and control.

What Forms of Control and Oversight Are Indicated, If Any?

Media research has described three proactive parental strategies for monitoring or curbing media exposure. As reviewed by Padilla and Coyne,[115] the first, *cocooning* (also called restrictive mediation), involves parental effort to restrict certain media at home (e.g., rules about content viewed, location of media source in the home, or time spent). Cocooning is more effective with younger children and cannot be a parent's sole strategy given the ubiquity of wireless access at home, at school, and with peers. *Prearming* (also called active mediation) encourages parent-child discussion regarding children's exposure to questionable media content or (in the case of digital media) online behavior. The objective of prearming is to assist the child in thinking critically about media and taking an active role in consuming and understanding media. The third type of proactive media monitoring is *co-viewing*, where parents view media with their children. This strategy is less relevant to hand-held devices such as smartphones. In contrast to these proactive strategies for oversight and control, another approach is called *deference*, whereby parents actively choose to do nothing in response to conflicting values as a means of showing trust for the child. This approach is more appropriate for use with older adolescents, where family rules are already understood.

Although research is limited on which strategy is most effective for digital media, parents who were more likely to use prearming with print media at 1-year follow-up had closer bonds with their adolescents.[115] Prearming is associated with greater parental effort but also greater efficacy for adolescents.[116] There may also be associations between parents' general level of monitoring, unrelated to digital media, and adolescents' online behavior. A study of US adolescents (aged 12−17 years) and their parents reported that when adolescents perceived that their parents monitored them in general, outside of digital media, they engaged in instant messaging/chat, online social networking, video streaming, and massive multiplayer online gaming activities at lower rates. Put another way, teens who reported that their parents had greater awareness of their whereabouts, activities, and friend group engaged less in these online behaviors, compared to their peers who were less-monitored by their parents.[108]

In our experience, use of cocooning with adolescents may be futile since teens are likely to respond to restrictive gatekeeping by migrating to different platforms (e.g., creation of fake accounts, using a laptop for Facetime when a phone is taken away). One exception is the importance of restricting teens' mobile phone access at night, or what is referred to as a digital curfew. In addition to previous correlational research on the disruptive effects of nighttime mobile phone use on adolescents' sleep,[117,118] a recent longitudinal study of US adolescents found that as nighttime mobile phone use increased over time, so did poor sleep behavior—which predicted decreases in well-being across domains (e.g., depressed mood, externalizing behavior, low self-esteem, and poor coping).[119] Digital curfews for younger children are easier to implement at the time they first obtain a smartphone. This helps create a default family rule for no mobile phone at bedtime.

Another monitoring strategy parents commonly use is becoming "friends" with their teen on social networking sites. Although many teens create multiple social networking sites to which parents may not have access, parents' online social networking with the children has nonetheless been associated with increased self-reported connection between parents and adolescents.[120] Self-reported connection also mediated the relationship between social networking with parents and behavioral outcomes, including higher prosocial behavior and lower relational aggression and internalizing behavior among youth. Conversely, adolescent social networking use without parents was associated with increased relational aggression, internalizing behaviors and delinquency, and decreased feelings of connection.[120] Results suggest that online social networking with parents could strengthen parent-child relationships and then lead to positive outcomes for adolescents, or could be a proxy for a healthier parent-child bond independent of digital media. Study authors emphasize that connecting via social networking is only one of many ways to build such connection[120]; ensuring connections "in real life" is obviously even more important.

Deference, or parents actively choosing to do nothing in response to conflicting values as a means of showing trust, is an effective strategy with older adolescents.[115] Parents must respond with appropriate limits; however, when teens engage in behavior suggesting more adult containment is needed. There certainly are situations where digital media should be restricted, and psychiatrists are most likely to be consulted at such times. Complete restriction should be reserved for situations where behavior is frankly unsafe (e.g., online sexual communication with adults; ongoing harassment, bullying, or digital abuse as a perpetrator, victim, or both; use that interferes with daily functioning). Occasionally this level of behavior will require more containment and intervention than parents can provide, in which case out-of-home placement may be necessary for crisis stabilization and safety planning.[34]

Meaning

Parents are often concerned about the meaning of adolescents' use of digital media both with respect to present and future well-being. In this chapter, we have emphasized the correspondence between children's offline functioning and digital media use, and we encourage clinicians to help parents also to think developmentally about devices.[95] This means considering the child's developmental stage and the "work" that corresponds with this period (e.g., peer relationships, sexual identity, and individuation from parents), and how the use of digital media may support or inhibit this process.[31] Another aspect of meaning to consider is whether the behavior of concern relates to technology at all:

> *A technology-focused conflict can be about the expressed content, or it can be a metaphor for relational issues. Therapists must first sort out if the conflict is simply about too much technology or if the technology is fertile ground for some other conflict between parent and child.[96]*

Often parents are able to make this determination on their own, but other times professional help from a child psychiatrist or psychologist is required. Our review of activities associated with the greatest risk provides a framework for making these determinations.

Conclusions

Examined together, the 4Ms offer a starting point to help facilitate challenging parent-child conversations, which we suggest are likely to help teens make more self-protective digital choices as they mature. The lack of research on the long-term effects of digital media use cannot be overstated, and this must temper the certainty with which we consult with parents, schools, and our child and adolescent patients. However, grounding our approach to these digital challenges in the broader literature on child development, including parenting, parental monitoring, risk-taking, and developmental psychopathology, is both parsimonious and promising. Psychiatrists should remember the ways that online risk is deeply intertwined with offline adjustment and well-being and should use this knowledge to educate families, teens themselves, and the media when popular representations promote a simplified or misleading narrative.

REFERENCES

1. Lenhart A. *(2015) Social Media and Technology Overview.* Pew Research Center; 2015. Available at: http://www.pewinternet.org/2015/04/09/teens-social-media-technology-2015.
2. Lenhart A, Purcell K, Smith A, Zickuhr K. *Social Media and Young Adults.* Pew Research Center Internet and Technology; 2010. Available at: http://www.pewinternet.org/2010/02/03/social-media-and-young-adults/.
3. Turkle S. Always-on/always-on-you: the tethered self. In: Katz JE, ed. *Handbook of Mobile Communication Studies.* Cambridge, MA: MIT Press; 2008:121−137.
4. Turkle S. *Alone Together: Why We Expect More from Technology and Less from Each Other.* New York: Perseus; 2011.
5. Draper N. Is your teen at risk? Discourses of adolescent sexting in United States television news. *J Child Media.* 2012;6:221−236.
6. Hasinoff AA. *Sexting Panic: Rethinking Criminalization, Privacy and Consent.* Chicago, IL: University of Illinois Press; 2015.
7. Richtel M. Are teenagers replacing drugs with smartphones? *N Y Times;* 2017. Available at: https://www.nytimes.com/2017/03/13/health/teenagers-drugs-smartphones.html.
8. Twenge J. Have smartphones destroyed a generation? *Atlantic.* Available at: https://www.theatlantic.com/magazine/archive/2017/09/has-the-smartphone-destroyed-a-generation/534198/.
9. boyd d. *It's Complicated: The Social Lives of Networked Teens.* New Haven: Yale University Press; 2014.
10. Herring SC. Questioning the generational divide: technological exoticism and adult constructions of online youth identity. In: Buckingham D, ed. *Youth, Identity and Digital Media.* Cambridge: MIT Press; 2008:71−92.
11. Marvin C. *When Old Technologies Were New: Thinking about Electric Communication in the Late Nineteenth Century.* New York: Oxford; 1988.
12. Cicchetti D, Toth SL. Transactional ecological systems in developmental psychopathology. In: Luthar SS, Burack JA, Cicchetti D, Weisz JR, eds. *Developmental Psychopathology: Perspectives on Risk, Adjustment and Disorder.* Cambridge: Cambridge University Press; 1997: 317−349.
13. Subrahmanyam K, Smahel D, Greenfield P. Connecting developmental constructions to the Internet: identity presentation and sexual exploration in online teen chat rooms. *Dev Psychol.* 2006;42:395−406.
14. Greenfield PM. Developmental considerations for determining appropriate Internet use guidelines for children and adolescents. *J Appl Dev Psychol.* 2004;25: 751−762.
15. boyd d, Hargittai E, Schultz J, Palfrey J. Why parents help their children lie to Facebook about age: unintended consequences of the 'children online privacy protection act'. *First Monday.* 2011;16(2011). Available at: http://journals.uic.edu/ojs/index.php/fm/article/view/3850/3075.
16. Common Sense Media. *The Common Sense Census: Media Use by Tweens and Teens;* 2015. Available at: https://www.commonsensemedia.org/research/the-common-sense-census-media-use-by-tweens-and-teens.
17. The Associated Press-NORC Center for Public Affairs Research. *New Survey Reveals Snapchat and Instagram Are the Most Popular Social Media Platforms Among American Teens;* 2017. Available at: http://www.apnorc.org/projects/Pages/Instagram-and-Snapchat-are-Most-Popular-Social-Networks-for-Teens.aspx.
18. Gimelli R. *Normal Child and Adolescent Development.* Washington, DC: American Psychiatric Press; 1996.
19. Smahel D, Subrahmanyam K. Adolescent sexuality on the Internet: a developmental perspective. In: Saleh FM, Grudzinskas A, Judge AM, eds. *Adolescent Sexual Behavior in the Digital Age: Considerations for Clinicians, Legal Professionals and Educators.* New York: Oxford; 2014:62−88.
20. Wolak J, Finkelhor D, Mitchell KJ, Ybarra M. Online predators and their victims: myths, realities and implications for prevention and treatment. *Am Psychol.* 2008; 63(2):111−128.
21. Finkelhor D. *The Internet, Youth Safety and the Problem of "Juvenoia".* University of New Hampshire, Crimes Against Children Research Center; 2011, 2015. Available at: http://www.unh.edu/ccrc/pdf/Juvenoia%20paper.pdf.
22. Finkelhor D. Commentary: cause for alarm? Youth and internet risk research − a commentary on Livingstone and Smith. *J Child Psychol Psychiatry.* 2014;55: 655−658.

23. Livingstone S, Smith PK. Annual research review: harms experienced by child users of online and mobile technologies: the nature, prevalence and management of sexual and aggressive risks in the digital age. *J Child Psychol Psychiatry.* 2014;55:635−654.

24. Schoon I. *Risk and Resilience: Adaptations in Changing Times.* New York: Cambridge University Press; 2006.

25. Elhai JD, Dvorak RD, Levine JC, Hall BJ. Problematic smartphone use: a conceptual overview and systematic review of relations with anxiety and depression psychopathology. *J Affect Disord.* 2017;207:251−259.

26. van den Eijnden RJ, Meerkerk GJ, Vermulst AA, Spijkerman R, Engels EC. Online communication, compulsive Internet use, and psychosocial well-being among adolescents: a longitudinal study. *Dev Psychol.* 2008;44:655−665.

27. Yen JY, Cheng-Fang Y, Chen CS, Chang YH, Yeh YC, Ko CH. The bidirectional interactions between addiction, behaviour approach and behaviour inhibition systems among adolescents in a prospective study. *Psychiatry Res.* 2012;200:588−592.

28. Ybarra ML, Mitchell KJ. Youth engaging in online harassment: associations with caregiver-child relationships, Internet use, and personal characteristics. *J Adolesc.* 2004;27:319−326.

29. Cooper A. Sexuality and the Internet: surfing into the new millennium. *Cyberpsychol Behav.* 1998;1:181−187.

30. Giedd JN. The digital revolution and adolescent brain evolution. *J Adolesc Health.* 2012;51:101−105.

31. Valkenburg PM, Peter J. Online communication among adolescents: an integrated model of its attraction, opportunities, and risks. *J Adolesc Health.* 2011;48:121−127.

32. Carson NJ, Ganser M, Khang J. Assessment of digital media use in the adolescent psychiatric evaluation. *Child Adolesc Psychiatr Clin N Am.* 2018;27(2):133−143.

33. Judge AM. "Sexting" among U.S. adolescents: psychological and legal implications. *Harv Rev Psychiatry.* 2012;20:86−96.

34. Pridgen B. Navigating the Internet safely: recommendations for residential programs targeting at risk adolescents. *Harv Rev Psychiatry.* 2010;18:131−138.

35. Patchin JW, Hinduja S. Bullies move beyond the schoolyard: a preliminary look at cyberbullying. *Youth Violence Juv Justice.* 2006;4:148−169.

36. Willard NE. *Cyberbullying and Cyberthreats: Responding to the Challenge on Online Social Aggression, Threats, and Distress.* Champaign: Research Press; 2007.

37. O'Brennan LM, Bradshaw CP, Sawyer AL. Examining developmental differences in the social-emotional problems among frequent bullies, victims, and bully/victims. *Psychol Sch.* 2009;46:100−115.

38. Pontzner D. A theoretical test of bullying behavior: parenting, personality, and the bully/victim relationship. *J Fam Violence.* 2010;25:259−273.

39. Kowalski RM, Giumetti GW, Schroeder AN, Lattanner MR. Bullying in the digital age: a critical review and meta-analysis of cyberbullying research among youth. *Psychol Bull.* 2014;140:1073−1137.

40. Kowalski RM, Giumetti GW, Schroeder AN, Reese H. Cyberbullying among college students: evidence from multiple domain of college life. In: Wankel C, Wankel L, eds. *Misbehavior Online in Higher Education.* Bingley: Emerald; 2012:293−311.

41. Mishna F, Khoury-Kassibri M, Gadalla T, Daciuk J. Risk factors for involvement in cyber bullying: victims, bullies and bully-victims. *Child Youth Serv Rev.* 2012;34:63−70.

42. Olweus D. School bullying: development and some important challenges. *Annu Rev Clin Psychol.* 2013;9:751−780.

43. Smith PK, Mahdavi J, Carvalho M, Fisher S, Russell S, Tippett N. Cyberbullying, its forms and impact in secondary school pupils. *J Child Psychol Psychiatry.* 2008;49:376−385.

44. Guo S. A meta-analysis of the predictors of cyberbullying perpetration and victimization. *Psychol Sch.* 2016;53:432−453.

45. Patton DU, Eschmann RD, Butler DA. Internet banging: new trends in social media, gang violence, masculinity and hip hop. *Comput Hum Behav.* 2013;29:A54−A59.

46. Solberg ME, Olweus D, Endresen IM. Bullies and victims at school: are they the same pupils? *Br J Educ Psychol.* 2007;77:441−464.

47. Lereya ST, Samara M, Dieter W. Parenting behavior and the risk of becoming a victim and a bully/victim: a meta-analysis study. *Child Abuse Negl.* 2013;37:1091−1108.

48. Sourander A, Klomej A, Ikonen M, et al. Psychosocial risk factors associated with cyberbullying among adolescents: a population-based study. *Arch Gen Psychiatry.* 2010;67:720−728.

49. Young R, Subramanian R, Miles S, Hinnant A, Andsager JL. Social representation of cyberbullying and adolescent suicide: a mixed-method analysis of news stories. *J Health Commun.* 2017;32(9):1082−1092.

50. Saleh FM, Feldman J, Grudzinskas A, Ravven S, Cody R. Cybersexual harassment and suicide. In: Saleh FM, Grudzinskas A, Judge AM, eds. *Adolescent Sexual Behavior in the Digital Age: Considerations for Clinicians, Legal Professionals and Educators.* New York: Oxford; 2014:139−160.

51. Hinduja S, Patchin J. Bullying, cyberbullying, and suicide. *Arch Suicide Res.* 2010;14:206−221.

52. Gianluca G, Espelage DL. Peer victimization, cyberbullying, and suicide risk in children and adolescents. *J Am Med Assoc.* 2014;312:545−546.

53. Russell ST, Joyner K. Adolescent sexual orientation and suicide risk: evidence from a national study. *Am J Public Health.* 2001;91(8):1276−1281.

54. Stone DM, Luo F, Ouyang L, Lippy C, Hertz M, Crosby AE. Sexual orientation and suicide ideation, plans, attempts, and medically serious attempts: evidence from local youth risk behavior surveys, 2001−2009. *Am J Public Health.* 2014;104:262−271.

55. Wilkinson L, Pearson J. School culture and the well-being of same-sex attracted youth. *Gend Soc.* 2009;23:542−568.

56. Mueller AS, James W, Abrutyn S, Levin ML. Suicide ideation and bullying among US adolescents: examining the intersections of sexual orientation, gender, and race/ethnicity. *Am J Public Health*. 2015;105:980−985.

57. Elsaesser C, Russell B, McCauley OC, Patton D. Parenting in a digital age: a review of parents' role in preventing adolescent cyberbullying. *Aggress Violent Behav*. 2017;35: 62−72.

58. Livingstone S, Helsper EJ. Parental mediation of children's Internet use. *J Broadcast Electron Media*. 2008; 52:581−599.

59. Mesch GS. Parental mediation, online activities, and cyberbullying. *Cyberpsychol Behav*. 2009;12:387−393.

60. Navarro R, Serna C, Martínez V, Ruiz-Oliva R. The role of Internet use and parental mediation on cyberbullying victimization among Spanish children from rural public schools. *Eur J Psychol Educ*. 2012;28:725−745.

61. Stattin H, Kerr M. Parental monitoring: a reinterpretation. *Child Dev*. 2000;71:1072−1085.

62. Ang RP. Adolescent cyberbullying: a review of characteristics, prevention and intervention strategies. *Aggress Violent Behav*. 2015;25:35−42.

63. Harris A, Davidson J. Teens, sex and technology: implications for educational systems and practice. In: Saleh FM, Grudzinskas A, Judge AM, eds. *Adolescent Sexual Behavior in the Digital Age: Considerations for Clinicians, Legal Professionals and Educators*. New York: Oxford; 2014: 262−292.

64. Wolak J, Finkelhor D. *Sexting: A Typology*. Crimes Against Children Research Center; 2011. Available at: http://www.unh.edu/ccrc/pdf/CV231_Sexting%20Typology%20Bulletin_4-6-11_revised.pdf.

65. Mitchell KJ, Finkelhor D, Jones LM, Wolak J. Prevalence and characteristics of youth sexting: a national study. *Pediatrics*. 2012;129:1−8.

66. Diamond LM, Savin-Williams RC. Adolescent sexuality. In: Lerner RM, Steinberg L, eds. *Handbook of Adolescent Psychology*. Hoboken: John Wiley; 2009:479−523.

67. Ponton LE, Judice S. Typical adolescent sexual development. *Child Adolesc Psychiatr Clin N Am*. 2004; 13:497−511.

68. Klettke B, Halliford DJ, Mellow DJ. Sexting prevalence and correlates: a systematic literature review. *Clin Psychol Rev*. 2014;34:44−53.

69. The Associated Press-NORC Center for Public Affairs Research and MTV. *The Digital Abuse Study*; 2009. Available at: http://www.athinline.org/pdfs/2013-MTV-AP-NORC%20Center_Digital_Abuse_Study_Full.pdf.

70. Dake JA, Price DH, Mazriaz L, Ward B. Prevalence and correlates of sexting behaviour in adolescents. *Am J Sex Educ*. 2012;7:1−15.

71. Dir AL, Coskunpinar A, Steiner JL, Cyders MA. Understanding differences in sexting behaviors across gender, relationship status, and sexual identity, and the role of expectancies in sexting. *Cyberpsychol Behav Soc Netw*. 2013;16:568−574.

72. Gordon-Messer D, Bauermeister JA, Grodzinski A, Zimmerman M. Sexting among young adults. *J Adolesc Health*. 2012;52:301−306.

73. Rice E, Rhoades H, Winetrobe H, et al. Sexually explicit cell phone messaging associated with sexual risk among adolescents. *Pediatrics*. 2012;130:667−673.

74. Temple JR, Paul JA, van den Berg P, Le VD, McElhany A, Temple BW. Teen sexting and its associations with sexual behaviours. *Arch Pediatr Adolesc Med*. 2012;166: 828−833.

75. Benotsch EG, Snipes DJ, Martin AM, Bull SS. Sexting, substance use, and sexual risk behaviour in young adults. *J Adolesc Health*. 2013;52:307−313.

76. Temple JR, Vi DL, van den Berg P, Ling Y, Paul JA, Temple BW. Brief report: teen sexting and psychosocial health. *J Adolesc*. 2014;37:33−36.

77. Temple JR, Choi H. Longitudinal association between teen sexting and sexual behavior. *Pediatrics*. 2014;134: 1−6.

78. Wolak J, Finkelhor D. *Sextortion: Key Findings from an Online Survey of 1,631 Victims*; 2016. Available at: http://www.unh.edu/ccrc/pdf/Key%20Findings%20from%20a%20Survey%20of%20Sextortion%20Victims%20revised%208-9-2016.pdf.

79. Weins WJ, Hiestand TC. Sexting, statutes and save by the bell: introducing a lesser change with an "aggravating factors" framework. *Tenn L Rev*. 2009;77:1−65.

80. Brown JD, D'Engle KL. X-rated: sexual attitudes and behaviors associated with U.S. early adolescents' exposure to sexually explicit media. *Commun Res*. 2009; 36:129−151.

81. Lippman JR, Campbell SW. Damned if you do, damned if you don't…if you're a girl: relational and normative contexts of adolescent sexting in the United States. *J Child Media*. 2014:1−16.

82. Ringrose J, Harvey L, Gill R, Livingstone S. Teen girls, sexual double standards and "sexting" gendered value in digital image exchange. *Fem Theor*. 2013;14: 305−323.

83. Wolak J, Finkelhor D, Mitchell KJ. How often are teens arrested for sexting? Data from a national sample of police cases. *Pediatrics*. 2012;129:4−12.

84. Walsh W, Wolak J, Finkelhor D. *Sexting: When Are State Prosecutors Deciding to Prosecute? The Third National Juvenile Online Victimization Study (NJOV-3)*. University of New Hampshire Crimes Against Children Research Center; 2013. Available at: https://scholars.unh.edu/cgi/viewcontent.cgi?referer=https://www.google.com/&httpsredir=1&article=1042&context=ccrc.

85. Angelides S. 'Technology, hormones and stupidity': the affective politics of teenage sexting. *Sexualities*. 2013;16: 665−689.

86. Strohmaier H, Murphy M, DeMatteo D. Youth sexting: prevalence rates, driving motivations, and the deterrent effect of legal consequences. *Sex Res Soc Policy*. 2014;11: 245−255.

87. Jones LM, Mitchell KJ, Walsh WA. *A Systematic Review of Effective Youth Prevention Education: Implications for Internet Safety Education*. Durham, NH: Crimes Against Children Research Center, University of New Hampshire; 2014. Available at: https://scholars.unh.edu/ccrc/42/.

88. Jones LM, Mitchell KJ, Walsh WA. *A Content Analysis of Youth Internet Safety Programs: Are Effective Prevention Strategies Being Used?* Durham, NH: Crimes Against Children Research Center, University of New Hampshire; 2014. Available at: https://scholars.unh.edu/cgi/view content.cgi?article=1040&context=ccrc.

89. Walter HJ, Vaughan RD, Gladis MM, Ragin DF, Kasen S, Cohall AT. Factors associated with AIDS risk behaviors among high school students in an AIDS epicenter. *Am J Public Health*. 1992;82:528−532.

90. Chia SC, Gunter AC. How media contribute to misperceptions of social norms about sex. *Mass Commun Soc*. 2006;9:301−320.

91. Metzler CW, Noell J, Biglan A, et al. The social context for risky sexual behavior among adolescents. *J Behav Med*. 1994;17:419−438.

92. Millstein SG, Moscicki AB. Sexually-transmitted disease in female adolescents: effects of psychosocial factors and high risk behaviors. *J Adolesc Health*. 1995;17:83−90.

93. Schroeder CM, Prentice DA. Exposing pluralistic ignorance to reduce alcohol use among college students. *J Appl Soc Psychol*. 1998;28:2150−2180.

94. Brofenbrenner U. *The Ecology of Human Development*. Cambridge: Harvard University Press; 1979.

95. Judge AM. Rethinking social media: low-tech solutions to high-tech dilemmas. In: *Annual Harvard Medical School Conference on School Mental Health Boston, MA*. 2015.

96. Choice T, Rubin D, Danforth N, Gorrindo T. Building bridges in a fractured family: developing new conversations around technology and sexual orientation. *Harv Rev Psychiatry*. 2015;23:201−211.

97. Fasula AM, Miller KS. African-American and Hispanic adolescents' intentions to delay first intercourse: parental communication as a buffer for sexually active peers. *J Adolesc Health*. 2006;38:193−200.

98. Akers AY, Holland C, Bost J. Interventions to improve parental communication about sex: a systematic review. *Pediatrics*. 2011;127:494−510.

99. Lefkowitz ES, Kahlbaugh P, Au TK, Sigman M. A longitudinal study of AIDS conversations between mothers and adolescents. *AIDS Educ Prev*. 1998;10:351−365.

100. Whalen CK, Henker B, Hollingshead J, Burgess S. Parent adolescent dialogues about AIDS. *J Fam Psychol*. 1996;10:343−357.

101. Lefkowitz ES, Sigman M, Au TK. Helping mothers discuss sexuality and AIDS with adolescents. *Child Dev*. 2000;71:1383−1394.

102. Gunter B. *Media Sex: What Are the Issues?* Mahwah: Lawrence Erlbaum Associates; 2002.

103. Malamuth NM, Billings V. The functions and effects of pornography: sexual communication versus the feminist models in light of research findings. In: Bryant J, Zillmann D, eds. *Perspectives on Media Effects*. Hillsdale: Lawrence Erlbaum; 1986:83−108.

104. Brown JD, Halpern CT, L'Engle KL. Mass media as a sexual super peer for early maturing girls. *J Adolesc Health*. 2005;36:420−427.

105. Kirschner PA, Bruyckere P. The myth of the digital native and the multitasker. *J Teach Educ*. 2017;67:135−142.

106. Davison KK, Francis LA, Birch LL. Links between parents' and girls' television viewing behaviors: a longitudinal examination. *J Pediatr*. 2005;147:436−442.

107. Bandura A. *Social Foundations of Thought and Action: A Social Cognitive Theory*. Englewood Cliffs: Prentice Hall; 1986.

108. Vaala SE, Bleakley A. Monitoring, mediating, and modeling: parental influence on adolescent computer and internet use in the United States. *J Child Media*. 2015;9:40−57.

109. Radesky J, Miller AL, Rosenblum KL, Appugliese D, Kaciroti N, Lumeng JC. Maternal mobile device use during a structured parent−child interaction task. *Acad Pediatr*. 2015;15:238−244.

110. Hiniker A, Soobel K, Suh H, Sung Y, Lee CP, Kienz JA. *Texting While Parenting: How Adults Use Mobile Phones While Caring for Children Art the Playground*. University of Washington; 2015. Available at: http://citeseerx.ist.psu.edu/viewdoc/download?doi=10.1.1.725.8178&rep=rep1&type=pdf.

111. McDaniel BT, Radesky JS. Technoference: parent distraction with technology and associations with child behavior problems. *Child Dev*. 2018;89:100−109.

112. Dishion TJ, McMahon RJ. Parental monitoring and the prevention of child and adolescent problem behavior: a conceptual and empirical formulation. *Clin Child Fam Psychol Rev*. 1998;1:61−75.

113. Cohen DA, Rice JC. A parent-targeted intervention for adolescent substance abuse prevention: lessons learned. *Eval Res*. 1995;19:159−180.

114. Otto LB, Atkinson MP. Parental involvement and adolescent development. *J Adolesc Res*. 1997;12:68−89.

115. Padilla-Walker LM, Coyne SM. "Turn that thing off!" parent and adolescent predictors of proactive media monitoring. *J Adolesc*. 2011;34:705−715.

116. Nathanson AI. The unintended effects of parental mediation of television on adolescents. *Media Psychol*. 2002;4:207−230.

117. Oshima N, Nishida A, Shimodera S, et al. The suicidal feelings, self-injury, and mobile phone use after lights out in adolescents. *J Pediatr Psychol*. 2012;7:1023−1030.

118. Lemola S, Perkinson-Gloor N, Brand S, Dewald-Kaufmann JF, Grob A. Adolescents' electronic media use at night, sleep disturbance, and depressive symptoms in the smartphone age. *J Youth Adolesc*. 2015;44:405−418.

119. Vernon L, Modecki K, Barber B. Mobile phones in the bedroom: trajectories of sleep habits and subsequent adolescent psychosocial development. *Child Dev*. 2017;0:1−12.

120. Coyne SM, Padilla-Walker LM, Day RD, Harper J, Stockdale L. A friend request from dear old dad: associations between parent−child social networking and adolescent outcomes. *Cyberpsychol Behav Soc Netw*. 2014;17:8−13.

CHAPTER 4

Dystopian Movies and YA Novels

STEVEN C. SCHLOZMAN, MD

INTRODUCTION

Perhaps the most poignant irony of dystopian fiction is that it could never be enjoyed in an actual dystopia. This fact provides a key ingredient for the dystopian menu that has continually enticed adolescents when they visit the bookstore, library, or movie theater. If the world were truly a dystopia, there would of course be no time for the dour speculations that books like *1984* or *The Hunger Games* provoke. We'd all be too busy fighting "the man."

And *that* is exactly the point. What if "the man" is everywhere, and no one seems to care? Doesn't that sound like a typical adolescent complaint? Teenagers, through a combination of cultural forces and incomplete brain development, often see the world in stark and sullen colors. No one understands what really matters, they argue. No one allows free expression or (safe enough) experimentation. If it is such a free world, teens ask, then why doesn't it *feel* that way. Adolescents devour one dystopian tale after another as they wrestle with their developmentally appropriate drive for more independence and leeway than we adults are prepared to offer. Indeed, some have argued that the Young Adult (YA) dystopian market has almost single handedly revived an interest among teens in reading and telling stories. Others wring their hands over the perceived nihilistic gasoline that these stories pour on an already smoldering adolescent fire.

As child psychiatrists and psychologists, we owe it to ourselves and to our patients to better understand the draw that these stories have for young people. A review of all dystopian narratives is well beyond the scope of a single article. There are entire books and entire college courses devoted to this topic. Therefore, this article will instead use some of the most prominent dystopian stories to illustrate the potency of these themes among emerging adolescents. Importantly, it is of course not only disaffected youth who enjoy a good apocalyptic or dystopian fable. We can use dystopian tropes to delve into the psychological and biological intricacies of normal development as well as the many psychopathological challenges that accompany coming of age. In order to do this, though, we must first define what a dystopian tale involves.

DEFINING DYSTOPIA

An agreed upon definition of dystopia is more elusive than one might expect. Formally, the term dystopia has been used to describe both real and fictional circumstances where freedom is severely restricted. In other words, a dystopia exists within a totalitarian framework, with pervasive and unchallengeable limits on basic human rights.[1] When referring to dystopian fictions, scholars have noted that dystopian narratives serve as cautionary tales. Once we allow totalitarian rule, these authors argue in their stories, we cannot turn back.[2] Others have further noted that dystopian tales warn us that we will not even be aware that our freedoms have been taken. Indeed, this is the focus of Eric Fromm's afterward to George Orwell's dystopian classic, *1984*.[3] Finally, there is growing consensus that one cannot identify the features of dystopian depiction without also considering the much sought-after characteristics of utopian settings. This school of thought notes that many imagined and real dystopian societies emerged from a genuine desire to create something good.[4] In this sense, both utopias and dystopias are literally social constructs. They are imagined or real societies that are created and maintained by potent social forces. From these various conceptualizations of dystopian narratives, we can start to appreciate the potency of the dystopian tale for the emerging adolescent.

DYSTOPIAN STORIES AS ADOLESCENT PROTESTS

Studies of adolescent creative writing read like primers for dystopian novels. The creative fiction from a large sample of teen storytellers describes intense competition, misplaced rewards for aberrant behavior, and a pervasive suspicion that teachers are fraudulent in their knowledge but confident in their power.[5] Any one of these thematic consistencies is ripe material for dystopian stories. Competition, for example, figures prominently in *The Hunger Games*. Suzanne Collins' immensely popular novel involves teens who must literally compete to the death using physical prowess as well as cunning intellect. Similarly, the theme of misplaced rewards abounds in the popular *Divergent* series. These books describe a post-apocalyptic American city where teens are classified at the emergence of adolescence into categories that dictate their behavior for the rest of their lives. The "Dauntless" teens are rewarded for acts of recklessness that are deemed brave rather than risky. The teens assigned to "Amity" are praised for avoiding all acts of altercation even when lives are at stake. A further example is present in the science fiction dystopian novel, *The Knife of Never Letting Go*. Here the teen protagonist is aware that his newfound adolescent friend is savvier than his adult superiors, but because his thoughts are literally broadcast into the minds of others due to a strange infection, he strives to keep his romantic and heroic aspirations as quiet as possible despite the fact that the hapless adults will necessarily know what he is thinking.

Central to all of these thematic consistencies is the tensioned dialectic that adolescence creates between individuals and the groups to which they belong. The "jock" is obviously more than "just a jock" at a given high school, but in stories like *Divergent*, people are locked into narrow and confining identities. The key adolescent task of identity formation is threatened by the totalitarian rules and definitions that govern the social landscape of dystopian stories. Teens therefore turn to these tales for the literary comradery that what appear to be otherwise outlandish stories conveniently and empathically afford.[6]

NEUROBIOLOGY OF DYSTOPIAN TALES

Is there something particularly dystopian about the way that the adolescent brain makes sense of the world? Recall that dystopias are by definition notoriously misleading. In dystopian stories, often what appears to be a calm and functional society is in fact a world of violence and paranoia. Things are not as they seem. Consider the classic dystopian novel *The Giver*. The protagonist sees no option but to escape his rigid and controlled community. He can see no other path toward authentically affirming his values and beliefs.

Over and over, we are told that his emotions are experienced intensely despite the artificially managed affect that his society forcibly maintains. This is very much like the now well-established fact that adolescent cognitions are dominated by limbic activation at the expense of higher order contemplation. In the classic dystopian tale, the combination of limbic excitement is necessary for the higher brain to take notice of the injustices that are allowed to persist. In this sense, the adolescent brain is both primed for and affirmed by dystopian ideas.

PSYCHOPATHOLOGY AND DYSTOPIAN NARRATIVES

Much of the themes associated with classic dystopian narratives are easily grasped and even embraced throughout normal adolescent development. The question remains, however, whether dystopian literature is associated with worrisome psychopathology. This is a potentially controversial conjecture. The very potency of dystopian regimes is often wielded in the guise of adults calling others psychologically unbalanced. For example, classics like Huxley's *Brave New World* describe those who do not agree with the tenets of the highly rigid society as "savages."

Therefore, associating an affinity for dystopian stories with risk factors for psychopathology risks utilizing the very tools that we are warned against in many dystopian tales. In fact, bioethicists have used dystopian language in describing certain psychotherapeutic interventions. The use of β-blockers to alter affect during pathologically harmful memories for individuals with posttraumatic stress disorder has been called a dystopian endeavor.[7] Michael Moore considered his film, *Bowling for Columbine*, an apt depiction of a particularly American dystopia.[8]

Still, one can appreciate how any teen who reads nothing but dystopian stories, sees nothing but dystopian movies, and listens to nothing but dystopian music might be at risk for an underlying psychiatric syndrome. Certainly, adolescents who demonstrate an overreliance on any single narrative theme deserves further investigation. Nevertheless, there exists virtually no studies correlating obsessive attention to dystopian stories with psychopathological states. There are published studies involving the highly controversial associations between violent video games and violent music with dangerous psychopathology. These studies are not the purview of this essay, but it is worth noting that there are multiple confounders for these findings that seem to better explain the correlated psychiatric concerns.[9] In fact, Drs Olson and Kutner argued in their ground-breaking book *Grand Theft Childhood* that video games, including those with violently dystopian narratives, provide connection rather than isolation among otherwise vulnerable youth.[10]

To this end, any conjecture about dystopian literature as a potential source for adolescent suffering and concomitant dangerous behavior is not well founded. This has not, however, stopped schools all over the world from attempting to ban these stories for fear of the influence that they might have on their young readers. As recently as this year, school districts in the United States considered banning *1984* for "its violent and sexually charged language".[11] Similar concerns were expressed over the popularity of *The Hunger Games* when its popularity was peaking.[12] Teens typically appreciate the irony that books about censorship are often the first to be censored. This connection, consistent with the higher order thinking that characterizes the normally developing brain, is the best means by which clinicians can utilize the displacement that dystopian literature affords to help their patients to negotiate the bumpy waters that threaten the emergence into adulthood.

THERAPEUTIC USES OF DYSTOPIAN LITERATURE

There is a rich literature detailing the use of fiction in psychotherapeutic work with children and adolescents. Much of this literature focuses on the particular potency of dystopian narratives. The dystopian best seller *Never Let Me Go* has been discussed as a vector through which therapists can help their young patients to explore themes of personhood and shifting identity.[13] Similarly, *The Hunger Games* has been used to help parents to better understand the extent to which their children are exposed in real life to the complexities of a violent world.[14] In both instances, these books have helped therapists and caregivers to understand and relate to the adolescents they encounter. Importantly, these works have also allowed these same adolescents to convey their anxieties about the world in the safe place that displacement affords. Psychotherapeutic literature is ripe with examples of fantasy, science fiction, and speculative narratives, being used as windows into the concerns of otherwise aloof teens.[15] Dystopian stories are merely a subset of the narratives that have long been utilized by teens in helping us to understand their concerns.

CONCLUSION

The most pressing issue regarding the popularity of dystopian literature is why it has become so incredibly popular and profitable. This inquiry can yield important insight into the societal concerns that plague teens who will soon become the adults of our world. Many scholars have noted that these kinds of stories are not at all new, but that they seem to increase during strife-ridden times. "Without discontent, there can be no utopia," argues Jack Zipes in his forward to the collection of essays titled *Utopian and Dystopian Writing for Children and Young Adults*.[16] In other words, teens gravitate to these kinds of stories so that they make clear to us what they find lacking in the world that they stand to inherit. With a 24-h news cycle covering an increasing divisive planet, perhaps teens have reason to worry. Perhaps this is why these books are experiencing such immense popularity. These stories help us to prepare for what teens hope to change in their troubled worlds. Our job is to help guide them toward the most efficient and satisfying means of effecting these changes.

REFERENCES

1. Claeys G. *Dystopia: A Natural History: A Study of Modern Despotism, Its Antecedents, and Its Literary Diffractions.* Oxford: Oxford University Press; 2017.
2. Gottlieb E. *Dystopian Fiction East and West: Universe of Terror and Trial.* Montreal, Canada: McGill-Queen's University Press; 2001.
3. Fromm E. Afterward. In: *1984*. London: Harcourt Brace; 1949:280−292.
4. Claeys G. News from somewhere: enhanced sociability and the composite definition of utopia and dystopia. *History.* 2013;98(330):146−173.
5. Olthouse J, Edmunds A, Sauder A. School stories: how do exemplary teen writers portray academics? *Roeper Rev.* 2014;36(3):168−177.
6. Miskec JM. Contemporary dystopian fiction for young adults: brave new teenagers ed. by Carrie Hintz, Balaka Basu, Katherine R. Broad (review). *Children's Lit Assoc Q.* 2014;39(3):442−445. The Johns Hopkins University Press.
7. Henry M, Fishman J, Youngner S. Propranolol and the prevention of post-traumatic stress disorder: it is wrong to erase the "sting" of bad memories? *Am J Bioeth.* 2007; 7(9):12−20.
8. Klawans S. Moore's dystopia. *Film Comment.* 2002;38(6): 32.
9. Richmond J, Wilson J. Are graphic media violence, aggression and moral disengagement related? *Psychiatry Psychol L.* 2008;15(2):350−357.
10. Kutner L, Olson CK. *Grand Theft Childhood: The Surprising Truth about Violent Video Games and What Parents Can Do.* New York: Simon & Schuster; 2008.
11. https://www.idahoednews.org/news/jefferson-county-administrators-consider-banning-classic-novel/.
12. https://verdict.justia.com/2012/04/16/a-spate-of-complaints-asking-libraries-to-censor-the-hunger-games-trilogy.

13. Rizq R. Copying, cloning and creativity: reading Kazuo Ishiguro's never let me go. *Br J Psychother*. 2014;30(4): 517–532.

14. Skinner M, McCord K. The hunger games: a conversation. *Jung J Cult Psyche*. 2012;6(4):106–113.

15. Ames M. Engaging "apolitical" adolescents: analyzing the popularity and educational potential of dystopian literature post-9/11. *High Sch J*. 2013;97(1):3–20.

16. Hintz C, Ostry E. *Utopian and Dystopian Writing for Children and Young Adults*. New York: Routledge; 2003.

CHAPTER 5

The Impact of Terrorism on Children and Adolescents: Terror in Their Eyes, Terror on Their Screens

ELIZA ABDU-GLASS, BA • WANDA P. FREMONT, MD • CAROLY PATAKI, MD • EUGENE V. BERESIN, MD

Terrorist attacks and their aftermath have powerful impacts on children, adolescents, and their families. Recent literature has documented the effects of direct and indirect exposure to terrorism. Media and social media exposure of terrorist events throughout the world has increased during the past few years. Images of terrorist attacks in the United States, including the Boston Marathon Bombing (BMB) and the World Trade Center, and those in the Middle East, Europe, Africa, South America, Asian countries, and other nations have been broadcast throughout the world. There is increasing concern about the effects of trauma exposure on children who experience violence and witness violent images. The immediacy and intensity of access to images, news, and commentary via social media has been particularly worrisome for adults who care for our youth. Parents, teachers, and healthcare providers are struggling to meet the challenges of helping youth cope with heightened anxiety, fear, sadness, and grief after exposure to traumatic events. To develop a proactive and strategic response to reactions to trauma in youth, clinicians, educators, and policy makers must understand the psychological effects of media coverage of terrorism on children. Moreover, efforts need to be focused on recognizing the compounded effects of trauma on youth who are exposed to repetitive accounts of traumatic events by private citizens and the media. Additionally, parents, caregivers, and teachers may need guidance in finding reliable and valid sources of information. Research in the past has focused largely on media coverage of criminal violence and war. Recent studies have examined the effect of immediate and remote exposure of terrorist attacks and other crisis situations and have shown a significant clinical impact on children and families.

DEFINITION OF TERRORISM

Terrorism is defined by the US Defense Department as "the calculated use of violence or threat of violence to inculcate fear: intended to coerce or to intimidate governments and societies in the pursuit of goals that are generally political, religious, or ideological."[1] The goal of terrorism is not only to cause visible disaster but also to inflict psychological fear and intimidation at any time, during periods of peace or conflict. Unlike family or community violence or the trauma resulting from war, terrorist activities are not confined to a specific geographic area or time. Terrorist events occur suddenly without any forewarning and frequently result in severe trauma. The threat persists indefinitely. Terrorism capitalizes on media coverage, whose powerful visual images create strong emotional responses. Terrorism can elicit emotions including fear, panic, despair, and rage even in individuals who live far away from the traumatic events.

Terrorism-induced trauma results in unique stressors and reactions in children. By its very nature, terrorism is likely to cause psychological stress. The unpredictable, indefinite threat of terrorist events, the profound effect on adults and communities, and the effect of extensive terrorist-related media coverage exacerbates underlying concerns and contributes to a continuous state of stress and anxiety. Research on the impact of terrorism on youth covers a range of violent acts, including isolated events in countries not at war and repeated terrorist attacks in areas of political conflict. Studies have examined the effects of direct exposure (e.g., physical presence, family or friend, or near-miss experiences) and remote exposure (through the media). Many of the effects of terrorism-induced trauma on children are much like the effects of man-made and natural disaster trauma, like coverage of Hurricane Katrina and the earthquake in Haiti.

Children vary in their reactions to traumatic events.[2,3] Some children suffer from worries and bad memories that dissipate with time and emotional support, while other children may be more severely traumatized and experience long-term problems. Children's responses include acute stress disorder, posttraumatic stress disorder (PTSD), anxiety, depression, regressive behaviors, separation problems, phobias, sleep difficulties, and behavioral problems. Children's emotional reactions may develop immediately after the trauma or may occur later. The Diagnostic and Statistical Manual of Mental Disorders, Fifth Edition, recognizes these two temporal categories of reaction.[4] Acute stress disorder is the most common psychiatric disorder to develop in the month following a traumatic event. PTSD is a similar symptomatic reaction that may occur after some time. Children and adolescents who suffer from acute stress disorder or PTSD may re-experience the trauma by having nightmares or recurring flashbacks of the event. In young children, repetitive play may occur in which themes or aspects of the trauma are expressed. Their dreams may be frightening, but without any recognizable content. Trauma-specific re-enactment may occur. Adolescents and children may feel numb and withdraw from the external world or avoid situations that arouse recollection of the trauma. They may displace their reactions to a terrorist attack to other forms of disasters, such as hurricanes or earthquakes. Symptoms of increased arousal may occur, including hypervigilance, sleep difficulties, irritability, difficulty concentrating, and outbursts of anger.

In addition to acute stress disorder and PTSD, children may develop comorbid disorders. These may include anxiety disorders (e.g., panic disorder, agoraphobia, generalized anxiety disorder, phobias, social phobia, obsessive-compulsive disorder), depression, and substance abuse—related disorders. Children may present with partial or variable symptoms of these disorders.[5–7]

RISK AND PROTECTIVE FACTORS FOR CHILDREN AND ADOLESCENTS

A child's reaction to trauma or terrorist events depends on multiple risk and protective factors, including prior histories of trauma exposure and psychiatric disorders, circumstances related to the history and terrorist event itself, and individual, family, and community strengths and vulnerabilities.

History and the Event

Children's responses vary in accordance to their level of exposure to the terrorist activities, either directly or indirectly. The degree of exposure to terrorist actions is related to the prevalence of PTSD. The more severe the traumatic event, the greater the risk of developing posttraumatic symptoms.[8,9] Children who experience loss directly are more symptomatic.[9–17] Physical injury or witnessing death and physical injury of others is associated with higher rates of PTSD and comorbid depression and anxiety.[12,18,19] The degree of personal loss (i.e., the child's relationship to the victim) also has been correlated with the number of posttraumatic stress symptoms in less exposed children. Knowing an injured or deceased person increases the risk of symptom development.[17] The highest rates of PTSD occur in children who have lost a parent.[20]

In addition to the level of trauma, the duration of exposure to violence predicts the risk for development of psychiatric problems in children.[13,16,21–23]

Individual Factors and Vulnerabilities

Individual factors that affect a child's differential response are related to developmental factors, including age and level of psychological maturity.[24–29] Neurobiological responses, predisposing risk factors, and effects of resiliency also influence a child's individual response to traumatic exposure.

DEVELOPMENTAL CONSIDERATIONS

What children understand during and after an exposure to a traumatic event is a function of their developmental level with respect to cognition, emotional, and social factors.

Preschool-Aged Children

Young children between the ages of 3 and 5 years are likely to express their concerns about safety in terms of separation from parents and other primary caretakers. They rely heavily on cues about danger from caretakers, and at this age, their cognitions indicate that they frequently do not understand the finality of death. Although preschoolers understand less of the actual events, they are more comforted than older children by parental behavior that is reassuring[30] and may have increased difficulties separating from their parents.[31] Children aged 5 years and younger may exhibit regressive behaviors, such as bed wetting, thumb sucking, or fear of the dark.[25,32–34] Additional symptoms may include fear, anxiety, sleep problems, and aggressive behaviors.[30]

Elementary School–Aged Children

Elementary school–aged children (6–11 years) derive a sense of security from clear-cut rules and are developmentally prone to polarizing even complex situations into "right" and "wrong." As children mature from 6 to 12 years of age, they increasingly develop a sense of empathy and altruism. For example, when faced with exposure to a terrorist act, children in this age group may fear for others and recognize death as final, although they only may be able to conceptualize it as remote. Elementary school–aged children are profoundly affected by exposure to a traumatic event, even if they are not involved directly. They may suffer from symptoms of anxiety, PTSD, and depression.[35] Signs of anxiety include school avoidance, somatic complaints (e.g., headaches, stomachaches), irrational fears, sleep problems, nightmares, irritability, angry outbursts, and obsessive thoughts about the news coverage.[17,36–38] Symptoms of depression may include sadness, feelings of hopelessness, and withdrawal.[39,40] They may have attention problems, and their school work may suffer.

Adolescents

Among early adolescents, although there is a cognitive awareness of the finality and inevitability of death, there is also a competing sense of immunity to being harmed. A sense of omnipotence may overpower a young teen's judgment regarding the actual danger that is present in his or her environment. At the same time, adolescents remain vulnerable to idealized notions. For example, the notion that if they helped the world's leaders to set up a meeting, the world's nations would likely be able to resolve their differences and end the threat of terrorism once and for all. When young teens are exposed to extraordinary events such as a terrorist attack, they may feel overly responsible for devising a plan that could protect them and their families from danger. Older adolescents are more able to separate personal fears of danger to themselves from world events that have resulted in harm to others. Adolescent (age 12–18 years) responses are more like adult responses and include intrusive thoughts, hypervigilance, emotional numbing, nightmares, sleep disturbances, and avoidance.[26,29] They are at increased risk of having problems with substance abuse, peer problems, and depression.[41] Trauma is often associated with intense feelings of humiliation, self-blame, shame, and guilt, which result from the sense of powerlessness and may lead to a sense of alienation and avoidance.[15,37,42,43] Adolescents may internalize the world as riskier and more dangerous.[44]

NEUROBIOLOGICAL CONSEQUENCES OF TRAUMA IN CHILDREN AND ADOLESCENTS

Evidence suggests that childhood exposure to traumatic events influences the neurobiological response to stress in the developing brain in such a way that it predisposes affected individuals to mood and anxiety symptoms later in life.[45] The finding that individuals who have sustained significant trauma during childhood have an increased risk of mood and anxiety disorders later in life may be related to changes in neurotransmitter systems that are stimulated by stress.[46] One important mediator of the stress response is corticotropin-releasing factor. In the presence of stress, this substance is increased in the brain. It is possible that children who have been exposed to chronic or severe stress have developed dysregulation of the corticotropin-releasing factor system. This may explain some of the symptomatology of traumatic syndromes, such as increased startle response, and symptoms of anxiety and mood disorder.[47]

PREDISPOSING RISK FACTORS

Some children are at greater risk of developing symptoms of anxiety and depression. Predisposing risk factors include exposure to past traumatic events during childhood,[48,49] childhood conduct problems,[50] childhood anxiety,[50] antisocial behavior, or a family history of psychiatric disorders.[41,51] All children's sense of safety and potential for personal danger is affected by a traumatic event, however. Each child reacts differently depending on sensitivity and temperament and whether he or she tends to internalize or externalize experiences and emotions.[52,53] Children may become fearful, distractible, anxious, or depressed. Their play and study may be affected, as can their pattern of sleep or eating.

History of trauma has been proven to increase the risk of PTSD for children following a terrorist attack, shooting, or other critical event. A graded dose-response relationship exists between adverse childhood experiences and poor health and overall well-being throughout life, highlighting the cumulative nature of trauma on lifetime psychological outcomes.[54]

Further studies found that sexual trauma victims had prolonged worsening of depressive symptoms following a school shooting, while their nonvictim peers showed more rapid symptom improvement. Students exposed to a school shooting with less preexisting trauma experiences demonstrated better resiliency than peers with trauma histories. This impact is pervasive, as sexual assault victims had worse PTSD and depressive symptoms than their peers at follow-up.[55] The cumulative impact of trauma predisposes children who are exposed to repeated or prolonged trauma to a variety of psychosocial difficulties throughout life.

RESILIENCE AMONG CHILDREN AND ADOLESCENTS

Many children and adolescents who are exposed to traumatic events, however, do not develop pervasive chronic posttraumatic syndromes. Factors associated with resilience among children and adolescents after exposure to severe traumatic events are related to biological and psychological characteristics. One hypothesis explains resilience in terms of the variability in emotional reaction and physiological arousal. There is variation in one's psychological interpretation of physiological arousal.[56] For example, when one encounters a fearful event, there is an initial increase in cortisol level in the brain and increase in heart rate in response to the initial fearful event. In this model, recovery from a traumatic event includes being able to respond to the event in a supportive environment without extreme avoidance and in the absence of persistent physiological arousal. Recovery is the normative path, whereas the development of a perpetual state of fear leads to posttraumatic symptoms. It is likely that early intervention might facilitate the process of recovery and reduce the risk for posttraumatic symptoms in vulnerable individuals.[56]

FAMILY FACTORS AND VULNERABILITIES

Children's response to violent events and their ability to cope with these disasters are influenced strongly by their parents' responses to the trauma.[57–61] A positive correlation between children's and parents' symptomatology has been noted.[62,63] The importance of parental involvement in mediating stress reactions in children has been studied in families exposed to terrorist attacks.[9] Parents may underestimate their children's reactions and need for support and care and unintentionally hinder their children's process of mastering the trauma.[7,64–66] Because terrorist incidents affect adults profoundly, parents and teachers may not be able to provide the support and reassurance needed to help avoid potential long-term emotional harm to their children. Increased levels of distress were noted in children whose parents responded to traumatic events with negative emotions. Positive coping responses in children were associated with parents who responded with positive emotional reactions to trauma.[9] Family protective factors that have been shown to buffer stress for children and increase resiliency include a stable, secure, emotional relationship with at least one parent, a parental model of constructive coping mechanisms,[24,57,62,67,68] and physical proximity of children to parents.[39]

Mothers play a decisive role in determining their children's reactions in times of crisis. During the scud missile crisis in Israel, children whose mothers retained better cognitive control of their reaction had better outcomes. How parents cognitively process a traumatic experience directly affects outcomes for children. It has also been shown that cohesive and supportive family structure was also related to improved outcomes for children. The better insulated, supported, and engaged parents are in their connections with other adults and within their community, the better they support their children in the face of terrorist attacks or other trauma situations. Adults who feel connected, protected, and supported can better themselves and help encourage better outcomes for their children.

COMMUNITY FACTORS

Responses of community members in populations exposed to terrorism have an important influence on children's coping skills. Children's resiliency to traumatic events is influenced by the degree of social support and positive community influences[69–74] around them. Community, educational, political, and religious support networks foster moral development in children.[70,71] The presence of a caring adult who can provide emotional support, encourage self-esteem, and promote competence has a moderating influence on acute and long-term mental health outcomes.[30,32,75,76] Community ideology, beliefs, and value systems also contribute to resiliency by giving meaning to dangerous events, allowing children to identify with cultural values and enabling children and adults to function under extreme conditions.[66,68,72,76–80]

CHILDREN'S RESPONSES TO MEDIA EXPOSURE OF TERRORIST EVENTS

The increased media and social media coverage of terrorist activities has had a significant impact on children's emotional responses. Research studies have shown consistently that one-third or more children watch the news,[81–84] and nearly half of the kids say they feel that following the news is important.[85] The media plays a central role in providing information to the public, especially during times of disaster. The images portrayed are powerful and intensely emotional and are often unedited and repeated frequently.

Terrorist organizations depend on media dissemination of such images to increase responses of fear and panic among the public. Along with the extensive use of social media, smart phones and tablets present increasing exposure to news events and to repeated exposure of images that may be disturbing.

For decades, research has examined the influence of violence and aggression on children and adolescents. With the recent increase in terrorist bombings and access to media coverage throughout the world, more studies have examined the effects of children's reactions to media coverage of terrorism. Research on the impact of media on children covers a range of violent acts that are classified as acts of terrorism, including the Oklahoma City bombings (1995), the Scud missile attacks, news coverage during the Persian Gulf War (1991), the attack on the World Trade Center (September 11, 2001), and the BMB (2013). Although the space shuttle Challenger disaster (1986) was not the result of a terrorist attack, studies of children who witnessed the explosion via television viewing provided valuable information on the effects of indirect trauma. The results of the research on children's responses to media coverage has shown that remote exposure, such as viewing terrorism on television, has a significant clinical impact.

The Challenger Disaster

Terr et al.[86,87] studied children's responses to the space shuttle Challenger explosion.[88] Children who watched the explosion on television were indirectly exposed to the traumatic event. Terr et al.[36] defined distant trauma as "the reaction (memory, thinking, symptoms) to a disastrous event, observed at the time of the event, but from a remote and safe distance." Children's responses included symptom patterns similar to PTSD. Children's reactions to distant trauma also included trauma-specific fear, fear of being alone, the habit of clinging to others, and event-specific fears. Children who lived on the East Coast were more symptomatic than children who lived on the West Coast. East Coast children had a significant increase in dreaming, drawing and behavioral re-enactment, trauma-specific fears (e.g., death and dying, taking risks, explosions, fires, airplanes), and clinging behaviors. Latency age children were more affected than adolescents. Children and adolescents throughout the United States had diminished expectations for the future. Most symptoms diminished within a year; however, for children with initial partial PTSD, symptoms (i.e., posttraumatic play for young children and hopeless attitudes about the future for adolescents) often would persist. Further studies have described a spectrum of trauma-related

conditions that resulted from remote exposure to violence, including viewing media coverage of disaster events.[13,15,17,37,57,89]

Oklahoma City Bombing

Pfefferbaum et al.[11,90] examined children's reactions to news coverage of the 1995 Oklahoma City bombing. More than 2000 middle school students in Oklahoma City were surveyed 7 weeks after the bombing. Television viewing of the bombing after the explosion was extensive. Children who experienced personal losses were at greater risk of watching significantly more terrorist-related television coverage than children without direct losses,[11,12] further exacerbating the traumatic experience. The degree of television exposure was related directly to posttraumatic stress symptomatology in children. In children who experienced a direct loss, the impact of viewing television was greater (increased initial arousal and fear); however, many nonbereaved youth experienced symptoms after TV exposure. Children who witnessed the bombing on television reported trauma-related stress for more than 2 years.[11] In addition to broadcast media (i.e., television and radio) exposure, print media (i.e., newspaper and magazine) exposure also was examined. Print media exposure correlated more strongly with enduring posttraumatic stress than broadcast media.[88]

Scud Missile Attacks and News Coverage During the Persian Gulf War

The effects of exposure to terrorism and the importance of parental involvement in mediating stress reactions in children have been studied in families exposed to the Scud missile attacks.[9,10,30,32,75] Bat-Zion and Levy-Shiff[9] noted that parents' responses were a central mediating factor for Israeli children's reactions to Scud missile attacks. Parental negative emotional expressions were associated with increased levels of distress in children, whereas positive emotional manifestations were associated with increased coping efforts. Laor et al.[30,32,75] studied the long-term consequences of the Scud missile attacks in Israeli children. Children of mothers with poor psychological functioning showed more stress symptomatology in families who were displaced. The association between children's and mothers' symptoms was stronger among younger children (aged 3 and 4 years). Unhealthy family interactions exacerbate children's stress, children manifest more symptoms, and their capacity to recover from the critical trauma is jeopardized.[32]

Parents' positive emotional responses may have a buffering effect on their children's reactions. Children with adequate family cohesion manifest less stress in reaction to trauma and are better able to recover from the initial impact of the trauma.[30,32,75] Unhealthy family interactions—either disengaged or enmeshed styles[91]—exacerbated children's stress. These children manifested more symptoms, and their capacity to recover from the critical trauma was jeopardized. Conversely, children with adequate family cohesion manifested less stress in reaction to trauma and were better able to recover from the initial impact.

World Trade Center (September 11, 2001)

Research on children's reactions to the terrorist attacks of September 11, 2001 corroborates the results of previous research studies. The degree of exposure, proximity to the disaster area, association with parental reactions, experience of distant trauma (including media coverage), and history of preexisting trauma were associated with increased stress symptoms. Children's reactions included symptoms of posttraumatic stress, depression, panic attacks, anxiety, separation anxiety, and agoraphobia. Children who were exposed to trauma before the attacks were more likely to experience PTSD and other psychiatric problems.[35] Halpern-Felsher and Millstein[44] studied adolescents in California 1 month after the September 11 attack. Adolescents experienced heightened perceptions of vulnerability to death, which extended beyond the terrorist attacks and generalized to unrelated risks. After exposure to the terrorist attacks, even from across the country, adolescents internalized a perception of the world as more risky and dangerous.

The media coverage of the September 11 terrorist attacks was extensive, and repeated coverage of the graphic images of planes striking the World Trade Center caused considerable concern about the added emotional effects of viewing the traumatic events. A national study conducted a few days after September 11, 2001 concluded that children (aged 5–18 years) watched 3 h of television news on the day of the attacks. Only 8% of children did not watch any coverage of the event.[92] Parents who reported that their children were upset restricted their children's television viewing. In children whose viewing of television was not restricted, the number of hours of television correlated with the number of stress symptoms. A study commissioned by the New York City board of education 6 months after the World Trade Center attacks noted that 62% of children spent much of their time and 33% of children spent some of their time learning about the September 11 attacks on television. Approximately 75% of children increased the amount of time they spent reading newspapers and magazines, and more than 30%

obtained information from the Internet. 10.5% (75,000) of students manifested symptoms of PTSD 6 months after September 11, including children who were not affected directly by the event. Among these children, the prevalence of stress was higher among children who spent more time watching television coverage of the events than children who spent less time. The author notes, however, that these results do not determine a direct causality between television viewing and PTSD rates. Although the images on television may have exacerbated children's stress responses, anxious children may have been more likely to seek information from the media than nondistressed children.[35]

The indirect exposure of September 11 via television, the Internet, and printed media was examined in a study of elementary school children in the southeast United States. More PTSD symptoms were reported in children who saw reports on the Internet (vs. television or printed material), saw images of death or injury, or feared that a loved one might have died in the attacks. There was no measurable benefit to seeing "positive" or "heroic" images. Older children and boys were noted to have greater media exposure and more trauma-specific PTSD symptoms.[93]

The correlation between television viewing of the September 11 attacks and an increased sense of insecurity and stress symptoms also was shown in a study of elementary school–aged children in Washington, DC.[94]

The effects of television viewing of the September 11 attacks also were examined in adults. Specific disaster-related television images were associated with PTSD and depression among persons who were exposed directly to the disaster.[95] The number of hours of television coverage viewed and an index of the content of that coverage were associated with PTSD symptoms.[96] Given the relationship between parental response and child reaction, parents should be aware if they themselves are sensitive to this type of coverage and be mindful of their own media exposure.

Palestinian Children Living in a War Zone

The impact of the media on children living in a war zone has been studied in Palestinian children and Kuwaiti children during the Gulf War. Palestinian children who were exposed to traumatic events indirectly by the media had a higher incidence of anticipatory anxiety and cognitive expressions of distress than children who were exposed directly, who in turn manifested more symptoms of PTSD.[89]

The effect of extensive terrorist-related media coverage further exacerbates the traumatic experience. Television coverage is a secondary source of exposure to trauma and creates a ripple effect. Large numbers of children not exposed directly to terrorist activities are affected. The unpredictable, indefinite threat of terrorist activities exacerbates underlying anxieties and contributes to a continuous state of stress and anxiety.

Boston Marathon Bombing

In the case of the BMB, in addition to children with direct exposure to the attack, children who experienced the subsequent manhunt were also vulnerable to developing PTSD. Comer et al.[97] found that on average, children watched 1.5 h of news coverage, but one-fifth of the children in their study watched more than 3 h of television coverage following the attack. Such prolonged exposure to media coverage of the attack and manhunt was found to be related to the development of PTSD symptoms, behavior problems, and total difficulties. Most parents did not limit their children's viewing of coverage of the attack or the manhunt.[97]

The effect of several marathon and manhunt exposures was assessed on probable PTSD and six additional outcomes.[97] When assessed individually, both marathon attendance and manhunt experience were strongly associated with three negative outcomes—posttraumatic stress, total difficulties, and conduct problems. Total manhunt exposure was also associated with an additional three outcomes—peer problems, hyperactivity and inattention, and emotional symptoms. The evident risk to community, an important protective and resiliency factor, may explain the large effect of manhunt and shelter-in-place experiences on children. Positive peer interaction and prosocial behavior were mitigating factors against negative outcomes related to attack exposure.[97]

The effects of indirect exposure on outcomes is further supported by findings that individuals who viewed 6 or more hours of BMB-related media exposure showed higher acute stress than people who had direct exposure to the attack.[98] This research also found a cumulative effect of community-related trauma events. Following the BMB, prior exposure to the 9/11 attacks and the Sandy Hook school shooting was clearly linked to high acute stress.[98]

TELEVISION, SOCIAL MEDIA, AND THE NEWS

The extent of children's exposure to television and the media is significant, although currently, most US youth spend many hours per day with social media. It is estimated that in 2017–18, 96.5% of American homes have a television,[99] and television is now prevalent in the lives of almost all children. By the age of 2 years,

74% of children have watched TV, and 43% of under-2-year-olds watch TV daily.

Estimates suggest that children aged 2–5 years watch about 25 h of television each week, and children aged 6–18 years log about 28 viewing hours weekly.[100] These viewing hours are mainly television, but about 4.5 h come from a multitude of additional media sources, including video games and online.[100,101]

Almost two-thirds of families have the television on during meals, and just less than half report that the TV is on "most of the time", regardless of whether someone is watching. About 70% of children have a TV in their room, and half say they have a gaming console in their bedroom as well.[101]

As of 2005, the percentage of television time that children aged 2–7 years spend watching television alone and unsupervised is 81%. Day care centers use television during a typical day 70% of the time.[102] The number of hours that the average American child spends in school per year is 900; far fewer than the average number of hours that a child spends watching television per year.

A survey of children and the media[83] noted that 65% of children reported watching a television news program, and 44% of children read a newspaper. More than 50% of the children reported feeling angry, sad, or depressed after watching the news.

CHILDREN'S INTERPRETATION OF THE MEDIA: DEVELOPMENTAL CONSIDERATIONS

Children's understanding and interpretation of television and digital media are related to their cognitive and psychological developmental level.[103–105] Children are less able than adults to regulate their emotions after watching traumatizing images. Preschool-aged children are most affected by visual images and emotional sounds.[106,107] They are more upset by images of dead bodies or bloodied survivors and crying victims or witnesses than falling buildings or announcer commentaries. They are not able to understand the extent of a tragedy. Preschool-aged children cannot distinguish between live pictures and replays. If events are shown repeatedly, they believe that the catastrophe is occurring repeatedly in real life. They are likely to believe that terrorism is happening while they are watching the coverage, and they believe that it is occurring near their home.[103] Children this age are likely to have an especially strong fright response to natural disasters and accidents.[108]

Elementary school–aged children (7–12 years) have a better understanding of the event but interpret it concretely.[103] They are more sensitive to injured children or children whose parents were killed. They have difficulty understanding the impact of the terrorist threats and adult responses to these threats. School-aged children are more likely to focus on their own safety and that of their family and be scared by coverage of crime and violence.

Adolescents are more capable of abstraction than younger children. They are equally affected by visual images; however, they also are concerned about community responses and the impact of threats on the future.[84] Their cognitive advances allow them to ponder the broader issues in terrorism, including complex philosophical and existential issues that involve social justice, politics, and theology. Their personal struggles with identity, meaning, and place in society may be compromised seriously or distorted by the perception of the world and its human interactions as dangerous, untrustworthy, and immoral. This world view may have a negative impact on their sense of hope for the future.

TELEVISION AND SOCIAL MEDIA: CONSTRUCTIVE AND DESTRUCTIVE EFFECTS

Media coverage of terrorist events has positive and negative consequences. Although there has been extensive research about children's exposure to the entertainment media, there is far less scientific research about children's exposure to the news, especially exposure to terrorist media coverage.

Positive Effects

Several constructive effects of the media have been emphasized.[109,110] The media plays a vital role in disseminating information quickly to local, national, and international regions. Media coverage may facilitate family and community cohesion. It facilitates the dissemination of educational information and may serve as a vehicle for discussion in older children and adolescents. Klingman[109] noted that the media, the Internet, and the telephone serve as extensive support systems. Television stations and the Internet can broadcast advice on how to help children cope with stress and anxiety related to disastrous events.

Negative Effects

The increased incidence of stress-related symptoms in children exposed to media coverage of terrorist events has been mentioned previously. Repeated media exposure is especially detrimental for young children because of their cognitive immaturity. The ubiquitous presence of televisions, smart phones, tablets, and computers may compromise further our youths' ability to integrate their exposure given the amount of material they experience alone without adult supervision and guidance. The effect of the repeated coverage of events, specifically designed to invoke psychological and emotional distress, may promote the trauma and increase the duration and intensity of the effects. This is particularly true of using portable digital media as it provides a means of instant access, often without adult supervision. The media may have a continued negative impact on parents and caregivers, which directly affects the coping abilities of their children. More research is needed to measure the effects of media coverage of terrorist events and determine whether they have detrimental or positive effects on mental health outcomes.

Social and Mobile Media as News Sources

There has been a significant rise in the use of mobile media. As of 2017, 98% of households with children younger than 8 years have mobile devices like tablets and smartphones—a significant increase from 52% in 2011.[111] Forty-two percent of children younger than 8 years have a personal tablet device, jumping from under 1% in 2011.[111] Television remains a popular screen for children, but mobile devices now account for one-third of total screen use. Accompanying the rise in availability of mobile devices, the amount of time spent on mobile screens has increased from 5 min in 2011 to 48 min in 2017.[111] Although actual television screen time has decreased, the amount of time children spend watching television has increased by watching on other types of screens, like phones, tablets, or computers.[101] In addition, 42% of children younger than 8 years now have their own personal tablet, compared to just 1% in 2011.[111]

Pew Research Center[112] reports that almost three-fourths of teens report owning a smartphone with access to mobile Internet, mobile, and apps. Armed with this mobile technology, about 25% of teens report being almost always connected online. Facebook is the most popular social media site among this age group, although over 70% of teens say they have multiple social media accounts online and on apps. Half also report using Instagram, in addition to 40% also using Snapchat.[112]

The widespread access to nontraditional online media sources has changed how both young people and adults get the news. Data from 2017 reports that two-thirds of adults in the United States receive at least some portion of the news from social media.[113] About 66% of American adults use Facebook, indicating that about 45% of US adults get news from the site.[113] In addition to Facebook, Twitter, YouTube, and Snapchat are now regular sources of news for a growing number of people. All three social media platforms saw an increase in news sourcing, and the sites have invested in this capability. For instance, Snapchat features news and "breaking news" stories from CNN, NBC, and the New York Times in their Discover section.[113] Although these data reflect adult consumption of news via social media, it is easy to assume that tweens and teens will be similar. The popularity and major use of social media by this population indicates that they will also receive news information on social media platforms.

Online platforms are the preferred news source for young people.[114] Teens[13-18] are slightly more likely to get their news from social media sites than from family, but tweens[10-12] still heavily rely on family instead of social media. Tweens favor YouTube and Facebook while teenagers heavily prefer Facebook above other social media sites.[114] Given that reports following the September 11 attacks revealed that children who had higher Internet, rather than television, media exposure had increased symptoms and risk for PTSD,[93] this rise in the Internet as a news source for young people is a crucial development.

Reliance on social media and mobile media as news sources can contribute to the psychological distress and after effects of traumatic events. Following a school lockdown, Jones et al.[115] found that students who turned to social media for information during the crisis were subject to rumors and conflicting information. A week after the lockdown event, those students who had outside contact with others via social media, text, phone, or other means during the lockdown and received incorrect information reported more acute distress.[115] Given the growing dependence and prevalence of social and mobile media as news outlets, this finding should be considered for guidelines for caregivers on how to handle such events and prevent posttraumatic outcomes. In the immediate aftermath of an event, and until facts can be verified, social media is an unofficial information channel with potentially negative effects on mental health outcomes. This is notable because of the strong influence of media images and news, coupled with people's inability to discern between true and false reports.[116] To combat the circulation of rumors and conflicting stories, officials should also release updated information online frequently and as soon as possible, albeit this is difficult given the multiple modalities of social media today.

The rapid rise in media consumption, media access, and mobile media means that news information is more readily available, in a larger variety of ways, more rapidly than before, and from a wider range of sources. This development makes coverage of terrorist attacks, crisis events, or natural disasters more widespread and pervasive and may raise the potential for posttraumatic stress reactions. People no longer need to seek out the news. Rather, news information finds its way to peoples' home or mobile screens, almost immediately following an event. This instantaneous barrage of coverage increases the indirect exposure of young children, tweens, and teens and may raise questions about the validity of information spreading before being fact checked. News may be shared at school, or viewed privately on screens, limiting the opportunity of trusted caregivers to comfort and process trauma with their children. This is important considering reports stating over 40% of children believe, incorrectly, they can discriminate between true and untrue news stories[116] and research showing that receiving false information or rumors in times of crisis may worsen mental health outcomes.[115] Concerns about the validity of reporting on social media outlets is yet another variable that might add to traumatic responses, particularly if exaggerated or, at worst, transmitted in the effort to promote intense emotional responses. Thus, the actual reporting of news through social media, itself may be another form of terrorism. The impact of cyberterrorism is a new arena that merits research.

Clinical Interventions and Treatment

The effectiveness and comparative advantages of specific interventions and treatment modalities for children exposed to terrorism have yet to be sufficiently studied. Only recently have researchers developed rigorously designed studies to examine the effectiveness of treatments in children exposed to non−terrorism-induced trauma (e.g., single-incident traumas, natural disasters, sexual abuse, community violence, and war-induced trauma). The results of this research are promising. Children exposed to terrorist activities often manifest similar symptoms to children who have experienced other types of trauma. The results of research on the acute and chronic reactions of children to trauma may have significant implications for intervention strategies and treatment of children exposed to terrorism. No research has addressed the issues of treatment and interventions that are helpful to children who have been traumatized specifically by media coverage of terrorist events. Several recommendations can be inferred from the literature on treatment of trauma, however. A general review of community, school-based, individual, and family interventions and treatments is provided, followed by guidelines and suggestions specifically related to media coverage of terrorist events.

The application of trauma-focused interventions addresses several protective and risk factors that have useful implications for treatment of children exposed to terrorism. They emphasize the importance of parental and community reactions. Assisting parents and caregivers and including them in treatment is considered a crucial component of treatment. Psycho-education, cognitive restructuring, exposure, and coping skills management are emphasized. The importance of the effects of distant trauma and media coverage is taken into consideration.

Coping and Media Literacy (CML) training is effective at reducing the reactionary stress and anxiety responses in both children and parents when faced with news clips depicting the possibility of future terror attacks.[117] CML training educates parents in verbal and nonverbal methods of reacting to and discussing terrorism with children, as well as the media and media literacy skills. These skills are effective, and given the strong influence of parental reaction on the child's feelings, this training is doubly important for reducing acute stress and posttraumatic stress.[117]

Essential intervention strategies for dealing with community-wide acts of terrorism include early community-based intervention, clinical needs assessment to identify children at risk, multimodal, trauma-loss-focused treatment programs, and program evaluation of treatment efficacy.[64] Early community-based interventions focus on safety and protection. Restoration of rest and sleep, emotional support by parents and caregivers in the community, and stress-related symptom reduction are emphasized. Community-wide screening—conducted in schools, primary care settings, or neighborhood centers—identifies children at risk. Although there is no consensus on the most effective method of assessment, numerous structured interviews and self-reports are available.[118,119] Screening identifies children at risk and children in need of acute, trauma-related service. An essential component of the screening process is differentiating expected, developmentally appropriate reactions to trauma from more severe and persistent reactions. Screening information may be used to develop specialized treatment programs based on the unique needs of a child, family, or community. Screening results also serve to provide pretreatment data for evaluating outcome studies of treatment effectiveness. Triage and referral, based on knowledge of psychopathology and risk factors, are essential components of intervention.

Family therapy, individual trauma-informed therapy, group therapy, and school and community interventions have been used to treat traumatized children and families, provide them with coping skills, and address issues related to trauma and loss. No systematized studies have proved their effectiveness.[120–123] Psychoeducational group meetings (i.e., parent or community meetings) reduce symptoms of individual, family, and community fear and arousal levels.[124] School-based interventions to treat PTSD symptoms have received empirical support in the literature.[125–127] Several manuals on treatment programs for use after community traumatic events, including acts of terrorism, have been developed and distributed internationally.[128–133] These intervention programs and materials include active involvement of children's parents, caregivers, healthcare providers, community leaders, and educators. They present educational materials on basic safety skills, psychological stress responses, and treatment exercises to address symptoms and behavioral difficulties associated with trauma and loss. The preliminary results of the interventions and manuals developed to aid children after terrorist attacks are promising. Outcome data have not been examined, however, and further research is needed to evaluate their effectiveness. Children and families who manifest significant psychiatric impairment and dysfunction need more intensive mental health interventions treatment. Cognitive behavioral therapy has been the most rigorously studied treatment for traumatized children.[134–142] Studies by March[142] and Goenjian's[140] suggested that cognitive restructuring (i.e., reprocessing the traumatic event and identifying traumatic triggers), relaxation training, anger management training, teaching of proactive coping skills, and grief management are important methods for treating PTSD after disasters. Neither study addressed problems faced by children exposed to chronic trauma, comorbid disasters, history of trauma exposure, and serious family dysfunction, however.

There is some data available on the effectiveness of pharmacotherapy to treat symptoms that occur in children exposed to trauma. Selective serotonin reuptake inhibitors have been shown to have therapeutic effects on symptoms of depression and anxiety disorders in children,[143,144] however, trauma-informed therapy is the first line of treatment for PTSD. However, since symptoms of anxiety and depression are common in children after trauma, treatment with selective serotonin reuptake inhibitors provides an option for these symptoms. β-Blockers have been effective in reducing PTSD symptom ratings for adults who actively evoked trauma recall, up to 6 weeks after the drug administration.[145,146] Both short- and long-acting, given this positive result, new studies can investigate whether children and adolescents may benefit from these pharmacological treatment options.

Certain limitations exist when applying trauma-specific interventions to children who have experienced ongoing violence and the continual threat of terrorism. Crisis intervention alone does not prevent the long-lasting effects of children exposed to terrorism.[8,19] Compounded effects of multiple traumas have not been addressed. The unpredictability of terrorist attacks, indefinite nature of violent threats, lack of specific geographic boundaries, and effects of media coverage result in unique stressors and pose specific challenges for treatment of terrorism-induced trauma in children.

GUIDELINES FOR PARENTS, HEALTHCARE PROVIDERS, AND EDUCATORS: TRAUMA AND THE MEDIA

Helping children and adolescents overcome psychological problems in the aftermath of terrorist events is an important challenge for families and communities. Proactive and preventive methods to help children cope with loss and anxiety may help facilitate positive posttraumatic adjustment and allow for healthier outcomes in children's growth and development. Because the media plays a major role in informing the public about terrorism and may be a causative agent in symptom formation, it is critical for parents and families to have guidance about the use and misuse of media in traumatic times. What follows are media-related suggestions for healthcare providers, educators, and parents when dealing with children in the aftermath of terrorist attacks.

Parents, Educators, Healthcare Providers, Politicians, and Journalists Must Increase Their Awareness About the Potentially Harmful Effects of Media Exposure on Children

Disaster-related television viewing by children should be monitored closely by parents. Children's exposure should be limited. Adults also benefit from limiting their own exposure to reduce their stress reactions so that they and their children are better able to cope. Vulnerable persons who have risk factors, such as young children and individuals with previous traumatic experiences, should be especially cautious. When children are permitted to watch television, parents and caregivers are advised to watch the coverage with them. This

supervision provides adults with the opportunity to observe children's signs of distress and be available to answer questions and discuss relevant topics. School staff also must be aware of the importance of monitoring media exposure and should consider policies related to viewing coverage of traumatic events.

Adult awareness of children's exposure to media coverage must now expand to include social and mobile media. These technologies increase the amount of coverage children may see, possibly unbeknownst to parents or other adults. It is important for parents, caregivers, and teachers to know what young people see online, on smartphones, and using apps so the topics can be addressed. Parents should know what types of media kids are using and where they use it. In modern times, the jobs of parents, teachers, and health professionals are to educate kids about proper and improper use of digital media and encourage healthy use of it.

Parents and caretakers may also want to perform a media inventory with their children. This can include knowing what devices they have access to, where they are located, and what apps and sites they use to allow parents to accurately and directly address the media their children see. This is especially important to mediate stress reactions during times of crisis and fear. Additionally, parents and children should use mobile media together, whether it be online YouTube streaming, Facebook, Snapchat, or any other media news source. Although this may not be common practice, during times of crisis it is important for parents and children to watch coverage together so they can process, discuss, and understand what they are seeing.

Adults Benefit from Seeking Positive Ways of Understanding and Coping With Their Own Responses to Terrorist Events to Optimally Help Their Children to Cope

Since September 11, 2001, many resources have been made available to help parents cope with the terrorism-related fears and anxieties.[147−149] A constructive use of the media may be helpful in this situation to access information to help parents. Any parent who is overwhelmed by the effects of the disaster should seek help from primary healthcare providers, educators, mental health agencies, and clergy. If parents are not able to manage their own responses to the trauma, they are not effective in reassuring their children and helping them discuss their concerns, particularly when their children see graphic images on television, hear stories on the news, and read about current events in newspapers and magazines.

Children Cannot Be Sheltered Entirely from Knowing About or Reacting to a Disturbing Event

In the modern world, children of all ages are almost guaranteed to have exposure to media, particularly digital media. For the youngest children, parents may opt to shelter and limit a child from exposure to frightening and disturbing media images. When possible, young children should be encouraged to express their feelings in words, and parents' answers should be honest and developmentally appropriate. One should not provide more information than is requested. For children in late elementary school, who are exposed to some images in school, programs may be previewed by parents and then watched together as a family. Long after an event, children may watch shows with parents to help them understand terrorism, for example, "Through a child's eyes: September 11, 2001," which is an Emmy Award–winning HBO children's special that deals with young school-age children's responses to the September 11 attacks.[150] Children's fears of not knowing or understanding what has happened may be more disturbing than the truth. It is important for parents to present information to children according to a child's developmental level. Listening is more important than talking. Children should be encouraged to express their concerns, and their feelings should be validated. All questions should be treated with respect, not ignored or dismissed. Responses should be made with calm reassurance and empathy. If a child's question causes anxiety or discomfort, the adult should not remain silent, because a child may interpret the silence as a sign of danger. It is permissible to tell a child that his or her question cannot be answered immediately but will receive a response after the adult has time to think about it.

Because older children are exposed to media accounts of terrorism at home and most likely also in the classroom, discussing terrorist activities—without overwhelming them—and encouraging questions or correcting misperceptions is the key. Exposure to news and mobile media is almost universal in today's world; it is incredibly difficult to completely shelter school-age children and teens from the news. The best practice may be for parents to assume their child will see media coverage of an event, and use these situations as an opportunity for meaningful discussion with their children.

Although all children are individuals and have unique developmental needs, some questions and basic needs are universal in trauma situations. In the event of a crisis or terror attack, all children need to know that they are safe, that the adults who care for them are safe, and how this event will affect their daily lives. Even though this type of thing is out of the ordinary, it is important to keep life feeling ordinary and stick to normal routines as much as possible.

Some children's and adolescent's Responses May Be Confusing

Children and adolescents may initially cover up fears and anxieties. For example, they may make comments such as "We should not be upset, nothing has happened to us." Just as adults should be aware of their own defenses and coping styles, they should be sensitive to children's defenses and ways of coping. This awareness may involve judicious use of media chosen at a child's developmental level. Young children should not watch adult-oriented shows. For example, older elementary school–aged children may tolerate being exposed to news "briefs" in which simple concise statements of the facts are made (e.g., reports that occur on major networks between television shows) but may not be ready to watch broadcasts that spend 30 min or more with interviews, photos, and more detailed discussion of a devastated building or land.

If a Child Chooses Not to Talk About the Events, Parents Should Respect That Decision While Monitoring for Any Emerging Symptoms

Children may not be ready to share their experiences immediately; they may wait days or weeks. Adults should ensure that children know that they are available to listen and discuss children's feelings whenever the children need them. Conversely, some children are interested in listening and watching and are paying attention to media exposure although they are not ready for discussion. Parents should continue to monitor and guide a child's exposure to media reports that contain frightening information and not assume that a child is unaware, unaffected, or disinterested in an event simply because the child is not ready to talk about it.

Finally, and important clinically, parents need to appreciate who their kids are, that they are the experts when it comes to their kids, and then tailor an approach to the strengths and weaknesses of their kids. If a child is very anxious, it may be wise to limit access, not by prohibition but by having conversations. Similarly, if a child/teen has difficulty with self-regulation of mood, that is another variable that needs addressing. When a child is ready to discuss, parents can provide open, honest answers and support.

Adults Need to Reassure Children That They Are Safe and Will Be Protected

Media reports can be used to help reassure children and adolescents that many adults are working to maintain a safe and protected environment for them. Parents may choose to offer taped news reports or specific types of media discussion that will help a child to feel secure in the knowledge that adults are taking charge and responding in ways that are protective. Films about resilience, survival, family and community consolidation, and triumph over adversity may play a constructive role by giving children a reasonable sense of hope for the future. Maintaining familiar routines helps children know what to expect and is comforting to them. Reassuring children that they are loved and that they will be cared for gives them a sense of security. They should not be offered false assurance, however. Parents should teach children to manage their fears and anger constructively by showing them how to handle their emotions in healthy ways. They can be made to feel more in control by allowing them to make decisions (e.g., what to eat at mealtime, what to wear, what movie to see).

FURTHER RECOMMENDATIONS

The continuing frequency of terrorism-related events around the world underscores the urgent need for an effective public health approach for children and families. The media have a responsibility to balance their professional goals of delivering news and preventing potentially untoward effects. With the rising dependence on and use of social media, leaders in this area must also explore methods to monitor the spread of information in times of crisis and help limit the spread of false accounts and attempt to reduce trauma responses. This may be a complex challenge to undertake but is necessary as adults and children increasingly use social media as a news source. It is important for journalists and editors to understand the impact of their reporting on children. Mental healthcare leaders and providers must be educated and prepared to deal with children who need care in the aftermath of terrorist activities. DuFour (Frederick DuFour, PhD, personal communication) has noted that "terrorism is a community mental health issue" because terrorism is "psychological warfare." Collaboration among community, educational, primary care, and mental healthcare organizations has been initiated and is likely to continue to grow and develop. General healthcare and primary pediatric organizations like the American Academy of Pediatrics, not just mental health specialists, have power to educate the public and promote good mental health practices for all. Further collaboration among these agencies and the media is necessary. Advocacy for program development and funding to help children is needed. Efforts should be focused on increasing community services for children affected by terrorism and encouraging further research on terrorism and its unique impact on children and families. Public policy to limit media coverage is a controversial issue but must be addressed. Increased public education about responsible and reliable coverage is essential to ensure that mental healthcare providers, primary care providers, organizations, journalists, educators, spiritual leaders, and community organizations are better prepared to prevent retraumatizing experiences and help children cope. Better public education about responsible and validated media coverage can also help people discern facts from fiction and evaluate any inaccuracies or confusion in media coverage. In turn, this will minimize long-term psychological problems and enhance healthier outcomes and growth.

REFERENCES

1. United States Department of Defense. Department of Defense Combating Terrorism Program (Department of Defense Directive Number 2000.12). Available from: http://www.defenselink.mil/pubs/downing_rpt/annx_e.html.
2. Yehuda R, McFarlane AC, Shalev AY. Predicting the development of posttraumatic stress disorder from the acute response to a traumatic event. *Biol Psychiatry*. 1998;44: 1305–1313.
3. Smith EM, North CS. Posttraumatic stress disorders in natural disasters and technological accidents. In: Wilson JP, Raphael B, eds. *Internatioanl Handbook of Traumatic Stress Syndromes*. New York: Plenum Press; 1993: 405–419.
4. American Psychiatric Association. *Diagnostic and Statistical Manual of Mental Disorders* (DSM-5). 5th ed. Washington, DC: American Psychiatric Association; 2013.
5. Almqvist K, Broberg AA. Mental health and social adjustment in young refugee children 3O years after their arrival in Sweden. *J Am Acad Child Adolesc Psychiatry*. 1999;38: 723–730.
6. Ayalon O. Children as hostages. *Practitioner*. 1982;226: 773–781.
7. Macksoud M, Dyregrov A, Raundalen M. Traumatic war experiences and their effects on children. In: Raphael B, Wilson JP, eds. *International Handbook of Traumatic Stress Syndromes*. New York: Plenum Press; 1993:625–633.
8. Almqvist K, Brandell-Frosberg M. Refugee children in Sweden: post-traumatic stress disorder in Iranian preschool children exposed to organized violence. *Child Abuse Negl*. 1997;21:351–366.

9. Bat-Zion N, Levy-Shiff R. Children in war: stress and coping reactions under the threat of Scud missile attacks and the effect of proximity. In: Leavitt L, Fox N, eds. *The Psycho- Logical Effects of War and Violence on Children.* Hillsdale, NJ: Lawrence Erlbaum Associates, Inc; 1993: 143−179.

10. Klingman A, Sagi A, Raviv A. The effect of war on Israeli children. In: Leavitt L, Fox N, eds. *The Psychological Effects of War and Violence on Children.* Hillsdale, NJ: Lawrence Erlbaum Associates, Inc; 1993:75−92.

11. Pfefferbaum B, Nixon SJ, Tucker RM, et al. Post traumatic stress responses in bereaved children following the Oklahoma City bombing. *J Am Acad Child Adolesc Psychiatry.* 1999;39:1372−1379.

12. Pfefferbaum B, Gurwitch R, McDonald N, et al. Posttraumatic stress among young children after the death of a friend or acquaintance in a terrorist bombing. *Psychiatr Serv.* 2000;51:386−388.

13. Allwood MA, Bell-Dolan D, Husain SA. Children's trauma and adjustment reactions to violent and nonviolent war experiences. *J Am Acad Child Adolesc Psychiatry.* 2002;41:450−457.

14. Dyregrov A, Gupta L, Gjestad R, et al. Trauma exposure and psychological reactions to genocide among Rwandan children. *J Trauma Stress.* 2000;13:3−21.

15. Goenjian AK, Pynoos R, Steinberg AM, et al. Psychiatric comorbidity in children of the 1988 earthquake in Armenia. *J Am Acad Child Adolesc Psychiatry.* 1995;34: 1174−1184.

16. Goldstein RD, Wampler NS, Wise PH. War experiences and distress symptoms of Bosnian children. *Pediatrics.* 1997;100:873−878.

17. Nader K, Pynoos R, Fairbanks L, et al. Children's reactions one year after a sniper attack at their school. *Am J Psychiatry.* 1990;147:1526−1530.

18. Desivilya H, Gal R, Ayalon O. Long-term effects of trauma in adolescents: comparison between survivors of a terrorist attack and control counterparts. *Anxiety Stress Coping.* 1996;9:1135−1150.

19. Trappler B, Friedman S. Posttraumatic stress disorders of the Brooklyn Bridge shooting. *Am J Psychiatry.* 1996;153: 705−707.

20. Elbedour S, Baker A, Shalhoub-Kevorkian N, et al. Psychological responses in family members after the Hebron massacre. *Depress Anxiety.* 1999;9:27−31.

21. Gabarino J, Kosteleny K. The effects of political violence on Palestinian children's behavior problems: a risk accumulation model. *Child Dev.* 1996;67:33−45.

22. Macksound M. Assessing war trauma in children: a case study of Lebanese children. *J Refug Stud.* 1992;5:1−15.

23. Pynoos RS, Nader K. Prevention of psychiatric morbidity in children after disaster. In: Shaffer D, Philips I, Enzer NB, eds. *OSAP Prevention Monograph-2: Prevention of Mental Disorders, Alcohol and Other Drug Use in Children and Adolescents.* Washington, DC: US Government Printing Office; 1989:535−549.

24. Hanford HA, Mayes SD, Mattison RE, et al. Child and parent reaction to the Three Mile Island nuclear accident. *J Am Acad Child Adolesc Psychiatry.* 1986;25: 346−356.

25. Osofsky JD. The effects of exposure to violence on young children. *Am Psychol.* 1995;50:782−788.

26. Realmuto GM, Masten A, Carole LF, et al. Adolescent survivors of massive childhood trauma in Cambodia: life events and current symptoms. *J Trauma Stress.* 1992;5: 589−599.

27. Terr LC. What happens to early memories of trauma? A study of twenty children under age five at the time of the documented traumatic events. *J Am Acad Child Adolesc Psychiatry.* 1988;27:96−104.

28. Vogel JM, Vernberg EM. Psychological responses of children to natural and human-made disasters. 1. Children's psychological responses to disasters. *J Clin Child Psychol.* 1993;22:464−484.

29. Weisenberg M, Schwartzwald J, Waysman M, et al. Coping of school-age children in the sealed room during the scud missile bombardment and postwar stress reactions. *J Consult Clin Psychol.* 1993;61:462−467.

30. Laor N, Wolmer L, Mayes L, et al. Israeli preschool children under scuds: a 30-month follow-up. *J Am Acad Child Adolesc Psychiatry.* 1997;36:349−356.

31. Terr LC. Childhood traumas: an outline and overview. *Am J Psychiatry.* 1996;148:10−20.

32. Laor N, Wolmer L, Mayes L, et al. Israeli preschoolers under the scud missile attacks. *Arch Gen Psychiatry.* 1996;53:416−423.

33. Scheeringa MS, Zeanah CH, Drell MJ, et al. Two approaches to the diagnosis of posttraumatic stress disorder in infancy and early childhood. *J Am Acad Child Adolesc Psychiatry.* 1995;34:191−200.

34. Davidson J, Smith R. Traumatic experiences in psychiatric outpatients. *J Trauma Stress.* 1990;3:459−475.

35. Hoven CW, Duarte CS, Lucas CP, et al. *Effects of the World Trade Center Attack on NYC Public School Students. Initial Report to the New York City Board of Education.* New York: Columbia University Mailman School of Public Health and New York State Psychiatric Institute and Applied Research and Consulting; 2002.

36. Terr LC, Bloch DA, Michel BA, et al. Children's symptoms in the wake of Challenger: a field study of distant-traumatic effects and an outline of related conditions. *Am J Psychiatry.* 1999;156:1536−1544.

37. Pynoos RS, Frederick C, Nader K, et al. Life threat and posttraumatic stress in school-age children. *Arch Gen Psychiatry.* 1987;44:1057−1063.

38. Kandemir-Ozdinc N, Erdur-Baker O. Children and television news. *Procedia Soc Behav Sci.* 2013;84:351−355.

39. Garbarino J. The experience of children in Kuwait: occupation, war and liberation. *Child Youth Fam Serv Q.* 1991;14:2−3.

40. Terr LC. Psychic trauma in children and adolescents. *Psychiatr Clin North Am.* 1985;8:815−835.

41. Giaconia RM, Reinherz HZ, Silverman AB, et al. Trauma and posttraumatic stress disorder in a community population of older adolescents. *J Am Acad Child Adolesc Psychiatry*. 1995;34:1369−1380.

42. Cicchetti D, Toth S, Lynch M. The developmental sequelae of child maltreatment: implications for war-related trauma. In: Leavitt L, Fox N, eds. *The Psychological Effects of War and Violence on Children*. Hillsdale, NJ: Lawrence Erlbaum Associates, Inc; 1993:41−74.

43. van der Kolk B, McFarlane A. The black hole of trauma. In: Van der Kolk BA, Weisaeth L, eds. *Traumatic Stress*. New York: Guilford Press; 1996:3−23.

44. Halpern-Felsher BL, Millstein GM. The effects of terrorism on teens' perception of dying: the new world is riskier than ever. *J Adolesc Health*. 2002;30:308−311.

45. Nemeroff CB. Neurobiological consequences of childhood trauma. *J Clin Psychiatry*. 2004;65(1):18−28.

46. Nemeroff CB. The preeminent role of early untoward experience on vulnerability of major psychiatric disorders: the nature-nurture controversy revised and soon to be resolved. *Mol Psychiatry*. 1999;4:106−108.

47. Heim C, Nemeroff CB. Neurobiology of early life stress: clinical studies. *Semin Clin Neuropsychiatry*. 2002;7:147−159.

48. Breslau N, Chilcoat HD, Kessler RC, et al. Previous exposure to trauma and PTSD effects of subsequent trauma. *Am J Psychiatry*. 1999;156:902−907.

49. Garrison CZ, Wwinrich MW, Hardin SB, et al. Posttraumatic stress disorder in adolescents after a hurricane. *Am J Epidemiol*. 1993;138:522−530.

50. Breslau N, Davis GC. Traumatic events and posttraumatic stress disorder in an urban population of young adults. *Arch Gen Psychiatry*. 1991;48:216−222.

51. Breslau N, Davis GC. Posttraumatic stress disorder in an urban population of young adults: risk factors for chronicity. *Am J Psychiatry*. 1992;152:529−535.

52. Lonigan CJ, Shannon MP, Taylor CM, et al. Children exposed to disaster. II: risk factors for the development of post-traumatic symptomatology. *J Am Acad Child Adolesc Psychiatry*. 1994;33:94−105.

53. Tyano S, Iancu I, Solomon Z, et al. Seven-year follow-up of child survivors of a bus-train collision. *J Am Acad Child Adolesc Psychiatry*. 1996;35:365−373.

54. Centers for Disease Control and Prevention, Kaiser Permanente. *The ACE Study Survey Data: Major Findings*. 2016.

55. Lowe SR, Galea S. The mental health consequences of mass shootings. *Trauma Violence Abuse*. 2015;18(1):62−82.

56. Yehuda R. Risk and resilience in posttraumatic stress disorder. *J Clin Psychiatry*. 2004;65(suppl 1):29−36.

57. Breton J, Valla J, Lambert J. Industrial disaster and mental health of children and their parents. *J Am Acad Child Adolesc Psychiatry*. 1993;32:438−445.

58. Bromet EJ, Goldgaber D, Carlson G, et al. Children's well-being 11 years after the Chernobyl catastrophe. *Arch Gen Psychiatry*. 2000;57:563−571.

59. Deblinger E, Steer R, Lipmann J. Maternal factors associated with sexually abused children's psychosocial adjustment. *Child Maltreat*. 1999;4:13−20.

60. Korel M, Green BL, Gleser GC. Children's responses to a nuclear waste disaster: PTSD symptoms and outcome prediction. *J Am Acad Child Adolesc Psychiatry*. 1999;38:368−375.

61. McFarlane AC. Family functioning and overprotection following a natural disaster: the longitudinal effects of posttraumatic morbidity. *Aust N Z J Psychiatry*. 1987;21:210−218.

62. Bryce J, Walker N, Ghorayeb F, et al. Life experiences, response styles and mental health among mothers and children in Beirut, Lebanon. *Soc Sci Med*. 1989;28:685−695.

63. McFarlane AC. Posttraumatic phenomena in a longitudinal study of children following a natural disaster. *J Am Acad Child Adolesc Psychiatry*. 1987;26:764−769.

64. Gurwitch RH, Sitterle KA, Young BH, et al. The aftermath of terrorism. In: La Greca AM, Silverman WK, Vernberg EM, et al., eds. *Helping Children Cope with Disasters and Terrorism*. Washington, DC: American Psychological Association; 2002:327−357.

65. Rigamer EF. Psychological management of children in a national crisis. *J Am Acad Child Adolesc Psychiatry*. 1986;25:364−369.

66. Sack WH, Angell RH, Kinzie JD, et al. The psychiatric effects of massive trauma on Cambodian children: II. The home and the school. *J Am Acad Child Adolesc Psychiatry*. 1986;25:377−383.

67. Losel F, Bliesener T. Resilience in adolescents: a study on the generalizability of protective factors. In: Hurrelmann K, Losel F, eds. *Health Hazards in Adolescence*. New York, NY: Walter de Gruyter; 1990:299−320.

68. Kinzie JD, Sack W, Angell RH, et al. The psychiatric effects of massive trauma on Cambodian children. *J Am Acad Child Adolesc Psychiatry*. 1986;25:370−376.

69. Fergusson DM, Linskey TL. Physical punishment/maltreatment during childhood and adjustment in young adulthood. *Child Abuse Negl*. 1997;21:617−630.

70. Gabarino J, Kostelny K. Child maltreatment as a community problem. *Child Abuse Negl*. 1992;16:455−464.

71. Gabarino J, Dubrow N, Kostelny K, et al. *Children in Danger*. San Francisco, CA: Jossey - Bass; 1992.

72. Miller KE. Child Dev. The effects of state terrorism and exile on indigenous Guatemalan refugee children: a mental health assessment and an analysis of children's narratives. *Child Dev*. 1996;1996(67):89−106.

73. Smith P, Perin S, Yule W, et al. War exposure and maternal reactions in the psychological adjustment of children from Bosnia-Herzegovina. *J Child Psychol Psychiatry*. 2001;42:395−404.

74. Udwin O, Boyle S, Yule W, et al. Risk factors for long term psychological effects of a disaster experienced in adolescence: predictors of posttraumatic stress disorder. *J Child Psychol Psychiatry*. 2000;41:969−979.

75. Laor N, Wolmer L, Cohen D. Mother's functioning and children's symptoms 5 years after a SCUD missile attack. *Am J Psychiatry.* 2001;58:1020−1026.

76. Melville MB, Lykes MB. Guatemalan Indian children and the sociocultural effects of government sponsored terrorism. *Soc Sci Med.* 1992;34:533−548.

77. Baker A. Effects of political and military traumas on children: the Palestinian case. *Clin Psychol Rev.* 1999;19: 935−950.

78. Punamaki RL. Psychological stress response of Palestinian mothers and their children in conditions of military occupation and political violence. *Q Newsl Lab Comp Hum Cogn.* 1987;9:76−79.

79. Sack WH, McSharry S, Clarke GN, et al. The Khmer adolescent project: I. Epidemiologic findings in two generations of Cambodian refugees. *J Nerv Ment Dis.* 1994; 182:387−395.

80. Sack WH, Gregory C, Seeley M. Posttraumatic stress disorder across two generations of Cambodian refugees. *J Am Acad Child Adolesc Psychiatry.* 1995;34:1160−1166.

81. Atkin C. Broadcast news programming and the child audience. *J Broadcast.* 1978;22:47−61.

82. Drew D, Reeves B. Children and TV news. *J Broadcast.* 1978;57:45−54.

83. Fairbank, Maslin, Maullin, and Associates. Children now: children and the media. Tuned in or tuned out? America's children speak out on the news media. Available from: http://www.childrennow.org/media/mc94/news.html.

84. Smith SL, Wilson BJ. Children's comprehension and fear reactions to television news. *Media Psychol.* 2002;4:1−26.

85. Common Sense Media Research. *News and America's Kids − How Young People Perceive and Are Impacted by the News.* San Francisco, CA: Common Sense Media; 2017.

86. Terr LC, Bloch DA, Michel BA, et al. Children's memories in the wake of Challenger. *Am J Psychiatry.* 1996;153: 618−625.

87. Terr LC, Bloch DA, Michel BA, et al. Children's thinking in the wake of Challenger. *Am J Psychiatry.* 1997;154: 744−751.

88. Pfefferbaum B, Seale T, Brandt E, et al. Media exposure in children one hundred miles from a terrorist bombing. *Ann Clin Psychiatry.* 2003;15(1):1−8.

89. Thabet AM, Abed Y, Vostanis P. Emotional problems in Palestinian children living in a war zone: a cross-sectional study. *Lancet.* 2002;359:1801−1804.

90. Pfefferbaum B, Nixon SJ, Yivis R, et al. Television exposure in children after a terrorist incident. *Psychiatry.* 2001;4:202−211.

91. Minuchin S. *Families and Family Therapy.* Cambridge, MA: Harvard University Press; 1974.

92. Schuster MA, Stein BD, Jaycox LH, et al. A national survey of stress reactions after the September 11, 2001 terrorist attacks. *N Engl J Med.* 2001;345:1507−1512.

93. Saylor CF, Cowart BL, Lipovsky JA, et al. Media exposure to September 11: elementary school students' experiences and posttraumatic symptoms. *Am Behav Sci.* 2003; 46(12):1622−1642.

94. Phillips D, Prince S, Schiebelhut L. Elementary school children's responses 3 months after the September 11 terrorist attacks: a study in Washington, DC. *Am J Orthopsychiatry.* 2004;74(4):509−528.

95. Ahern J, Galea S, Resnick H, et al. Television images and psychological symptoms after the September 11 terrorist attacks. *Psychiatry.* 2002;65:289−300.

96. Schlenger WE, Caddell JM, Ebert L, et al. Psychological reactions to terrorist attacks: findings from the national study of Americans' reactions to September 11. *JAMA.* 2002;288:581−588.

97. Comer JS, Dantowitz A, Chou T, et al. Adjustment among area youth after the Boston marathon bombing and subsequent manhunt. *Pediatrics.* 2014;134(1):1−8.

98. Holman AE, Garfin DR, Cohen Silver R. Media's role in broadcasting acute stress following the Boston Marathon bombings. *Proc Natl Acad Sci.* 2013;111(1):93−98.

99. Nielsen. Nielsen estimates 119.6 million TV homes in the U.S. for the 2017−18 TV season. Available from: http://www.nielsen.com/us/en/insights/news/2017/nielsen-estimates-119-6-million-us-tv-homes-2017-2018-tv-season.html.

100. McDonough P. Television and beyond a kid's eye view. Nielsen. Available from: http://www.nielsen.com/us/en/insights/news/2009/television-and-beyond-a-kids-eye-view.html.

101. Kaiser Family Foundation. Daily media use among children and teens up dramatically from five years ago. The Henry J. Kaiser Family Foundation. Available from: https://www.kff.org/disparities-policy/press-release/daily-media-use-among-children-and-teens-up-dramatically-from-five-years-ago/.

102. Kaiser Family Foundation. *Kids and the Media @ the New Millennium.* The Henry J. Kaiser Family Foundation; 2004.

103. Cantor J, Nathanson AI. Children's fright reactions to television news. *J Commun.* 1996;46(4):139−152.

104. Mommy Cantor J. *I'm Scared: How TV and Movies Frighten Children and What We Can Do to Protect Them.* San Diego, CA: Harvest/Harcourt Brace & Co; 1998.

105. Smith SL, Wilson BJ. Children's reactions to a television news story: the impact of video footage and proximity of the crime. *Communic Res.* 2000;2002(27):641−673.

106. Cantor J, Mares M, Oliver MB. Parents' and children's emotional reactions to TV coverage of the Gulf War. In: Greenberg BS, Gantz W, eds. *Desert Storm and the Mass Media.* Cresskill, NJ: Hampton Press; 1993:325−340.

107. Hoffner C, Cantor J. Developmental differences in responses to a television character's appearance and behavior. *Dev Psychol.* 1985;21:1065−1074.

108. Kaiser Family Foundation. Key facts: children and the news. Available from: https://kaiserfamilyfoundation.files.wordpress.com/2013/01/key-facts-children-and-the-news.pdf.

109. Klingman A. Children under the stress of war. In: La Greca AM, Silverman WK, Vernberg EM, et al., eds. *Helping Children Cope with Disasters and Terrorism.* Washington, DC: American Psychological Association; 2002:359−380.

110. Raviv A. The use of hotline and media interventions in Israel during the Gulf War. In: Leavitt LA, Fox NA, eds. *The Psychological Effects of War and Violence on Children.* Hillsdale, NJ: Lawrence Erlbaum Associates, Inc; 1993: 319–337.

111. Common Sense Media. The Common Sense Census: media use by kids age zero to eight. Common Sense Media. Available from: https://www.commonsensemedia.org/ sites/default/files/uploads/research/csm_zerotoeight_ fullreport_release_2.pdf.

112. Lenhart A. Teens, social media & technology overview 2015. Pew Research Center. Available from: http:// www.pewinternet.org/2015/04/09/teens-social-media- technology-2015/.

113. Shearer E, Gottfried J. News use across social media platforms 2017. Pew Research Center. Available from: http:// www.journalism.org/2017/09/07/news-use-across-social- media-platforms-2017/.

114. Common Sense Media. News and America's kids: how young people perceive and are impacted by the news. Info- graphic. Available from: https://www.commonsensemedia. org/research/news-and-americas-kids-infographic.

115. Jones NM, Thompson R, Schetter CD, et al. Distress and rumor exposure on social media during a campus lockdown. *PNAS.* 2017;114(4):11663–11668.

116. Common Sense Media. News and America's kids: how young people perceive and are impacted by the news. Available from: https://www.commonsensemedia.org/ sites/default/files/uploads/research/2017_commonsense_ newsandamericaskids.pdf.

117. Comer JS, Furr JM, Beidas RS, et al. Children and terrorism-related news: training parents in coping and media literacy. *J Consult Clin Psychol.* 2009;76(4): 568–578.

118. Cohen J. Practice parameters for the assessment and treat- ment of children with posttraumatic stress disorder. *J Am Acad Child Adolesc Psychiatry.* 1998;37(10):S4–S26.

119. Cohen JA, Berliner L, March JS. Treatment of children and adolescents. In: Foa EB, Keane T, eds. *Effective Treatmetns for PTSD: Practice Guidelines for the International Society for Traumatic Stress Studies.* New York: Guildford Press; 2000: 106–138.

120. Nader K. Treatment methods for childhood trauma. In: Wilson JP, Friedman M, Lindy J, eds. *PT Treating Psycho- logical Trauma and PTSD.* New York: Guilford Press; 2001:278–334.

121. Pope L, Campbell M, Kurtz P. Hostage crisis: a school- based interdisciplinary approach to posttraumatic stress disorder. *Soc Work Educ.* 1992;14:227–233.

122. Prinstein MJ, La Greca AM, Vernbert EM, et al. Children's coping assistance after a natural disaster. *J Clin Child Psy- chol.* 1996;25:463–475.

123. Terr LC. Childhood posttraumatic stress disorder. In: Gabbard GO, ed. *Treatment of Psychiatric Disorderes.* 3rd ed. Washington, DC: American Psychiatric Press; 2001: 293–306.

124. Nader K. Treating traumatic grief in systems. In: Wilson JP, Friedman M, Lindy J, eds. *Death and Trauma: The Traumatology of Grieving.* New York: Guildford Press; 1997:278–334.

125. La Greca AM, Silverman W, Vernberg EM, et al. Symp- toms of posttraumatic stress after Hurricane Andrew: a prospective study. *J Consult Clin Psychol.* 1996;64: 712–723.

126. Swenson CC, Saylor CF, Powell MP, et al. Impact of a nat- ural disaster on preschool children: adjustment 14 months after a hurricane. *Am J Orthopsychiatry.* 1996;66:122–130.

127. Vernberg EM, La Greca AM, Silverman WK, et al. Predic- tors of a child's post-disaster functioning following Hur- ricane Andrew. *J Abnorm Psychol.* 1996;105:237–248.

128. American Red Cross. *Facing Fear: Helping Young People Deal with Terrorism and Tragic Events.* Falls Church, VA: American Red Cross; 2001.

129. Gurwitch RH, Messenbaugh A. *Healing after Trauma Skills: A Manual for Professionals, Teachers, and Families Working with Children after Trauma/disaster.* Oklahoma City, OK: Children's Medical Research Foundation; 2001.

130. La Greca AM, Vernberg EM, Silverman WK, et al. *Helping Children Cope with Natural Disasters: A Manual for School Personnel.* Coral Gables, FL: University of Miami; 1994.

131. La Greca AM, Sevin S, Selvin EL. *Helping America Cope: A Guide to Help Parents and Children Cope with the September 11th Terrorist Attacks.* Coral Gables, FL: Dippity; 2001.

132. Storm V, McDermott B, Finlayson D. *The Bushfire and Me.* Newtown, Australia: VBD Publications; 1994.

133. Vernberg EM. Intervention approaches following disasters. In: La Greca AM, Silverman WK, Vernberg EM, et al., eds. *Helping Children Cope with Disasters and Terrorism.* Washington, DC: American Psychological As- sociation; 2002:55–72.

134. Berliner L, Saunders B. Treating fear and anxiety in sexu- ally abused children: results in a two-year follow up study. *Child Maltreat.* 1996;1:294–309.

135. Celano M, Hazzard A, Webb C, et al. Treating fear and anxiety in sexually abused girls and their mothers: an evaluation study. *J Abnorm Clin Psychol.* 1996;24:1–17.

136. Cohen JA, Marrarino AP. Factors that mediate treatment outcome of sexually abused preschool children: initial findings. *J Am Acad Child Adolesc Psychiatry.* 1996;35: 1402–1410.

137. Cohen JA, Marrarino A. Factors that mediate treatment outcome of sexually abused preschool children: a six and 12-month follow up. *J Am Acad Child Adolesc Psychi- atry.* 1998;37:44–51.

138. Deblinger E, Lippman J, Steer R. Sexually abused children suffering posttraumatic stress symptoms: initial treat- ment outcome findings. *Child Maltreat.* 1996;1:310–321.

139. Deblinger E, Steer RA, Lipmann J. Two-year follow-up study of cognitive behavioral therapy for sexually abused children suffering post traumatic stress symptoms. *Child Abuse Negl.* 1999;23:1371–1378.

140. Goenjian AK, Karayan I, Pynoos RS, et al. Outcome of psychotherapy among pre-adolescents after the 1988 earthquake in Armenia. *Am J Psychiatry*. 1997;154: 536−542.

141. King NJ, Tonge BJ, Mullen P, et al. Treating sexually abused children with posttraumatic stress symptoms: a randomized clinical trial. *J Am Acad Child Adolesc Psychiatry*. 2000;39:1347−1355.

142. March JS, Amaya-Jackson L, Murray MC, et al. Cognitive-behavioral psychotherapy for children and adolescents with PTSD after a single incident stressor. *J Am Acad Child Adolesc Psychiatry*. 1998;37:585−593.

143. Emslie GJ, Mayes TL. Mood disorders in children and adolescents: psychopharmacological treatment. *Biol Psychiatry*. 2001;49:1082−1090.

144. RUPP Anxiety Study Group. An eight-week placebo-controlled trial of fluvoxamine for anxiety disorders in children. *N Engl J Med*. 2001;344:1279−1285.

145. Brunet A, Saumier D, Liu A, et al. Reduction of PTSD symptoms with pre-reactivation propranolol therapy: a randomized controlled trial. *Am J Psychiatry*. 2018. https://doi.org/10.1176/appi.ajp.2017.17050481.

146. Tarsitani L, De Santis V, Mistretta M, et al. Treatment with β-blockers and incidence of post-traumatic stress disorder after cardiac surgery: a prospective observational study. *J Cardiothorac Vasc Anesth*. 2012;26(2):265−269.

147. National Mental Health Association. Available from: http://www.nmha.org/reassurance/secondanniversary/kidscopingtips.ctm.

148. Centers for Disease Control. Available from: http://www.bt.cdc.gov/masstrauma/copingpub.asp.

149. American Academy of Child and Adolescent Psychiatry. Available from: http://www.aacap.org/publications/factsfam/87.htm.

150. Schatz A. *Through a Child's Eyes: September 11, 2001*. HBO; 2002:30.

CHAPTER 6

Addicted Media: Substances on Screen

ALLISON OPTICAN, MD • PATRICIA A. CAVAZOS-REHG, PHD

INTRODUCTION

The 21st century media landscape poses unprecedented opportunities for drug and alcohol exposure. In addition to traditional media (e.g., movies, television, print), which are static and controlled, social networking sites (SNSs) provide a dynamic user interface, allowing for content to be accessible without cost and on demand. Additionally, shared content via SNSs is largely unregulated and user generated. As of 2015, nearly all young people in the United States have access to the Internet, and approximately 96% of 12- to 17-year-olds use SNSs.[1] In the face of targeted outreach to help curb adolescent substance use,[2] adolescents are exposed to more than $25 billion worth of media advertising for cigarette, alcohol, and prescription drugs each year through diverse media outlets.[3] Additionally, children and adolescents often observe favorable portrayals of substance use on popular television shows,[4] in movies,[5,6] and (increasingly) via SNSs.[7] Although most SNSs have policies in place to forbid direct marketing of illicit substances,[8,9] enforcement is challenging.[10] Further, youth exposure to peer-generated content portraying substance use behaviors is increasingly commonplace.[11,12] Whether from traditional media or SNSs, research suggests that exposure to substance use on screen increases the likelihood that young people will engage in substance use.[11,13,14]

This chapter provides a comprehensive review of current peer-reviewed literature related to portrayal of substances in the media and its potential impact on children and adolescents. The review will expand upon the related chapter[15] from the 2005 edition of this book, specifically highlighting the influence and scope of SNSs. "Substances" hereafter refers to tobacco, alcohol, and marijuana, which are identified by the National Survey on Drug Use and Health as the most common addictive substances that are consumed by young people.[16]

ALCOHOL

Alcohol is the most commonly used and abused substance among children and adolescents.[17] Despite targeted public health outreach, underage drinking remains a major public health threat associated with increased morbidity and mortality.[18] Efforts to reduce and prevent underage drinking are impeded by the favorable portrayal of alcohol use on traditional media platforms and SNSs.[19,20] Regarding the former, a recent Center on Alcohol Marketing and Youth report demonstrated that youth exposure to alcohol advertising on US television increased 71% between 2001 and 2009[21]; similarly, a 2017 content analysis of popular movies found that alcohol brand placements have nearly doubled over the past 2 decades, with a high frequency of brand placements identified in G-, PG-, and PG-13-rated movies.[22] SNSs reflect an expanding medium through which youth may be exposed to alcohol use. Content analyses of user data drawn from SNSs demonstrate pervasive references to alcohol among youth, with over 95% of sampled profiles containing picture references to alcohol use.[12] There is also evidence of alcohol marketing on SNSs, specifically targeting youth.[23]

The role of traditional media in influencing drinking-related norms and expectancies has long been studied. Mechanistically, identification of more positive affective responses to alcohol portrayals is associated with more favorable drinking expectancies, perceived greater social approval for drinking, beliefs that drinking is more common among peers and adults, and intention to drink more as adults.[24] Results from several experimental studies from the 1980s[25,26] suggest that exposure to drinking on screen (as scripted into television shows and movies) can influence children's beliefs about the appropriateness and normalization of drinking. For instance, a dual-controlled study of children exposed to a drinking scene on the hit television series *M.A.S.H.* demonstrated that exposed children had increased propensity to choose whiskey over water when asked immediately postexposure to offer a drink to an adult.[25] Experimental data from Atkin similarly indicates that adolescent exposure to alcohol advertising is associated with increased likelihood to drink, drink heavily, and drink in hazardous situations (e.g., while driving).[26]

Expanding on early experimental work, the question of whether exposure to alcohol advertising influences actual alcohol use among young people has been addressed through large prospective cohort studies and has recently been systematically reviewed.[27] Of 13 studies reviewed that controlled for potential confounders (e.g., age, ethnicity, and social influences), 12 have found evidence that exposure to alcohol-related ads predicts both the onset of drinking among nondrinkers and increased levels of consumption among existing drinkers. Jernigan et al. find that youth exposure to alcohol marketing is also associated with binge drinking and hazardous drinking (e.g., drinking and driving).[28] Alcohol advertisements perceived as favorable, memorable, and/or effective at engaging consumers with brand merchandise have also been shown to positively influence adolescents' intention to purchase the brand and products promoted.[29] Despite alcohol industry's calls to limit youth exposure to alcohol advertisements,[30] the industry has a documented record of directing ads to those under the minimum legal drinking age.[31] King et al. have shown, for example, that beer and liquor advertisements occur more frequently in magazines with higher adolescent readerships.[32] Additionally, alcohol advertisements on television are overrepresented during programs with high percentage of youth viewership.[33]

Beyond formal advertising from alcohol retailers, drinking behavior is commonly scripted into television shows and movies. Actors who drink on screen are often regular, relatable, and glamorous characters, of high socioeconomic status and/or physically attractive.[34] Likewise, negative consequences of alcohol use that would counter the notion that drinking is always a safe, virtuous, and/or common activity are seldom mentioned or portrayed.[20,35] As Wallack et al. from the Prevention Research Center at UC Berkeley notes, *"The sheer frequency of alcohol on television and the manner in which drinking is portrayed raise serious questions as to the role that television may play in the development and reinforcement of beliefs and behaviors regarding alcohol and its appropriate use."*[35]

Increasingly, there has been a shift toward online marketing of alcohol through SNSs as well as brand-specific Web sites. In 2011, alcohol brands were shown to have the third-highest consumer "engagement rate" on Facebook, after automobiles and retail.[36] McCreanor et al. identified 93 commercial pages with more than 1 million "friends" for top beer brands and 334 pages for top spirit brands with more than 3 million "friends" of Facebook.[37] The Facebook pages of Smirnoff and Victoria Bitter promote their brand by explicitly asking their followers to post comments about their drinking behavior.[38] Since 2012, there has been an explosion in user engagement with alcohol brands on SNSs (for an example, see Fig. 1 in Ref. 23).

Unlike traditional advertising, social media marketing relies on consumer interaction and dialog, making regulation a challenge. Given that children and adolescents are among the heaviest users of SNSs,[39] the potential impact of SNSs advertising on alcohol use attitudes and behaviors is significant. In an experimental study to assess this concern, Barry et al. developed and tracked a series of fictitious youth profiles on Instagram and Twitter over 1 month and found that all profiles (with reported ages 13–21 years) could fully access, view, and interact with alcohol industry content.[40] On Instagram, all profiles were allowed to follow alcohol brand pages and, within the 30-day study period, received an average 362 directed advertisement posts. While Twitter did block users younger than 21 from following alcohol brands, the two fictionalized 21-year-old profiles were allowed to follow brand pages and collectively received 1836 alcohol-related posted (or "tweets") within the study period.[40]

Peer-to-peer engagement with alcohol-related content via SNSs may involve sharing drinking events and experiences through posts, status updates, check-ins, likes, photos, and videos.[34] Studies have shown that sharing drinking events on SNSs functions to solidify friendships, create drinking cultures which are "airbrushed," and minimize the visibility of negative consequences.[41–43] In evaluating user-generated data on SNSs, studies have identified frequent depictions of risky drinking-related behaviors among youth (e.g., binge drinking, co-usage of other illicit substances, and drunken sexual encounters).[44–47] Alcohol-related displays may include texts (e.g., *"Matt got drunk last night"*), photographs depicting alcohol consumption, or links to alcohol-related groups or companies—all of which contribute to normalizing risky drinking behavior.[48–50] In a study of alcohol-related posts on Facebook, MySpace, and YouTube, 75% of youth reported that they had seen a picture posted by a friend of another friend drinking alcohol, 30% had a friend post a picture of them drinking, and 26% had self-posted a drinking photo.[49] On Twitter, Cavazos-Rehg et al. identified nearly 12 million drinking-related posts over a 1-month period of analysis (nearly 400,000 drinking-related posts per day).[42] As depicted in Fig. 6.1, a content analysis of these Tweets reflected a disproportionately positive sentiment toward alcohol use (i.e., normalizing and/or promoting drinking behaviors) peaking on weekends and when heavy drinking is popular (e.g., St Patrick's Day).[42]

The culture of intoxication fueled by SNSs reflects a serious public health challenge.[51] Studies have shown that users who display alcohol references on their SNS profile are more likely to demonstrate poor health literacy as well as engage in risky drinking behaviors.[13,16,52] As shown by Moreno and Whitehill, older adolescents whose Facebook posts suggested problem drinking behaviors were more likely to score as "at risk" on a problem-drinking screen.[13] Further, viewing normalized alcohol portrayals on SNSs has been associated with higher levels of risk-promoting cognitions (e.g., more willingness to drink, increased proalcohol use attitudes), as well as actual engagement in risky alcohol use and other drug use.[52,53]

TOBACCO

Tobacco use is the leading cause of preventable mortality in the United States. Recent data suggest that 40 million Americans still smoke, and each day approximately 2500 youth try their first cigarette.[54] Ninety percent of adult smokers begin smoking in their teens, or earlier; of these, two-thirds become regular, daily smokers before they reach the age of 19 years.[55] Exposure to smoking on traditional media, either formally via advertising or as depicted by Hollywood actors on screen, is directly associated with smoking initiation.[56-60] Although restrictions on tobacco marketing have been in place since the 1970s,[61] each year tobacco companies continue to allocate significant resources on protobacco advertising, such that nearly 8.5 billion dollars was spent on tobacco advertising and promotional materials in 2014 alone.[62] The rapidly evolving (and unregulated) sphere of new media (e.g., the Internet and SNS) have allowed for a resurgence of tobacco promotion, particularly targeting youth.[63] Through embedding powerful, positive messages online, and actively engaging with consumers, the tobacco industry can foil the decades-long public health campaign to denormalize smoking.[64]

Smoking is commonly portrayed on television and movies.[65-67] According to the 2016 Surgeon General's report, 47% of new PG-13-rated films depict smoking—a finding unchanged since 2010.[68] Smoking rates in movies and television are often exaggerated compared to actual smoking rates in the population.[69] According to content analysis by Glantz et al., smoking appeared in movies at a rate of 10.7 smoking incidents per hour of film time in the 1950s; this is similar to the rate observed in 2002, despite a near 50% reduction in the smoking rate among US adults in the 2000s versus the 1950s.[69] Studies have shown that portrayals of smoking on cinema and television influence youth perceptions about tobacco. For nonsmoking adolescents, exposure to tobacco in movies has potential for increasing positive emotions, excitement, and happiness and heightens the likelihood that they will associate smoking with status and vitality.[70] Actors smoking on

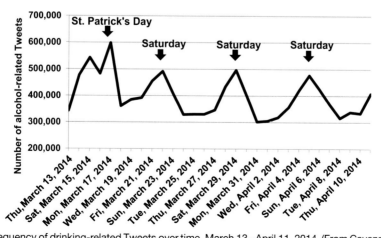

FIG. 6.1 Frequency of drinking-related Tweets over time, March 13–April 11, 2014. (From Cavazos-Rehg PA, Krauss MJ, Sowles SJ, Bierut LJ. "Hey everyone, I'm drunk." An evaluation of drinking-related Twitter chatter. *J Stud Alcohol Drugs.* 2015;76(4):635–643; with permission.)

screen may also convey sexuality (Sharon Stone in *Basic Instinct*), toughness (John Travolta in *Broken Arrow*), romance (Charlie Sheen in *The Chase*), and adolescent acts of rebellion (Leonardo DiCaprio in *Romeo + Juliet*), as well as a way to relieve stress (Winona Ryder in *Girl Interrupted*).[71] A number of studies have examined the relationship between smoking in movies and television, and adolescent smoking initiation, controlling for sociodemographic factors (gender and ethnicity),[72] personality characteristics (sensation-seeking), direct tobacco marketing (ad receptivity),[73] peer influence (exposure to friends who smoke),[70] and parenting.[74] According to a National Cancer Institute report, *"The total weight of evidence from cross-sectional, longitudinal, and experimental studies indicates a causal relationship between exposure to depictions of smoking in movies and youth smoking initiation."*[75]

Despite the 1998 Master Settlement Agreement's prohibition of youth-targeted tobacco advertisement,[32] there is continued evidence of online promotional activities initiated by tobacco companies.[76] Tobacco companies are able to directly advertise online and may interact with SNS users through brand-specific fan pages.[77] Tobacco brands, including Winston, Black Devil, Camel, and British American Tobacco, have been implicated in directly marketing to youth by providing links to Web-based cigarette shops on their fan pages.[78] According to a 2015 Facebook content analysis, 43 unique cigarette brand-specific pages were identified with a cumulative total of 1,189,976 page likes and 19,022 posts.[79] Fan pages often included images of fashionable, confident young men and women smoking, thereby promoting the view that smoking is normative among a young and educated group that contrasts with current smoking demographics (e.g., obtained high school education or less and living in poverty).[80] In an analysis of 163 popular YouTube videos retrieved from a search of the top five non-Chinese tobacco brands, a majority (71.2%) of the content was classified as being "protobacco," with at least 20 of the videos appearing to be industry driven.[81] Further, Cavazos-Rehg et al. found that 11% of underage adolescents who took part in the 2012 National Youth Tobacco Survey reported having received direct promotions from tobacco companies through SNSs on at least one occasion during the 30 days prior to taking the survey.[63] Of particular concern was that tobacco ads/promotions exposure via SNSs occurred among highly susceptible youth (i.e., minorities, very young youth, and youth who have not yet used tobacco) and was associated with a number of favorable attitudes toward tobacco (Table 6.1).[63]

A major challenge for tobacco control has been the rise of noncigarette tobacco products (fruit- and candy-flavored cigars, small cigars, waterpipe, and electronic nicotine delivery systems [ENDSs]),[82–85] in large part due to unrestricted promotion on traditional and new media.[86–88] ENDSs, or e-cigarettes, have amassed the largest following and mimic the sensation of smoking by delivering nicotine to users in the form of a vapor—an activity known as vaping.[89] The proportion of US adults who have ever used e-cigarettes increased rapidly from 1.8% in 2010 to 10.0% in 2013, with use rates highest among young adults and current cigarette smokers.[90] E-cigarettes are marketed via television,[91] print advertisements (that often feature celebrities),[92] and new media[93] as healthier alternatives to tobacco smoking, as useful for quitting smoking and reducing cigarette consumption, and as a way to circumvent smoke-free laws by enabling users to "smoke anywhere."[94] In the US, youth exposed to television e-cigarette advertisements increased by 256% from 2011 to 2013.[95] Facebook pages for e-cigarette brands include pictures of consumers posing with e-cigarettes with captions such as *"MAX-imum style"* and articles on *"10 ways to look cooler while vaping an e-cigarette".*[96]

Vapor stores, stores selling e-cigarette devices and liquids, also have a strong presence on the Internet and social media and are particularly popular with younger audiences. E-Cigarette Forum, marketed as *"the world's largest vape and e-cig website,"*[97] is sponsored by 81 e-cigarette companies, has over 600,000 active discussion pages, with nearly 18 million messages, and a current membership of more than 250,000. Posts on the Web site include product reviews discussing topics such as durability, battery life, thickness of vapor, device instructions, flavor, and evaluation criteria for good e-cigarettes. Promotional videos and images, directly from e-cigarette companies, can be found on SNSs such as YouTube[98] and Instagram.[99] Huang et al. have also identified a strong commercial presence on Twitter. Ninety percent of e-cigarette tweets from May to June 2012 were advertising related, with the majority including URLs for the direct promotion or sale of e-cigarettes.[94] Although existing scientific evidence has shown that e-cigarettes are less harmful than combustible cigarettes,[100] they still contain carcinogens and toxicants, and are regulated by the US Food and Drug Administration under the same remit as other tobacco products.[101] Further, e-cigarettes have not been approved as cessation devices.[101] Deceptive marketing may instill false reassurance that e-cigarettes are safe via advertising the absence of "tar" or "carcinogens" or

TABLE 6.1
Associations Between Exposure to New Media Tobacco Ads/Promotions and Tobacco Attitudes/Beliefs

Among Youth Who *Never* Used Tobacco

	Smokers Have More Friends aOR, 95% CI	Smoking Makes Young People Look Cool/Fit In aOR, 95% CI	Tobacco Products Are Dangerous aOR, 95% CI	Secondhand Smoke Is Harmful aOR, 95% CI	Would Smoke if a Friend Offered a Cigarette aOR, 95% CI[a]
TOBACCO ADS VIA…					
Text message	1.3, 0.95–1.7	1.6, 0.9–2.7	0.7, 0.5–0.95	0.4, 0.2–0.6	3.0, 1.4–6.4
Facebook/MySpace	1.3, 1.03–1.6	1.6, 1.1–2.2	0.8, 0.6–0.9	0.4, 0.3–0.7	1.9, 1.2–3.0

Among Youth Who *Ever* Used Tobacco

	Smokers Have More Friends aOR, 95% CI	Smoking Makes Young People Look Cool/Fit It aOR, 95% CI	Tobacco Products Are Dangerous aOR, 95% CI	Secondhand Smoke Is Harmful aOR, 95% CI	Intent to Quit aOR, 95% CI[a]
TOBACCO ADS VIA…					
Text message	1.9, 1.4–2.5	2.0, 1.5–2.9	0.8, 0.6–1.0	0.4, 0.3–0.6	0.7, 0.4–1.2
Facebook/MySpace	1.8, 1.5–2.2	1.8, 1.3–2.5	0.9, 0.7–1.1	0.5, 0.4–0.7	0.7, 0.5–1.1

Multivariable models control for demographic covariates. *aOR*, adjusted odds ratio; *CI*, confidence interval.
[a] Among current smokers only (N = 1178).

including pictorial and video representations of doctors.[102] Flavor has been broadly used, both in online-based advertisements[103] and offline store promotions,[104] to increase the appeal of e-cigarette products among youth. Exposure to e-cigarette advertisements has been associated with intention to use and actual use of e-cigarettes among adolescents.[91,105,106]

User-generated protobacco content has been observed on a plethora of SNSs such as YouTube,[107] Instagram,[88] Twitter,[108] and Facebook.[7] Content may include product reviews, informational how-to, videos, or sharing of personal experiences. On Twitter, posts about tobacco products frequently convey positive sentiments, with many users sharing information, personal opinion, and first-person use or intent. Positive content may further reflect a sense of invincibility and defiance, as exemplified by the following tweets: *"Smoking that good hookah with the bro Sultan! #GoodOld-Days #brotherforlife"* and, *"Beer ponggg/hookah round 2 with my goons waddduppppppp. I love when my parents rnt home!"*[86] It is less common for users to portray negative consequences of use.[3] Adolescents may even display images of "vape tricks" (e.g., blowing smoke ring) in an effort to appear "cool."[107,109] Smoking fetish imagery has also been observed—particularly on YouTube[110]—whereby tobacco content is associated with seduction and/or explicit sexual themes. In a large, representative sample of adolescents from Texas, authors report high level of engagement with both non-cigarette and combustible tobacco with girls, high school students, high sensation seekers, and students with friends who use tobacco, most likely to report writing, responding to, or re-blogging tobacco-related posts.[111] Over time, exposure to social media depictions of tobacco use have been shown to predict future smoking tendencies.[14]

MARIJUANA

Use of marijuana—a category I controlled substance per the US Controlled Substance Act—is common among youth.[112] In the US, more than half of adolescents will experiment with marijuana and, of those who try it more than once, approximately one-third will subsequently become regular users.[113] Chronic daily marijuana use in adolescence is associated with impaired educational attainment,[114] onset of primary psychiatric disorders (e.g., depression, mania, psychosis),[115] and use of other illicit substances (e.g., heroin and cocaine).[116] Lenient policies promoting increased accessibility, however, reflect the general public's

perception that cannabis use is not harmful. Although marijuana remains illegal under federal law per the Controlled Substances Act, in 2009, the Department of Justice advised US attorneys to not prosecute legitimate growers and distributors of medical marijuana where allowed by state law.[117] As of November 2016, recreational marijuana use is legal in eight states and the District of Columbia, and medical use is legal in numerous other states. The legal marijuana industry is one the fastest growing industries in the United States, expanding from $2.7 billion in wholesale and retail sales in 2014 to $6.9 billion in 2016.[118,119]

Mirroring legal shifts toward legalizing marijuana for recreational use, cultural shifts normalizing marijuana use have led to an increase in marijuana portrayals in Hollywood movies and television over recent years. Of all illicit drug use depicted on traditional media, marijuana is most frequently observed.[120] From the iconic cable television show *Weeds*, in which a widowed suburban housewife resorts to selling marijuana to provide for her family,[121] to movies such as *Harold and Kumar Go To White Castle* and *The Pineapple Express*, marijuana use on screen often projects levity, relaxation, excitement, and confidence. Negative consequences associated with marijuana use are frequently not portrayed.[3] Although there has been scientific conjecture that normalizing marijuana use on screen is associated with actual use among adolescents, at this time, research into this topic is scant.[122]

Young people may be exposed to direct marijuana advertising in states where recreational and medical marijuana are legal. Just as exposure to alcohol and tobacco advertising can shift attitudes toward normalization of use and increase likelihood of use, there is also emerging evidence demonstrating similar risks following exposure to marijuana advertising.[123,124] For example, a study of children in Southern California found that 30% of middle-school-age participants had seen a medical marijuana advertisement in the past 3 months (either in billboards, magazines, or via other sources), and there was a reciprocal cross-lagged association between this exposure and marijuana use or intentions to use in the future.[124] Cerdá et al. used longitudinal survey data from Monitoring the Future to examine changes in the perceived risks of occasional marijuana use and self-reported marijuana use among high school students in Colorado and Washington before and after legalization, comparing results to matched controls from other US states where marijuana is not legal.[123] They found an overall decrease in perceived risks of using marijuana in all states; however, the authors identified a larger decline in perceived risks and a larger increase in reported marijuana use among the 8th and 10th graders from Washington compared with Colorado or other states where marijuana is not legal. In light of increased accessibility and known risks of marijuana use among youth, there is increasing recognition that advertising regulations are needed.[125]

Many states explicitly prohibit the direct targeting of marijuana advertisements to children (Colorado Department of Revenue, 2013; New York State Department of Health, 2014; Washington State Legislature, 2013).[126,127] Illinois and Washington, for example, ban billboards within 1000 ft of schools/playgrounds. Connecticut, Massachusetts, New York, and Washington ban advertisements containing portrayals of underage use. Colorado and Washington ban the use of cartoon characters, and Colorado bans advertising on print, radio, and television when more than 30% of the audience is expected to be under the legal age. Montana has attempted to limit advertising on electronic media, albeit with enforcement limited to individuals with licenses and valid registry identification cards. There are, notably, several states with no advertising regulations in place (e.g., Arizona, Michigan, Minnesota, New Mexico, Rhode Island, Vermont).[128]

The legal marijuana industry increasingly utilizes the Internet to advertise dispensaries and products to the public.[129] Indeed, there are several marijuana-related online communities that have grown in popularity in recent years. Founded in 2013, MassRoots is a large network for marijuana users and sellers, allowing users and companies to create profiles, follow trending news, share images and other media, and advertise.[130] Weedmaps is another popular online directory of marijuana dispensaries, utilizing both Web site and app-based interfaces to attract users and promoting marijuana products by making various unsubstantiated health claims.[131] Research examining how youth may be impacted by exposure to marijuana-related content is in its infancy. Recent studies suggest that children and adolescents can not only engage with marijuana-related content online but also are able to procure marijuana products given that many online dispensaries lack age-verification restrictions and have easy mechanisms for online ordering and home delivery.[131,132]

SNSs have been recognized as a powerful modality for attracting marijuana consumers and promoting marijuana-related content.[132] Although SNSs have policies in place prohibiting direct advertising of marijuana,[8] there is still the potential for indirect advertising as well as dissemination of uncurated pro-marijuana content by users. On Twitter, for instance, Cavazos-Rehg et al. identified the popular profile "@stillblazingtho" with over 1 million followers, whereby approximately 82% of tweets associated with this account express positive sentiments toward the use of cannabis.[133] Using social analytic algorithms, the majority of account followers (73%) were found to be younger than 20 years, suggesting that younger users may be disproportionately exposed to marijuana-related content on SNSs. A separate Twitter content analysis identified a disproportionately high percentage of marijuana-related content posted by African-American users compared to other ethnicities.[134] On Instagram, a mobile-based photo- and video-sharing application, content analysis of 417,561 posts with marijuana-related hashtags found that advertisements sourced directly from dispensaries were present in 9% of the posts' images.[135] Further, alternative forms of marijuana were commonly portrayed, from marijuana concentrates to ingestibles or dabbing (Fig. 6.2).[135] On YouTube, videos about dabbing marijuana concentrates and marijuana edibles most commonly included instructional messages, product reviews, and demonstrations.[136–138] According to recent content analysis, YouTube videos referencing marijuana edibles were frequently encountered by adolescent users, with median view count similar to YouTube videos about alcohol intoxication and e-cigarettes.[7,137,139]

Exposure to pro-marijuana content on SNSs may influence use of marijuana and potentially normalize the use of high-potency marijuana products (i.e., marijuana "dabs" that contains up to 90% tetrahydrocannabinol). A recent content analysis of dabbing-related posts on Twitter identified multiple references to high-risk behaviors, including successive dabbing sessions, use of excessive amounts (e.g., using "fat" dabs, dabs ≥ 1 g), co-ingestion (e.g., use of dabs with other substances), and intense dabbing-related outcomes (e.g., passing out and feeling a loss of body control).[108] It is possible that exposure to this content may increase interest among individuals who have not yet initiated this behavior but use SNSs to learn more about expectancies following dabbing. Accordingly, a pilot study examining different types of exposure to marijuana content on Twitter found that both active exposure (e.g., following pro-substance Twitter feeds and/or generating one's own pro-substance content) and passive exposure (e.g., viewing peers' pro-substance content) to pro-marijuana content were positively associated with the likelihood of current marijuana use.[11]

Method of ingestion	n (%, 95% CI)	Example posts
Joints or blunts	283 (50%, 46%–54%)	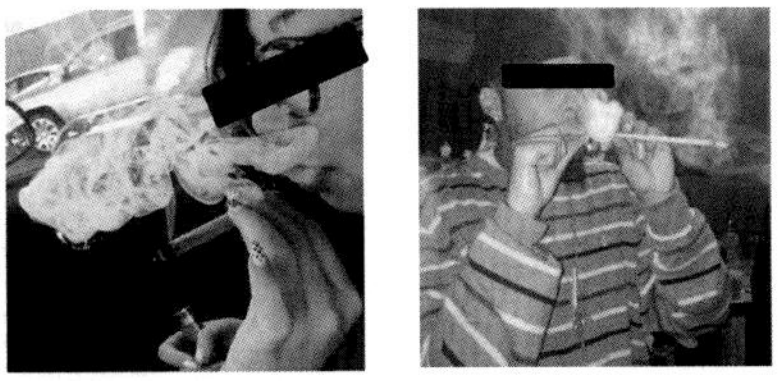
Bong or rig	263 (46%, 42%–50%)	
Marijuana concentrates (dabbing using rig)	113 (43%, 37%–49%)	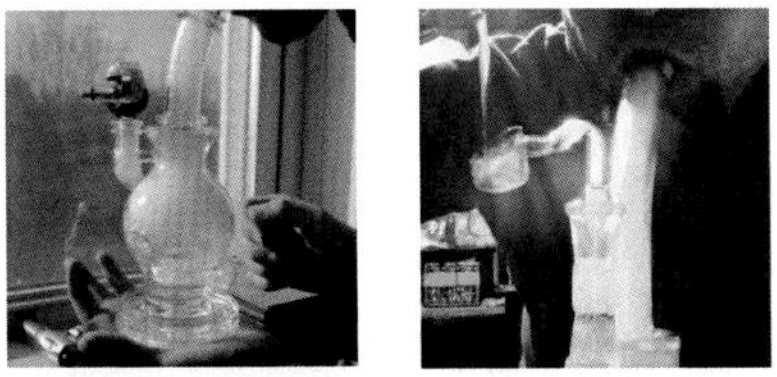
Plant-based marijuana (traditional bongs/pipes)	76 (29%, 23%–35%)	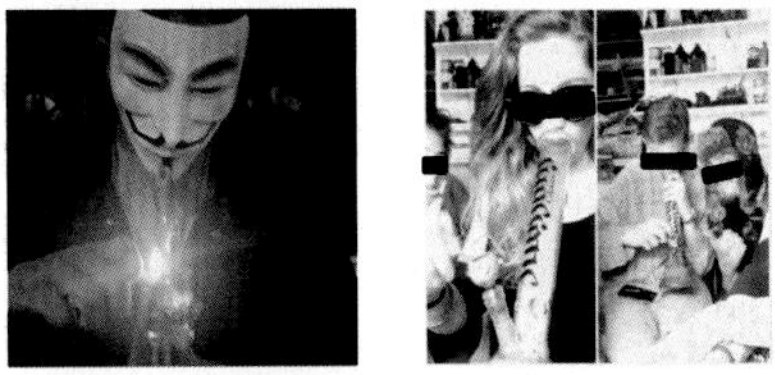
Vape pen (marijuana concentrates)	20 (4%, 2%–6%)	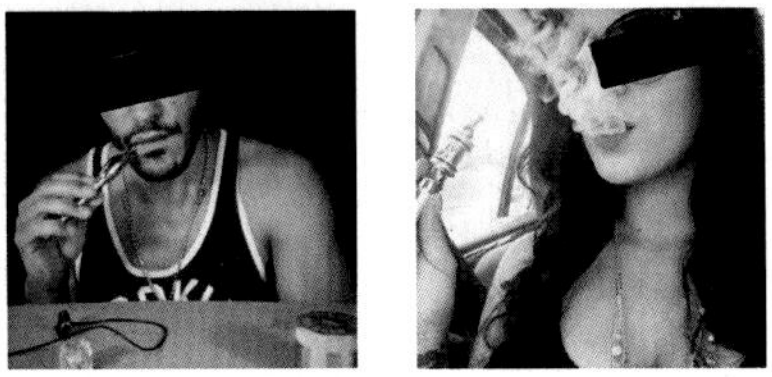

FIG. 6.2 Instagram posts portraying a person using marijuana (N = 568/2136, 27% 95% confidence interval [CI] 25%–29%). (Data from Cavazos-Rehg PA, Krauss MJ, Sowles SJ, Bierut LJ. Marijuana-related posts on Instagram. *Prev Sci.* 2016;17(6):710–720.)

OTHER SUBSTANCES

While less common than alcohol, tobacco, and marijuana, discussions about the nonmedical use of prescription medications (NUPMs) can be easily found on SNSs and mirror the concerning misuse patterns among young people. Per the Centers for Disease Control and Prevention, 20.7% of high school students reported having engaged in NUPM (OxyContin, Percocet, Vicodin, Adderall, Ritalin, or Xanax) in 2011.[140] In 2014, more than 1700 young adults died from prescription (mostly opioid) overdoses.[141] Prescription opiates can be a gateway drug for some individuals as multiple studies demonstrate that those who abuse opiate medications are at higher risk for initiation of heroin use, in part because it is cheaper and/or easier to obtain than opiates.[142,143] Evaluating a cross-section of publicly available tweets pertaining to prescription opiates, Chan et al. find that the majority of messages of a personal nature contained references to aberrant opioid behaviors. For example, of the 125 personal messages retrieved, 70% contained themes of opioid prescription misuse, and 21% explicitly mentioned using opioids to obtain a "high."[144]

Abuse of Adderall, a prescription stimulant, is also commonly portrayed on Twitter, particularly among college students.[145–150] Analyses have shown that Adderall is frequently used as a college study aid, with activity peak during college exam periods, and a clear pattern of multisubstance use is apparent in many tweets.[145] There is also concern about co-ingestion, as members of the social networks of prescription drug abusers on Twitter typically also post about abusing multiple prescription drugs.[151] Tweets extracted by

Hanson et al. include contemporary keywords which identify risk behaviors (e.g., pop, crush, steal, inhale, and mimosa).[150] Tweets also conveyed evidence of medication abuse via intoxication: "*Adderall + Benadryl has put me in a weird awake/tired haze. Relatively certain that I'm saying things i wont [sic] remember in the morning,*"[150] and seeking statements: "*Seriously. Need adderall. Will pay $$$. Help me.*" and "*looking to buy ~20–40 mg adderall, email ***".*[150]

FUTURE DIRECTIONS

Methodological surveillance of SNSs has become an important research tool to identify health trends. Compared to traditional epidemiologic methods (e.g., population health surveys, cohort studies, registries), real-time data collection through the Internet and SNS allows for swifter health data consolidation and analysis. New fields of study such as "infodemiology" and "infoveillance" have emerged and represent "the science of distribution and determinants of information in an electronic medium, specifically the Internet, or in a population, with the ultimate aim to inform public health and public policy."[152] For health topics fraught with stigma, such as illicit substance use, analysis of publically available data on social media allows for study of free-living interactions and activities without the inherent limitations of an experimental protocol. Evolving information and communication patterns on the Internet can be harbingers of change on a population health level.

As adolescents increasingly turn to social media for health information, therein lies an important opportunity for the healthcare community to engage adolescents regarding their health outside of the traditional office setting. The National Institutes of Health Collaborative Research consortium with National Institute on Drug Abuse has recently appropriated funding to support research utilizing social media to advance the scientific understanding, prevention, and treatment of substance use and addiction.[153] Promising engagement programs such as Above the Influence have amassed a large following on social media (with over 1.4 million "friends" on Facebook vs. 155 "friends" for the average Facebook user[154]), promoting narratives related to the marijuana abstinence.[155] Relatively little has been published demonstrating the effectiveness of social media-based prevention tools. A new program, Living the Example (LTE), uses social media-based branding efforts to reframe youth perceptions about substance use; according to a recent pilot study, participants found the LTE program to be engaging and convincing and generally "liked" the posts. Further,

positive receptivity to LTE messages was associated with evidence of reduced self-reported drug use intentions, specifically for marijuana, use of sedatives/sleeping pills, and reports of intent to use any drug.[156]

CONCLUSION

The rapidly evolving media landscape raises concerns for the health and well-being of children and adolescents. As Web-based applications and SNSs expand, so too has the scope of drug and alcohol exposure. Once limited to advertising and scripted exposure on television and movies, youth exposure to illicit substance is now as easy as opening Facebook or Twitter on any Internet-connected device. The significant extent to which illicit substances are portrayed on social media has promoted the concept of "intoxigenic" digital spaces.[157] Substances abuse may be portrayed on SNSs via pictures, videos, or text, leading to the normalization of high-risk behavior. As we have demonstrated, adolescents who view tobacco-, alcohol-, or marijuana-related posts by members of one's peer group are at increased risk for actual substance use. New and creative approaches will be important to mitigate the risk of adolescent engagement with such content on social media.

FUNDING SOURCE

This study was funded by the National Institutes of Health (grant numbers R01DA039455 and K02DA043657 [PAC-R]).

REFERENCES

1. *Social Media Fact Sheet*. Pew Research Center: Internet, Science & Tech; 2017. http://www.pewinternet.org/fact-sheet/social-media/.
2. Inman DD, van Bakergem KM, Larosa AC, Garr DR. Evidence-based health promotion programs for schools and communities. *Am J Prev Med*. 2011;40(2):207–219.
3. Strasburger VC, American Academy of Pediatrics, Council on Communications and Media. Policy statement—children, adolescents, substance abuse, and the media. *Pediatrics*. 2010;126(4):791–799.
4. Long JA, O'Connor PG, Gerbner G, Concato J. Use of alcohol, illicit drugs, and tobacco among characters on prime-time television. *Subst Abus*. 2002;23(2):95–103.
5. Dal Cin S, Worth KA, Dalton MA, Sargent JD. Youth exposure to alcohol use and brand appearances in popular contemporary movies. *Addiction*. 2008;103(12): 1925–1932.
6. Dal Cin S, Stoolmiller M, Sargent JD. When movies matter: exposure to smoking in movies and changes in smoking behavior. *J Health Commun*. 2012;17(1):76–89.

7. Morgan EM, Snelson C, Elison-Bowers P. Image and video disclosure of substance use on social media websites. *Comput Hum Behav.* 2010;26(6):1405−1411.

8. *Advertising Policies.* https://www.facebook.com/policies/ads/.

9. *Drugs and Drug Paraphernalia.* Twitter Help Center. https://support.twitter.com/articles/20170437.

10. Mart S, Mergendoller J, Simon M. Alcohol promotion on Facebook. *J Glob Drug Policy Pract.* 2009;3(3):1−8.

11. Cabrera-Nguyen EP, Cavazos-Rehg P, Krauss M, Bierut LJ, Moreno MA. Young adults' exposure to alcohol- and marijuana-related content on Twitter. *J Stud Alcohol Drugs.* 2016;77(2):349−353.

12. Beullens K, Schepers A. Display of alcohol use on Facebook: a content analysis. *Cyberpsychol Behav Soc Netw.* 2013;16(7):497−503.

13. Moreno MA, Whitehill JM. Influence of social media on alcohol use in adolescents and young adults. *Alcohol Res.* 2014;36(1):91−100.

14. Depue JB, Southwell BG, Betzner AE, Walsh BM. Encoded exposure to tobacco use in social media predicts subsequent smoking behavior. *Am J Health Promot.* 2015;29(4):259−261.

15. Thompson KM. Addicted media: substances on screen. *Child Adolesc Psychiatr Clin N Am.* 2005;14(3):473−489, ix.

16. *Results from the 2013 National Survey on Drug Use and Health: Summary of National Findings.* https://www.samhsa.gov/data/sites/default/files/NSDUHresultsPDFWHTML2013/Web/NSDUHresults2013.pdf.

17. Fishman M, Bruner A, Adger Jr H. Substance abuse among children and adolescents. *Pediatr Rev.* 1997;18(11):394−403.

18. Hingson RW, Zha W, Weitzman ER. Magnitude of and trends in alcohol-related mortality and morbidity among U.S. college students ages 18−24, 1998−2005. *J Stud Alcohol Drugs Suppl.* 2009;(16):12−20.

19. Dadich AM, Burton SM, Soboleva A. Promotion of alcohol on Twitter. *Med J Aust.* 2013;199(5):327−329.

20. Van Den Bulck H, Simons N, Gorp BV. Let's drink and be merry: the framing of alcohol in the prime-time American youth series The OC. *J Stud Alcohol Drugs.* 2008;69(6):933−940.

21. *Youth Exposure to Alcohol Advertising on Television, 2001−2008.* Baltimore, MD: Center on Alcohol Marketing and Youth; 2010. http://www.camy.org/_docs/resources/reports/youth-exposure-alcohol-advertising-magazine-01-08-full-report.pdf.

22. Alcohol marketing in popular movies doubles in past two decades: highest increase in alcohol brand placements found in movies rated for children. *ScienceDaily.* https://www.sciencedaily.com/releases/2017/05/170504083144.htm.

23. Jernigan DH, Rushman AE. Measuring youth exposure to alcohol marketing on social networking sites: challenges and prospects. *J Public Health Policy.* 2014;35(1):91−104.

24. Grube JW, Waiters E. Alcohol in the media: content and effects on drinking beliefs and behaviors among youth. *Adolesc Med Clin.* 2005;16(2):327−343, viii.

25. Rychtarik RG, Fairbank JA, Allen CM, Foy DW, Drabman RS. Alcohol use in television programming: effects on children's behavior. *Addict Behav.* 1983;8(1):19−22.

26. Atkin CK. Effects of televised alcohol messages on teenage drinking patterns. *J Adolesc Health Care.* 1990;11(1):10−24.

27. Smith LA, Foxcroft DR. The effect of alcohol advertising, marketing and portrayal on drinking behaviour in young people: systematic review of prospective cohort studies. *BMC Public Health.* 2009;9:51.

28. Jernigan D, Noel J, Landon J, Thornton N, Lobstein T. Alcohol marketing and youth alcohol consumption: a systematic review of longitudinal studies published since 2008. *Addiction.* 2017;112(suppl 1):7−20.

29. Chen M-J, Grube JW, Bersamin M, Waiters E, Keefe DB. Alcohol advertising: what makes it attractive to youth? *J Health Commun.* 2005;10(6):553−565.

30. *Self-regulation in the Alcohol Industry: A Federal Trade Commission Report to Congress.* Federal Trade Commission; 1999. https://www.ftc.gov/reports/self-regulation-alcohol-industry-federal-trade-commission-report-congress.

31. Garfield CF, Chung PJ, Rathouz PJ. Alcohol advertising in magazines and adolescent readership. *JAMA.* 2003;289(18):2424−2429.

32. King 3rd C, Siegel M, Jernigan DH, et al. Adolescent exposure to alcohol advertising in magazines: an evaluation of advertising placement in relation to underage youth readership. *J Adolesc Health.* 2009;45(6):626−633.

33. Centers for Disease Control and Prevention (CDC). Youth exposure to alcohol advertising on television−25 markets, United States, 2010. *Morb Mortal Wkly Rep.* 2013;62(44):877−880.

34. Moewaka Barnes H, McCreanor T, Goodwin I, Lyons A, Griffin C, Hutton F. Alcohol and social media: drinking and drunkenness while online. *Crit Public Health.* 2016;26(1):62−76.

35. Wallack L, Grube JW, Madden PA, Breed W. Portrayals of alcohol on prime-time television. *J Stud Alcohol.* 1990;51(5):428−437.

36. Socialbakers. *What Brand Categories Lead Marketing on Facebook.* Socialbakers.com. https://www.socialbakers.com/blog/266-what-brand-categories-lead-marketing-on-facebook/.

37. McCreanor T, Lyons A, Griffin C, Goodwin I, Moewaka Barnes H, Hutton F. Youth drinking cultures, social networking and alcohol marketing: implications for public health. *Crit Public Health.* 2013;23(1):110−120.

38. Brodmerkel S, Carah N. Alcohol brands on Facebook: the challenges of regulating brands on social media. *J Public Aff.* 2013;13(3):272−281.

39. Lenhart A, Madden M. *Social Networking Websites and Teens.* Pew Research Center: Internet, Science & Tech; 2007. http://www.pewinternet.org/2007/01/07/social-networking-websites-and-teens/.

40. Barry AE, Bates AM, Olusanya O, et al. Alcohol marketing on twitter and Instagram: evidence of directly advertising to youth/adolescents. *Alcohol Alcohol.* 2016;51(4):487−492.

41. Niland P, Lyons AC, Goodwin I, Hutton F. "Everyone can loosen up and get a bit of a buzz on": young adults, alcohol and friendship practices. *Int J Drug Policy.* 2013;24(6):530−537.

42. Cavazos-Rehg PA, Krauss MJ, Sowles SJ, Bierut LJ. "Hey everyone, I'm drunk." An evaluation of drinking-related Twitter chatter. *J Stud Alcohol Drugs.* 2015;76(4):635−643.

43. Niland P, Lyons AC, Goodwin I, Hutton F. "See it doesn't look pretty does it?" Young adults' airbrushed drinking practices on Facebook. *Psychol Health*; 2014. http://www.tandfonline.com/doi/abs/10.1080/08870446.2014.893345.

44. Hinduja S, Patchin JW. Personal information of adolescents on the Internet: a quantitative content analysis of MySpace. *J Adolesc.* 2008;31(1):125−146.

45. McGee JB, Begg M. What medical educators need to know about "Web 2.0". *Med Teach.* 2008;30(2):164−169.

46. Moreno MA, Parks M, Richardson LP. What are adolescents showing the world about their health risk behaviors on MySpace? *MedGenMed.* 2007;9(4):9.

47. Moreno MA, Parks MR, Zimmerman FJ, Brito TE, Christakis DA. Display of health risk behaviors on MySpace by adolescents: prevalence and associations. *Arch Pediatr Adolesc Med.* 2009;163(1):27−34.

48. Egan KG, Moreno MA. Alcohol references on undergraduate males' Facebook profiles. *Am J Mens Health.* 2011;5(5):413−420.

49. Moreno MA, Briner LR, Williams A, Brockman L, Walker L, Christakis DA. A content analysis of displayed alcohol references on a social networking web site. *J Adolesc Health.* 2010;47(2):168−175.

50. Westgate EC, Neighbors C, Heppner H, Jahn S, Lindgren KP. "I will take a shot for every 'like' I get on this status": posting alcohol-related Facebook content is linked to drinking outcomes. *J Stud Alcohol Drugs.* 2014;75(3):390−398.

51. Ridout B, Campbell A, Ellis L. "Off your Face(book)": alcohol in online social identity construction and its relation to problem drinking in university students. *Drug Alcohol Rev.* 2012;31(1):20−26.

52. Litt DM, Stock ML. Adolescent alcohol-related risk cognitions: the roles of social norms and social networking sites. *Psychol Addict Behav.* 2011;25(4):708−713.

53. Huang GC, Unger JB, Soto D, et al. Peer influences: the impact of online and offline friendship networks on adolescent smoking and alcohol use. *J Adolesc Health.* 2014;54(5):508−514.

54. Jamal A, Gentzke A, Hu SS, et al. Tobacco use among middle and high school students − United States, 2011−2016. *Morb Mortal Wkly Rep.* 2017;66(23):597−603.

55. Bonnie RJ, Stratton K, Kwan LY, Committee on the Public Health Implications of Raising the Minimum Age for Purchasing Tobacco Products, Board on Population Health and Public Health Practice, Institute of Medicine. *Patterns of Tobacco Use by Adolescents and Young Adults.* US: National Academies Press; 2015.

56. Centers for Disease Control and Prevention (CDC). Cigarette smoking among adults−United States, 2004. *Morb Mortal Wkly Rep.* 2005;54(44):1121−1124.

57. DiFranza JR, Wellman RJ, Sargent JD, et al. Tobacco promotion and the initiation of tobacco use: assessing the evidence for causality. *Pediatrics.* 2006;117(6):e1237−e1248.

58. Wellman RJ, Sugarman DB, DiFranza JR, Winickoff JP. The extent to which tobacco marketing and tobacco use in films contribute to children's use of tobacco: a meta-analysis. *Arch Pediatr Adolesc Med.* 2006;160(12):1285−1296.

59. Wakefield M, Flay B, Nichter M, Giovino G. Role of the media in influencing trajectories of youth smoking. *Addiction.* 2003;98(suppl 1):79−103.

60. Sargent JD. Smoking in movies: impact on adolescent smoking. *Adolesc Med Clin.* 2005;16(2):345−370, ix.

61. Jacobson PD, Wasserman J, Anderson JR. Historical overview of tobacco legislation and regulation. *J Soc Issues.* 1997;53(1):75−95.

62. *Federal Trade Commission Cigarette Report for 2014 and Federal Trade Commission Smokeless Tobacco Report for 2014.* Federal Trade Commission; 2016. https://www.ftc.gov/reports/federal-trade-commission-cigarette-report-2014-federal-trade-commission-smokeless-tobacco.

63. Cavazos-Rehg PA, Krauss MJ, Spitznagel EL, Grucza RA, Bierut LJ. Hazards of new media: youth's exposure to tobacco ads/promotions. *Nicotine Tob Res.* 2014;16(4):437−444.

64. Fairchild AL, Bayer R, Colgrove J. The renormalization of smoking? E-cigarettes and the tobacco "endgame". *N Engl J Med.* 2013;370(4):293−295.

65. Worth KA, Cin SD, Sargent JD. Prevalence of smoking among major movie characters: 1996−2004. *Tob Control.* 2006;15(6):442−446.

66. Jamieson PE, Romer D. Portrayal of tobacco use in prime-time TV dramas: trends and associations with adult cigarette consumption−USA, 1955−2010. *Tob Control.* 2015;24(3):243−248.

67. Jamieson PE, Romer D. Trends in US movie tobacco portrayal since 1950: a historical analysis. *Tob Control.* 2010;19(3):179−184.

68. Smoking CO on Health. *Smoking and Tobacco Use; Fact Sheet; Smoking in the Movies*; July 2017. http://www.cdc.gov/tobacco/data_statistics/fact_sheets/youth_data/movies/.

69. Glantz SA, Kacirk KW, McCulloch C. Back to the future: smoking in movies in 2002 compared with 1950 levels. *Am J Public Health.* 2004;94(2):261−263.

70. Song AV, Ling PM, Neilands TB, Glantz SA. Smoking in movies and increased smoking among young adults. *Am J Prev Med.* 2007;33(5):396–403.

71. Sargent JD, Beach ML, Dalton MA, et al. Effect of seeing tobacco use in films on trying smoking among adolescents: cross sectional study. *BMJ.* 2001;323(7326):1394–1397.

72. Sargent JD, Dalton MA, Beach ML, et al. Viewing tobacco use in movies: does it shape attitudes that mediate adolescent smoking? *Am J Prev Med.* 2002;22(3):137–145.

73. Morgenstern M, Sargent JD, Engels RCME, et al. Smoking in movies and adolescent smoking initiation: longitudinal study in six European countries. *Am J Prev Med.* 2013;44(4):339–344.

74. Charlesworth A, Glantz SA. Smoking in the movies increases adolescent smoking: a review. *Pediatrics.* 2005;116(6):1516–1528.

75. Davis RM, Gilpin EA, Loken B, Viswanath K, Wakefield MA. *The Role of the Media in Promoting and Reducing Tobacco Use*; 2008. http://www.tobaccocontrol.org.pk/Resources/books/The%20Role%20of%20the%20Media%20on%20Promoting%20and%20Reducing%20Tobacco%20Use.pdf.

76. Freeman B, Chapman S. Is "YouTube" telling or selling you something? Tobacco content on the YouTube video-sharing website. *Tob Control.* 2007;16(3):207–210.

77. Liang Y, Zheng X, Zeng DD, Zhou X, Leischow SJ, Chung W. Exploring how the tobacco industry presents and promotes itself in social media. *J Med Internet Res.* 2015;17(1):e24.

78. Freeman B. New media and tobacco control. *Tob Control.* 2012;21(2):139–144.

79. Richardson A, Ganz O, Vallone D. Tobacco on the web: surveillance and characterisation of online tobacco and e-cigarette advertising. *Tob Control.* 2015;24(4):341–347.

80. Centers for Disease Control and Prevention. *Smoking and Tobacco Use; Fact Sheet; Adult Cigarette Smoking in the United States.* http://www.cdc.gov/tobacco/data_statistics/fact_sheets/adult_data/cig_smoking/.

81. Elkin L, Thomson G, Wilson N. Connecting world youth with tobacco brands: YouTube and the internet policy vacuum on Web 2.0. *Tob Control.* 2010;19(5):361–366.

82. Regan AK, Promoff G, Dube SR, Arrazola R. Electronic nicotine delivery systems: adult use and awareness of the "e-cigarette" in the USA. *Tob Control.* 2011. https://doi.org/10.1136/tobaccocontrol-2011-050044.

83. Schuster RM, Hertel AW, Mermelstein R. Cigar, cigarillo, and little cigar use among current cigarette-smoking adolescents. *Nicotine Tob Res.* 2013;15(5):925–931.

84. Kostygina G, Glantz SA, Ling PM. Tobacco industry use of flavours to recruit new users of little cigars and cigarillos. *Tob Control.* 2016;25(1):66–74.

85. Smith-Simone S, Maziak W, Ward KD, Eissenberg T. Waterpipe tobacco smoking: knowledge, attitudes, beliefs, and behavior in two U.S. samples. *Nicotine Tob Res.* 2008;10(2):393–398.

86. Myslín M, Zhu S-H, Chapman W, Conway M. Using Twitter to examine smoking behavior and perceptions of emerging tobacco products. *J Med Internet Res.* 2013;15(8):e174.

87. Cole-Lewis H, Pugatch J, Sanders A, et al. Social listening: a content analysis of e-cigarette discussions on Twitter. *J Med Internet Res.* 2015;17(10):e243.

88. Allem J-P, Chu K-H, Cruz TB, Unger JB. Waterpipe promotion and use on Instagram: #Hookah. *Nicotine Tob Res.* 2017:ntw329.

89. Grana R, Benowitz N, Glantz SA. E-cigarettes. *Circulation.* 2014;129(19):1972–1986.

90. Kim AE, Arnold KY, Makarenko O. E-cigarette advertising expenditures in the US, 2011–2012. *Am J Prev Med.* 2014;46(4):409–412.

91. Farrelly MC, Duke JC, Crankshaw EC, et al. A randomized trial of the effect of e-cigarette TV advertisements on intentions to use e-cigarettes. *Am J Prev Med.* 2015;49(5):686–693.

92. Richardson A, Ganz O, Stalgaitis C, Abrams D, Vallone D. Noncombustible tobacco product advertising: how companies are selling the new face of tobacco. *Nicotine Tob Res.* 2014;16(5):606–614.

93. Kim AE, Hopper T, Simpson S, et al. Using Twitter data to gain insights into e-cigarette marketing and locations of use: an infoveillance study. *J Med Internet Res.* 2015;17(11):e251.

94. Huang J, Kornfield R, Szczypka G, Emery SL. A cross-sectional examination of marketing of electronic cigarettes on Twitter. *Tob Control.* 2014;23(suppl 3):iii26–iii30.

95. Duke JC, Lee YO, Kim AE, et al. Exposure to electronic cigarette television advertisements among youth and young adults. *Pediatrics.* 2014;134(1):e29–e36.

96. de Andrade M, Hastings G, Angus K. Promotion of electronic cigarettes: tobacco marketing reinvented? *BMJ.* 2013;347:f7473.

97. E-Cigarette Forum. *E-Cigarette Forum.* https://www.e-cigarette-forum.com/forum/.

98. Bromberg JE, Augustson EM, Backinger CL. Portrayal of smokeless tobacco in YouTube videos. *Nicotine Tob Res.* 2012;14(4):455–462.

99. Laestadius LI, Wahl MM, Cho YI. #Vapelife: an exploratory study of electronic cigarette use and promotion on Instagram. *Subst Use Misuse.* 2016;51(12):1669–1673.

100. Goniewicz ML, Gawron M, Smith DM, Peng M, Jacob 3rd P, Benowitz NL. Exposure to nicotine and selected toxicants in cigarette smokers who switched to electronic cigarettes: a longitudinal within-subjects observational study. *Nicotine Tob Res.* 2017;19(2):160–167.

101. Hartmann-Boyce J, Begh R, Aveyard P. Electronic cigarettes for smoking cessation. *BMJ.* 2018;360:j5543.

102. Grana RA, Ling PM. "Smoking revolution": a content analysis of electronic cigarette retail websites. *Am J Prev Med.* 2014;46(4):395–403.

103. Zhu S-H, Sun JY, Bonnevie E, et al. Four hundred and sixty brands of e-cigarettes and counting: implications for product regulation. *Tob Control.* 2014;23(suppl 3):iii3–iii9.

104. Vasiljevic M, Petrescu DC, Marteau TM. Impact of advertisements promoting candy-like flavoured e-cigarettes on appeal of tobacco smoking among children: an experimental study. *Tob Control.* 2016; 25(e2):e107−e112.

105. Agaku IT, Ayo-Yusuf OA. The effect of exposure to pro-tobacco advertising on experimentation with emerging tobacco products among U.S. adolescents. *Health Educ Behav.* 2013;41(3):275−280.

106. Villanti AC, Rath JM, Williams VF, et al. Impact of exposure to electronic cigarette advertising on susceptibility and trial of electronic cigarettes and cigarettes in US young adults: a randomized controlled trial. *Nicotine Tob Res.* 2016;18(5):1331−1339.

107. Forsyth SR, Malone RE. "I'll be your cigarette−light me up and get on with it": examining smoking imagery on YouTube. *Nicotine Tob Res.* 2010;12(8):810−816.

108. Krauss MJ, Sowles SJ, Moreno M, et al. Hookah-related twitter chatter: a content analysis. *Prev Chronic Dis.* 2015;12:E121.

109. Primack BA, Carroll MV, Shensa A, Davis W, Levine MD. Sex differences in hookah-related images posted on Tumblr: a content analysis. *J Health Commun.* 2016; 21(3):366−375.

110. Kim K, Paek H-J, Lynn J. A content analysis of smoking fetish videos on YouTube: regulatory implications for tobacco control. *Health Commun.* 2010;25(2): 97−106.

111. Hébert ET, Case KR, Kelder SH, Delk J, Perry CL, Harrell MB. Exposure and engagement with tobacco- and e-cigarette-related social media. *J Adolesc Health.* 2017. https://doi.org/10.1016/j.jadohealth.2017.04.003.

112. Redonnet B, Chollet A, Fombonne E, Bowes L, Melchior M. Tobacco, alcohol, cannabis and other illegal drug use among young adults: the socioeconomic context. *Drug Alcohol Depend.* 2012;121(3):231−239.

113. Primack BA, Douglas EL, Kraemer KL. Exposure to cannabis in popular music and cannabis use among adolescents. *Addiction.* 2010;105(3):515−523.

114. Hall W, Degenhardt L. Adverse health effects of non-medical cannabis use. *Lancet.* 2009;374(9698):1383−1391.

115. Moore THM, Zammit S, Lingford-Hughes A, et al. Cannabis use and risk of psychotic or affective mental health outcomes: a systematic review. *Lancet.* 2007; 370(9584):319−328.

116. Silins E, Horwood LJ, Patton GC, et al. Young adult sequelae of adolescent cannabis use: an integrative analysis. *Lancet Psychiatry.* 2014;1(4):286−293.

117. Endejan J. *Can Puff the Magic Dragon Lawfully Advertise His Wares*; 2015. Retrieved from: https://www.americanbar.org/content/dam/aba/publications/communications_lawyer/summer2015/CL_Sum15_v31n3_Endejan.auth checkdam.pdf.

118. *Executive Summary: The State of Legal Marijuana Markets.* Arcview Market Research; 2017.

119. Sola K. *Legal U.S. Marijuana Market Will Grow to $7.1 Billion in 2016: Report. Forbes;* 2016. https://www.forbes.com/sites/ katiesola/2016/04/19/legal-u-s-marijuana-market-will-grow-to-7-1-billion-in-2016-report/.

120. Primack BA, Kraemer KL, Fine MJ, Dalton MA. 1: association between media exposure and marijuana and alcohol use in adolescents. *J Adolesc Health Care.* 2008; 42(2):3.

121. Lavoie D. Smoking the other: marijuana and counterhegemony in Weeds. *Subst Use Misuse.* 2011;46(7): 910−921.

122. National Center on Addiction and Substance Abuse. *National Survey of American Attitudes on Substance Abuse IX: Teens and Parents.* Columbia University; 2005.

123. Cerdá M, Wall M, Feng T, et al. Association of state recreational marijuana laws with adolescent marijuana use. *JAMA Pediatr.* 2017;171(2):142−149.

124. D'Amico EJ, Miles JNV, Tucker JS. Gateway to curiosity: medical marijuana ads and intention and use during middle school. *Psychol Addict Behav.* 2015;29(3): 613−619.

125. Feeney KE, Kampman KM. Adverse effects of marijuana use. *Linacre Q.* 2016;83(2):174−178.

126. Ghosh T, Van Dyke M, Maffey A, Whitley E, Gillim-Ross L, Wolk L. The public health framework of legalized marijuana in Colorado. *Am J Public Health.* 2016;106(1):21−27.

127. *Frequently Asked Questions About Marijuana Advertising.* Washington State Liquor and Cannabis Board. http://lcb.wa.gov/mj2015/faq_i502_advertising.

128. Staff L. *State-by-State Guide to Cannabis Advertising Regulations.* Leafly; 2015. https://www.leafly.com/news/industry/state-by-state-guide-to-cannabis-advertising-regulations.

129. *Digital Ad Spending to Surpass TV Next Year.* eMarketer; 2016. http://www.emarketer.com/Article/Digital-Ad-Spending-Surpass-TV-Next-Year/1013671.

130. MassRoots. *MassRoots.* https://www.massroots.com/.

131. Bierut T, Krauss MJ, Sowles SJ, Cavazos-Rehg PA. Exploring marijuana advertising on Weedmaps, a popular online directory. *Prev Sci.* 2017;18(2):183−192.

132. Krauss MJ, Sowles SJ, Sehi A, et al. Marijuana advertising exposure among current marijuana users in the U.S. *Drug Alcohol Depend.* 2017;174:192−200.

133. Cavazos-Rehg P, Krauss M, Grucza R, Bierut L. Characterizing the followers and tweets of a marijuana-focused Twitter handle. *J Med Internet Res.* 2014;16(6):e157.

134. Cavazos-Rehg PA, Krauss M, Fisher SL, Salyer P, Grucza RA, Bierut LJ. Twitter chatter about marijuana. *J Adolesc Health.* 2015;56(2):139−145.

135. Cavazos-Rehg PA, Krauss MJ, Sowles SJ, Bierut LJ. Marijuana-related posts on Instagram. *Prev Sci.* 2016; 17(6):710−720.

136. Krauss MJ, Sowles SJ, Mylvaganam S, Zewdie K, Bierut LJ, Cavazos-Rehg PA. Displays of dabbing marijuana extracts on YouTube. *Drug Alcohol Depend.* 2015;155:45−51.

137. Krauss MJ, Sowles SJ, Stelzer-Monahan HE, Bierut T, Cavazos-Rehg PA. "It takes longer, but when it hits you it hits you!": videos about marijuana edibles on YouTube. *Subst Use Misuse.* 2017;52(6):709−716.

138. Cavazos-Rehg PA, Krauss MJ, Sowles SJ, Murphy GM, Bierut LJ. Exposure to and content of marijuana product reviews. *Prev Sci.* 2017. https://doi.org/10.1007/s11121-017-0818-9.

139. Huang J, Kornfield R, Emery SL. 100 million views of electronic cigarette YouTube videos and counting: quantification, content evaluation, and engagement levels of videos. *J Med Internet Res.* 2016;18(3):e67.

140. Mackey TK, Liang BA, Strathdee SA. Digital social media, youth, and nonmedical use of prescription drugs: the need for reform. *J Med Internet Res.* 2013; 15(7):e143.

141. National Institute on Drug Abuse. *Abuse of Prescription (Rx) Drugs Affects Young Adults Most;* 2016. https://www.drugabuse.gov/related-topics/trends-statistics/infographics/abuse-prescription-rx-drugs-affects-young-adults-most.

142. Grau LE, Dasgupta N, Harvey AP, et al. Illicit use of opioids: is OxyContin a "gateway drug"? *Am J Addict.* 2007;16(3):166–173.

143. *CBHSQ Data Review: Associations of Nonmedical Pain Reliever Use and Initiation of Heroin Use in the United States.* http://archive.samhsa.gov/data/2k13/DataReview/DR006/nonmedical-pain-reliever-use-2013.pdf.

144. Chan B, Lopez A, Sarkar U. The canary in the coal mine tweets: social media reveals public perceptions of non-medical use of opioids. *PLoS One.* 2015;10(8): e0135072.

145. Hanson CL, Burton SH, Giraud-Carrier C, West JH, Barnes MD, Hansen B. Tweaking and tweeting: exploring Twitter for nonmedical use of a psychostimulant drug (Adderall) among college students. *J Med Internet Res.* 2013;15(4):e62.

146. Sarker A, O'Connor K, Ginn R, et al. Social media mining for toxicovigilance: automatic monitoring of prescription medication abuse from twitter. *Drug Saf.* 2016;39(3): 231–240.

147. Seaman I, Giraud-Carrier C. Prevalence and attitudes about illicit and prescription drugs on twitter. In: *2016 IEEE International Conference on Healthcare Informatics (ICHI);* 2016:14–17. ieeexplore.ieee.org.

148. Scott KR, Nelson L, Meisel Z, Perrone J. Opportunities for exploring and reducing prescription drug abuse through social media. *J Addict Dis.* 2015;34(2–3): 178–184.

149. Shutler L, Nelson LS, Portelli I, Blachford C, Perrone J. Drug use in the Twittersphere: a qualitative contextual analysis of tweets about prescription drugs. *J Addict Dis.* 2015;34(4):303–310.

150. Hanson CL, Cannon B, Burton S, Giraud-Carrier C. An exploration of social circles and prescription drug abuse through Twitter. *J Med Internet Res.* 2013;15(9): e189.

151. Salimian PK, Chunara R, Weitzman ER. Averting the perfect storm: addressing youth substance use risk from social media use. *Pediatr Ann.* 2014;43(10):411.

152. Eysenbach G. Infodemiology and infoveillance: framework for an emerging set of public health informatics methods to analyze search, communication and publication behavior on the Internet. *J Med Internet Res.* 2009; 11(1):e11.

153. National Institute on Drug Abuse. *Using Social Media to Better Understand, Prevent, and Treat Substance Use;* October 16, 2014. https://www.drugabuse.gov/news-events/news-releases/2014/10/using-social-media-to-better-understand-prevent-treat-substance-use.

154. Aslam S. *Facebook by the Numbers (2018): Stats, Demographics & Fun Facts;* January 1, 2018. https://www.omnicoreagency.com/facebook-statistics/.

155. Evans WD, Holtz K, White T, Snider J. Effects of the above the influence brand on adolescent drug use prevention normative beliefs. *J Health Commun.* 2014;19(6): 721–737.

156. Evans W, Andrade E, Goldmeer S, Smith M, Snider J, Girardo G. The living the example social media substance use prevention program: a pilot evaluation. *JMIR Ment Health.* 2017;4(2):e24.

157. Griffiths R, Casswell S. Intoxigenic digital spaces? Youth, social networking sites and alcohol marketing. *Drug Alcohol Rev.* 2010;29(5):525–530.

CHAPTER 7

Media Literacy for Clinicians and Parents

CHERYL K. OLSON, SCD • EUGENE V. BERESIN, MD • STEVEN C. SCHLOZMAN, MD

Because of the astounding pace of this media revolution, the impact on children is not well understood. Does all of this media exposure prepare children for the world they will live in? Is it possible that this information deprives them of critical developmental opportunities such as play and more interpersonal activities with friends? Does the steady display of violence contribute to violent behavior? The answers are not as clear cut as some might think. Teenage crime rates are lower, for example.[1] Some children consider their time spent interacting with media as play, and there exists research to support this. This chapter presents a developmental context for the consumption of media, discusses current research, reviews the recommendations of major organizations, and takes a balanced perspective in the midst of a rising tide of media, technology, commercialism, and the inevitable and understandable controversy.

The growth of technology over the past decades has created an environment rich in media opportunities for children and adults. From the first popular radio broadcasts in the 1920s through the spread of the Internet in the 1990s, electronic media have clearly been established as a dominant global influence. Throughout this time, clinicians and researchers have studied and pontificated on the potential effects of various types of media on children and adolescents.[2] Findings have been heavily scrutinized and debated by the professional community, the manufacturers and creators of media, the government agencies charged with protecting children, and parents. Research in the field is complex; studies attempting to simulate everyday media exposure fail to capture the context of a child's life with its long list of individual, developmental, family, cultural, and economic variables.

The field of media literacy has emerged and been defined as the study of how and in what context individuals access, analyze, and evaluate media content.[3] Given this fairly broad definition, clinicians have struggled with how to integrate media literacy into clinical practice. Parents are torn between supporting the autonomy of their children, especially given the learning and narrative opportunities that electronic media make possible, and protecting their children from what might be harmful influences. The need to know how to integrate research findings and expert opinion into the everyday world of parenting is increasingly pressing.

This chapter will discuss media literacy for clinicians and parents through four lenses: the interaction between tasks of development and media exposure; the "socialization" of media through the family; special clinical circumstances and potential therapeutic uses of media; and ways to monitor or limit media use, including electronic media rating systems.

THE INTERACTION BETWEEN TASKS OF DEVELOPMENT AND MEDIA

How Young Children Perceive and Use Media

A basic understanding of developmental tasks at various ages helps to frame the debate about the utility of media in a child's life (see Chapter 16).

Infancy through toddlerhood

During infancy, from 0 to 6 months, the primary tasks are adjustment to the world outside the womb, eating and sleeping, and the beginning of social interaction through smiling, cooing, and reaching for people and objects. Physical touch is essential, with soft cuddling and comforting important to the actual facilitation of growth. Input to the brain as it is wiring itself and continuing to grow is crucial; it is highly likely that these early touch points with the environment influence neuronal pathways. The human voice and soft music are known to soothe and stimulate interaction, while loud voices and noises produce full-body startle response, interfere with the infant's ability to eat, and raise stress hormone levels. Media—especially music—may have a role in soothing and calming; parents naturally sing to their babies to quiet and comfort them.

From 6 months to 1 year, the infant is continuing to grow and interact with others. Exploration of the world around her through touch and feel is essential. Language is starting through reciprocal interactions, and the child is beginning to understand cause and effect. All of these tasks require an interactive process. The nonreciprocal way in which traditional media, such as television, operate does not provide the feedback loop necessary for children at this age. Infants need to explore through their senses, get immediate feedback, and then repeat these interactions over and over to learn from them. It is highly likely that, at this early age, cognitive and emotional learning are synergistic, that learning to pick up and eat "finger food' is developmentally optimized if this activity takes place with a warm, encouraging adult rather than in front of a screen presenting images and words unrelated to the infant's behavior or feelings.

Aside from music, and the occasional video chat with far-flung relatives,[4] the best use of electronic media at this stage may be none at all. The American Academy of Pediatrics discourages television watching for children younger than 2 years, encouraging adult-child interaction (such as talking, singing, or reading together) that promotes healthy brain development.[5] However, surveys of parents suggest that many infants and toddlers spend time in front of the television.[6] A 2012 survey[7] found that on a typical day, children aged 8 months to 8 years are exposed to almost 4 h a day of background television, which may harm the quality of parent-child interactions. (In the case of infants, it's difficult to know how "watching" is defined, since they don't seem to attend to television for more than brief periods.) The effects of television exposure may vary based on a child's temperament.

Moving on from 1 to 2 years, the development of motor skills and language with purpose continues. Children are beginning to scribble, throw a ball, feed themselves, and walk and run. Media can have a role in teaching language[8] (although print books appear to have an edge over electronic ones[9]) and again music has a role for soothing. Visual images are fascinating, and yet the ability to understand them is not developed and needs adult explanation; the ability to learn from a video image is limited.[10] Optimal learning at this stage

depends on interaction with someone else who is able to continuously modify his or her response, adjusting to what the child has just done and ideally how the child is feeling (frustrated, eager, tired, anxious, etc.). This allows the toddler to figure things out in small incremental ways, building a step at a time in knowledge and self-esteem at her own individual pace. Television, even if playing in the background, may disrupt this interaction and play with parents.[6] However, since toddlers will be surrounded by and using screens throughout childhood and adulthood, too much emphasis on "protecting" them from media could arguably be counterproductive.

Preschool years

As exploration continues from 2 to 5 years, the child is moving more into the world of socializing with others through play. The play skills of sharing, taking turns, and following simple rules begin to emerge. Many skills acquired gradually over these 3—4 years are actually school readiness skills. Some media content is specifically geared to promoting school readiness, such as programs from Sesame Workshop and PBS Kids. They often combine developmentally appropriate cognitive challenges, pacing, and repetition with characters that have feelings and values.[11,12] Many commercial-network programs are not geared to children's developmental stage. Frequent viewing of such programs can hinder later academic performance.[13] The accompanying commercial advertisements for food, toys, and games may also be detrimental. Children this age see little difference between program and commercial content, and don't understand the persuasive intent of advertising.[14] More time watching television[15] and the presence of television in a child's bedroom contribute to preschoolers' increasing risk of being overweight.[16]

As with television, effects of interactive media on cognitive development seem related to the appropriateness of software and parent involvement.[17] While interactive games have greater capacity to teach cause and effect, they may limit fantasy play within the structure of the software rather than being derived from or related to the child's own life. Children benefit in their social and emotional growth when their own experiences and feelings can be acted out with creative materials. Dress up, pretend worlds created with toys, drawings, paintings, and clay and cardboard creations are but a few examples of how play promotes self-expression at this stage. Still, many of these activities have proxies in the digital world.[18] While research is limited, interactive games and apps that support shared imaginative play have potential.[19]

One concern about children's media consumption is that youngsters aged 8 years and younger typically cannot reliably tell fantasy from reality and cannot comprehend complex motives and intentions. Studies by Cantor[20,21] have shown how children at this age become fearful upon seeing images that they think are real. Although these results are of concern, we also know from daily experience that children have a growing sense of what is real and what is not from an early age. When parents read fairy tales at bedtime, although there may be transient fright, few children suffer long-term harm or attempt the stunts related in the story. Few have jumped out of windows to mimic Superman or Spiderman. In our clinical experience, those children who have taken serious risks come from chaotic and often abusive or neglectful homes. They know reality and try to escape it. Research cannot easily capture the interplay between the developing child and the thousands of increasing complex and confusing images they see through television, apps, videogames, YouTube, and movies—some exciting, some fun, and some brutally realistic live coverage of a horrific event (see Chapter 5).

How School-Age Children and Adolescents Perceive and Use Media

A national survey of children's media use[22] found that children aged 8–10 years experience almost 8 h a day of total media exposure, and that 11- to 14-year-olds spend more time with media than any other age group. Children rapidly acquire new information during the early school age years with an accompanying understanding of time and motion, and greater understanding of cause and effect. During this time, they move from concrete thinking and the world of fantasy to abstract thinking and the ability to understand more complex thought, and thus a greater ability to learn from electronic media. There are also gains in academic and social skills, membership in peer groups, and development of important friendships. Entertainment media begins to shape children's understanding of social relationships and expectations about behavior and appearance, but the learning is limited since it does not occur through the child's personal interactions. There is also wide variability from child to child as to how they process information, particularly at the early phase of this stage from the age of 6–10 years, before the development of abstract thinking.

The role of temperament and traits

All of development occurs on the substrate of inborn temperament and traits. As established by Thomas et al.,[23] children come into this world with styles and traits that are persistent throughout childhood into adulthood. Some babies are easier to manage and learn self-regulation more quickly. Other babies become easily overwhelmed, overreact to stimuli, and require a longer time to be soothed. As infants grow to toddlers, their characteristics of shyness, natural curiosity and ready exploration, and even aggressiveness become more apparent. Thus, the effect of watching a scary movie on a shy 3-year-old or shy 7-year-old might be quite different from the effect on a 3-year-old who is already exhibiting aggressive tendencies or a 7-year-old who is known for her daring behavior.

Media researchers have tried to take traits into account, particularly in the area of aggression and violence. Some studies have found greater effects of violent content in video games for subjects who score high on measures of trait hostility or aggression; others have not.[24,25] More studies are needed to see how children's traits or temperament might moderate media effects. Children with trait hostility and aggression may be drawn to more violent activities, whether those be contact sports such as football or wrestling, more aggressive school yard play, or more violent media. And it is unclear whether playing football or a violent video game is a reinforcer of aggressive behavior for some children, or a "release" of hostility that is socially acceptable for others. Research data that describe risk factors for groups of children do not take into account individual variability, parental interactions, and a host of other factors that should be a part of parents' daily decision-making.

Summary

While this is not a comprehensive discussion of the interaction between media and the tasks of development, it highlights how the issues vary at different ages. Media literacy efforts need to take into account the age of the child and his/her developmental level. It is clear that electronic media have the power to teach; it is a matter of what the content and ads are teaching, the effects of these messages in the context of the child's life, and whether time spent with media unduly limits the necessary time for hands-on learning, first through play and later through age-appropriate social interactions. The reasonable balance between the passivity of television, interaction with electronic games, use of the Internet, one-to-one peer activities, group activities, and family time, probably varies with every child—based on age, personality, temperament, social or environmental factors, and more.

FAMILY CONTEXT AND MEDIA

American children now grow up surrounded by a seemingly limitless array of media content. As of 2010, the home of a typical child aged 8–18 years featured an average of four televisions, two game consoles, two computers, and multiple video and music recorders/players.[22] The rapid changes in media access are taking place within a family unit and culture that are also rapidly evolving. For example, between divorce and remarriage, death of a parent, out of wedlock births, foster care, and imprisonment, fewer children are raised from birth to 18 in a traditional, two-parent nuclear family. (During 2016, 65% of children younger than 18 years were living with two married parents, down from 77% in 1980.[26])

It's difficult for children to avoid the influence of mass media. They face peer expectations to keep up with most recent sports story or the hottest YouTube channel, and related fashion trend. Social media has become perhaps the most common means that children, adolescents, and young adults use to communicate with each other. In this digital age, it is almost impossible to find a young person (or adult) who is not texting or tweeting, on FaceBook, or using apps such as SnapChat or Instagram. This is the new mainstream. School assignments require them to search the Internet. Friends discuss the latest social media items before the school day starts. Children play video-simulated sports against each other, or join a worldwide game on the Internet.

National and local news is often obtained through social media or online news outlets rather than through traditional newspapers and magazines. The news audience has splintered. A 2018 Pew Research Center survey found that just 8% of 18- to 29-year-olds often get news from network television, compared with 49% of persons aged 65 years and older.[27] Times have changed. And they are changing at such a rapid pace that it is difficult for parents, caregivers, and grandparents to keep up with the rapid pace of media development and use.

What are reasonable family policies regarding the media? Parents may be tempted to bring it all to a halt, thinking, "I do not want my children exposed to all of these sights and sounds streaming into my home. I don't want their development harassed or hurried by media." They can try to severely restrict phone, tablet, and app usage. Yet, even if one could be successful in exerting the control necessary to limit media exposure, is this the approach that would optimize a child's development? Appropriately limiting autonomy and peer relationships is good parenting

when confronting substance use, gang behavior, delinquency, or protecting a younger child from a friend's irresponsible parents or a peer who is a bully or demeaning. How great does the danger have to be to rationalize limiting the child's developmental trajectory toward autonomy and the free flow of information among peers—preparation for the next stage of life, high school, and college? We know that prohibition and censorship do not work. In fact, limiting access to the very same digital media we as parents use every day would be hypocritical. The key question is how we and our children harness the use of digital media for better and not worse. How can we assume control of a world that has become embedded with digital media?

It is also tempting for a parent to say, "The horse is out of the barn. I have no control and they are going to see it and hear it no matter what. I want my child to have friends and not be 'out of it.' I want my child to like me. And who has the time for all this monitoring?" Parents can feel caught in the dilemma of overcontrolling their children's lives or surrendering control to the prevailing winds of our culture. Ultimately, each parent must decide what is best for his/her child based on knowledge of that particular child's strengths, weaknesses, or vulnerabilities, and the context of their chosen family values. Begin with a focus on health and safety, such as removing media from bedrooms at night to preserve sleep time and protecting personal information.

Family approaches and rules concerning media literacy and exposure should be consistent with what parents do to encourage autonomy in the many other areas of a child's life. Parents assess the child's readiness, strengths, and weakness; determine the risk associated with the developmental step; prepare the child; provide guidance; set rules or boundaries; cope with their own anxiety; and then launch the next step. For example, is the child ready to walk to school on her own? Can he find the way? Should she go with a friend? Does he understand the risk of going off the path or talking to a stranger? Can she follow traffic safety rules?

A reckless or impulsive child may not be ready and need to be older to safely accept this autonomy, whereas an anxious yet competent child may benefit from encouragement to be among the first in the class to achieve this landmark. For most middle-class children in the United States, it would certainly be "safer" to wait and maybe never allow a child to walk to school (or to be among the last in a class). And yet if a child is ready, many would take the risk; the act of walking away is a metaphor for growing up, being trustworthy, and ultimately gaining self-esteem. Thousands of these little gains form the basis of productive adulthood and generative parenting.

The same process of gradual movement toward autonomy, guided by parental involvement, applies to media decisions. Children benefit, given our culture and at the appropriate developmental step, from some decision-making authority about what they watch on television, what they do "to relax," how they balance leisure time with homework, what video games they play, and how they use smartphones, tablets, and the Internet. Parents who live in a safe neighborhood let a 6-year-old walk to school after initially walking with him, but do not let a child go downtown on a public bus. Similarly at this young age, a child would be allowed to go to a G-rated or maybe a PG movie, but not a PG-13 or R-rated movie. Parents set a range of acceptable options and let the child make some choices, the boundaries being set by the advantages of building autonomy and the risks of choices.

Understanding Media Content

The pervasive presence of violent or sexually inappropriate content in American media has unfortunately created a general negative tone regarding its influence on children and family life. One only has to look at the lineup of series on Netflix, HBO, and other networks to worry about the impact they have on our children. As researchers try to help parents manage the potential risks of excessive and unsupervised media use, the positive ways that media can be used within the family are often neglected. In fact, television can bring family members together, both for shared recreation and as a trigger for relevant discussions. On the recreational side, cheering on a favorite sports team or just spending time together is special and creates important shared memories. In terms of building character, rooting for a team that does not often win, but continues to play hard and embodies local pride can teach patience, anger management, and tolerance! On a more serious note, television can provide many hours of enjoyable time through educational shows, especially those on history, science, hobbies, or current issues relevant to families. But watching entertainment programs as a family can have unexpected benefits.

For example, it can be fun to watch a television talent competition with a teenager and to compare ratings of the contestants. But this is also an opportunity to discuss unrealistic expectations, being overdependent on other people's opinions or adoration, and coping with defeat. Discussion of the songs can lead to an appreciation of music favored by the younger or older

generation that would not otherwise have been heard. Similarly, watching family dramas and films set in the recent past can lead to Internet searches on the Vietnam War or the civil rights movement, and meaningful discussions of substance use, racism, premature and premarital sexuality, abortion, over- and undercontrolling parents, grief, anger, and forgiveness. In one national survey, one in three teens aged 15−17 years reported that television content had triggered a discussion about a sexual issue with a parent.[28]

Just as they learn the alphabet or English grammar, children in the elementary grades can start to understand both the technical and content aspects of television and movies.[29] The technical side includes the electronic workings of televisions, explained through interesting books (e.g., *The Way Things Work Now*), programs and Web sites (e.g., HowStuffWorks.com), and the commercial aspect of television, including how programs are paid for by companies selling their products. Children can also learn about the different types of programs (comedies, dramas, news, documentaries, etc.) and how to tell the "real" from the pretend. Finally, parents can describe the technical aspects of producing a program, from casting actors and making costumes and sets to camera angles and special effects. Again, parents can search for television programs and Web sites that explore topics such as these.

As children get older, they are more able to understand subtler aspects of program content, such as plots, themes, and historical or geographical setting, and how these combine with technical elements to affect how the program makes us feel. They can also explore motivations for characters' behaviors (from interpersonal relationships to substance use) and aspects of their appearance (such as clothing or weight), and identify common, perhaps harmful stereotypes (such the portrayal of grandparents, scientists, or "crazy people").

While many parents cringe at a series such as "Thirteen Reasons Why," focusing on a highly exaggerated portrayal of high school stress factors leading to a girl's suicide, it does raise important issues about bullying, misuse of drugs and alcohol, and sexual assault. These kinds of issues are openly discussed among our middle and high school students. We know that while many adolescents are binge watching, few parents watch with them. Some television content may be uncomfortable to watch with a teenager, but it's likely that these same scenes will be watched with peers in their homes, or at the movies, with no adult available to help put the behaviors and feelings in context. Discussion of these topics without the show as a substrate or facilitator would be difficult at best, and very unlikely to occur at all.

These sorts of questions can form the underpinnings of discussions with older children as you watch television and Internet videos together:[30]

- Who created this content and why are they sharing it? Who owns and profits from it?
- What techniques and issues are used to attract and hold attention?
- What lifestyles, values, and points of view are represented in this content?
- What (or who) is omitted from this content? Why was it left out?
- How might different people interpret this content?

As children begin to master abstract thinking and are able to explore more content on their own, it's important to talk about the credibility of Internet content and how to determine the quality or biases of what they find. The fragmenting of news media and increased consumption through social media means that children also need guidance on judging the credibility and possible biases of news sources. A 2016 Stanford study found that 82% of middle schoolers conflated online "sponsored content" (advertisements) and real news.[31] An online educational resource is available in conjunction with that study to teach adolescents how to evaluate news Web sites and claims on social media.[32] Parents need to be mindful of their own behavior. Recent research on children aged 12–17 years and their parents found that teens tend to imitate their parents' news consumption behavior; that is, they mirror what parents do, not what they recommend.[33]

Experience with the Internet should not just be viewed through the lens of harm reduction. While there is a real risk of unwanted exposure to X-rated material or solicitations from strangers,[34] when one weighs this potential risk versus the gains of autonomy, access to information, and communicating with a group of friends, the benefits greatly exceed the risk—provided the parent(s) have assessed the degree of autonomy their child is ready to manage and have discussed the dos and don'ts of online behavior. These include not giving out personal information such as phone numbers, account numbers, and passwords; recognizing that "free" stuff (games, ringtones, special content) might come with malware or demand information in return; and the importance of strong passwords.[35]

All of these media risks are happening in the home where there are opportunities to listen, observe (gently and at a distance), explain, and reassess. The key to media literacy is ongoing parental involvement that is geared to the child's developmental level, with gradual movement toward more and more autonomy as the child matures.

Sexual Content

For adolescents and younger children as well, easy access to Internet content has translated into easy access to sexual images, including pornography. What, if anything, could and should parents do? As with so many emotionally and culturally sensitive topics, the first step is to gain some perspective.

Peter and Valkenberg's review[36] of the English-language scientific literature from 1995 to 2015 on adolescents' use of pornography internationally found a wide range of prevalence rates. Part of that variation appears due to culture and country, and part due to differing questions asked by researchers, e.g., "ever exposed" versus "use within the past year." Even so, several patterns appear. The adolescents who used pornography the most tended to be male, in a later stage of puberty, were sensation-seekers, and had more weak or troubled family relations. However, it's important to recognize that viewing or reading pornography as a teenager is normative in many cultures and is not, by itself, a sign of a problem. For example, Häggström-Nordin et al.[37] found that 95% of Swedish boys and 50% of Swedish girls had read or viewed pornographic materials. An earlier study by Cowan and Campbell[38] found that 83% of American boys and 48% of American girls had seen pornographic videos.

Among the top concerns of parents is whether exposure to pornographic materials will lead a teenager to become sexually active at a younger age, and the potential consequences of such activity. Steinberg and Monahan[39] reanalyzed data from an earlier longitudinal study and found no evidence that exposure to what they referred to as "sexy media" resulted in earlier involvement with sexual intercourse.

That's not to say, however, that such exposure has no effects in other attitudes and behaviors. Sexual content in the media rarely includes portrayals of risks and responsibilities (e.g., condom use, pregnancy, STD transmission) that should be integral to adolescents' involvement in sexual activities.[40] However, this absence of information and perspective can provide a starting point for discussions with teenagers about not only those risks and responsibilities but also about how realistic those media relationships and gender portrayals are.[41]

SPECIAL CLINICAL CIRCUMSTANCES

Because of the focus on the potential negative effects of media, the special clinical circumstances where media can serve a specific therapeutic role for a child and the family are often neglected. Electronic media can be used as creative tools to address important issues such as the capacity for play and relaxation, the development of self-esteem, and the development of peer relationships.

The Striving Family

Some families are on overdrive in terms of work, daily schedules, expectations, and achievement orientation. Any time focused on an activity, either individual or group, has to be productive or a step to a more evolved "useful" activity. Even fun is defined as a lesson or practice that is part of making progress. These families are quite resistant to any "downtime" or "senseless fun." Often children in these families, if given a bit of permission, readily wish for or identify media opportunities through television, Internet, video games, or movies to take time off or feel more in tune with peers. These children state that their parents would never allow them to watch a desired television program or watch with them. Such parents assume a kind of elite status in their blanket condemnation of virtually all media.

These circumstances may call for a family prescription mandating a regular hour of senseless fun watching a comedy or drama to encourage a slight change in expectation or intensity of the striving. Sometimes families have rejected this single hour as the beginning of a moral decline, while others have discovered a series or a video game that has had a positive effect. (It is often an added benefit to have the child tutor the parent in a video game, reversing the common pattern in the striving family of parents constantly teaching and tutoring children.)

Difficulties with Peer Relations

Some children have difficulties with peer relationships and need some structure to facilitate time with friends. Often this structure can be an activity like a sports team, band, or Scouting. Some children do not participate in activities or groups, and media can serve this bridge function. In fact, for some isolated children or those with weaknesses in social skills, texting (and avoiding eye contact and nonverbal interaction) may be highly useful in developing relationships with peers. Going to a movie is among the most structured of activities, as is watching television or playing video games. Children who are quite socially awkward may be masters at certain video games and gain status by teaching others. Inviting a potential friend over for the newest version of a game can feel safe and facilitate a relationship.

The Child With Attention-Deficit/Hyperactivity Disorder

Children with attention-deficit/hyperactivity disorder (ADHD) are frequently particularly devoted to media, including television, video games, and computers. Many of these children find school stressful, demanding, and—even with a customized treatment plan—not very supportive of their self-esteem. Coming home from school and immediately starting on homework can be overwhelming. Children with ADHD seem to benefit from an after-school activity, especially a sport, and a little "down time" watching a television show as a transition to homework or as a break. Electronic games and the Internet are forgiving, can be reset, turned on and off, and do not criticize. The child is in control, errors are private and reversible, and there is always another chance. Some children with ADHD are very adept at video games and using computers, which can provide a highly valued source of self-esteem. Research suggests that judicious use of interactive games can enhance both social relationships and learning for children with ADHD.[42]

Children with Developmental Disorders

Children who are developmentally delayed often use media in ways similar to the child with ADHD. Television, videos, and computer games can occupy large amounts of time, filling the void of social contact. This population is at risk, however, of having difficulty distinguishing the fantasy world from the real world. Some children in particular will mimic what they have seen and heard in the wrong social context and thus put themselves potentially at risk. An example of this is the young teenager with Asperger's who watches the Comedy Central show "South Park," then enters school the next day and calls another student a name used in the show. The guiding principles for parents with developmentally delayed children are to be aware of their child's ability to tell fantasy from reality and tendency to mimic what is seen or heard in socially inappropriate ways. Children who are developmentally delayed may have trouble in these areas into their teenage years and beyond; parents must consider their child's developmental age versus chronologic age when using the age-based media rating systems.

UNDERSTANDING RATING SYSTEMS AND MONITORING

Rating Systems

The rating systems have been designed by each area of the entertainment industry for the ostensible purpose of helping parents choose age-appropriate media for their children. They have done so to stave off pressure for government regulation from policymakers and various interest groups. In most of the world, government regulation (e.g., the German Unterhaltungssoftware Selbstkontrolle [USK] system) or close cooperation between government, industry, and consumer groups (e.g., the Pan European Game Information [PEGI] age-rating system for interactive games) is the norm.[43] This section will first present the ratings systems for television, movies, computer/video games, and music/recordings. A discussion of the issues that have been debated between professional organizations, parents, and entertainment industry representatives will follow.

Television

The "TV Parental Guidelines" were developed in anticipation of V-chip technology, a device mandated by the Telecommunications Act of 1996 to be installed in television sets manufactured after January 2000. After the Act was passed, entertainment industry executives began to plan a ratings system, which went into effect in 1997. Information on guidelines is available at http://www.tvguidelines.org/ratings.htm.

The V-chip allows parents to program the set such that shows designated to have violent content are not shown. The ratings are: TV-Y (All Children), TV-Y7 (Directed to Older Children), TV-Y7-FV (Directed to Older Children-Fantasy Violence), TV-G (General Audience), TV-PG (Parental Guidance Suggested), TV-14 (Parents Strongly Cautioned), and TV-MA (Mature Audience Only; unsuitable for children younger than 17 years) (Table 7.1).

Note that programs in these last three categories may also have letter ratings, such as S for sexual situations, D for suggestive dialogue, L for coarse language, and V for violence. Confusingly, the meaning of these letters is not the same for TV-PG, TV-14, or TV-MA; they represent progressively stronger content.

Surveys suggest that parents are often unfamiliar with the ratings. For example, in a 2007 Kaiser Family Foundation survey, there was widespread confusion about the non-aged-based terms such as "FV."[44] The quality of industry ratings has also been questioned. A 2016 study in *Pediatrics* of 17 variously rated programs found the ratings accurately flagged sexual behavior and

gory violence but did less well with interpersonal violence or aggressive behaviors.[45]

Movies

The first modern US media ratings system, and the template for the rest, began in 1968 as a joint venture of the Motion Picture Association of America (MPAA) and the National Association of Theatre Owners.[46] The Classification and Ratings Administration (CARA) determines ratings and provides a brief explanation for those films not rated G (e.g., "rated R for violence and language"). The CARA rating board has 8–13 anonymous paid members; the MPAA President selects the chairman, but it's unclear how other members are selected. Producers or distributors who submit their movies for review pay fees that fund the board. According to the MPAA's Web site, "ratings are assigned by a board of parents who consider factors such as violence, sex, language and drug use and then assign a rating they believe the majority of American parents would give a movie."[47]

The ratings are G (General Audiences), PG (Parental Guidance Suggested), PG-13 (Parents Strongly Cautioned), R (Restricted: child younger than 17 years must be accompanied by an adult), and NC-17 (no one younger than 17 years admitted). Parents should be cautioned not to over-rely on ratings. Relative to other nations' movie rating systems, the US system has been criticized for placing far less weight on violence than on sexual content and profanity[48] (Table 7.2).

Computer/video games

In response to Congressional hearings and proposed legislation, a consortium of game producers founded the Interactive Digital Software Association (IDSA; now the Entertainment Software Association) in 1994. In turn, the IDSA created and funded a self-regulatory body called the Entertainment Software Rating Board (ESRB). According to the ESRB Web site,[49] each game's rating is based on the consensus of at least three trained raters who "typically have experience with children, whether through prior work experience, education or as parents or caregivers," have no ties to the industry, and are kept anonymous to avoid attempts to influence ratings (Table 7.3).

The rating system consists of two components: an age symbol to be placed on the front of the game and any of 30 "content descriptors" to be placed beside the age symbol on the back. More than 1000 games are now rated each year. According to the Entertainment Software Association,[50] 67% of titles rated in 2016

TABLE 7.1
TV Ratings

All Children

This program is designed to be appropriate for all children. Whether animated or live-action, the themes and elements in this program are specifically designed for a very young audience, including children from ages 2-6. This program is not expected to frighten younger children.

Directed to Older Children

This program is designed for children age 7 and above. It may be more appropriate for children who have acquired the developmental skills needed to distinguish between make-believe and reality. Themes and elements in this program may include mild fantasy violence or comedic violence, or may frighten children under the age of 7. Therefore, parents may wish to consider the suitability of this program for their very young children.

Directed to Older Children - Fantasy Violence

For those programs where fantasy violence may be more intense or more combative than other programs in this category, such programs will be designated TV-Y7-FV.

General Audience

Most parents would find this program suitable for all ages. Although this rating does not signify a program designed specifically for children, most parents may let younger children watch this program unattended. It contains little or no violence, no strong language and little or no sexual dialogue or situations.

Parental Guidance Suggested

This program contains material that parents may find unsuitable for younger children. Many parents may want to watch it with their younger children. The theme itself may call for parental guidance and/or the program may contain one or more of the following: some suggestive dialogue (D), infrequent coarse language (L), some sexual situations (S), or moderate violence (V).

Parents Strongly Cautioned

This program contains some material that many parents would find unsuitable for children under 14 years of age. Parents are strongly urged to exercise greater care in monitoring this program and are cautioned against letting children under the age of 14 watch unattended. This program may contain one or more of the following: intensely suggestive dialogue (D), strong coarse language (L), intense sexual situations (S), or intense violence (V).

Mature Audience Only

This program is specifically designed to be viewed by adults and therefore may be unsuitable for children under 17. This program may contain one or more of the following: crude indecent language (L), explicit sexual activity (S), or graphic violence (V).

TABLE 7.2
Voluntary Movie Rating System

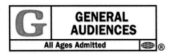

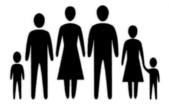

Nothing that would offend parents for viewing by children.

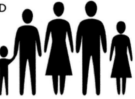

Parents urged to give "parental guidance." May contain some material parents might not like for their young children.

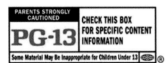

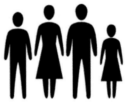

Parents are urged to be cautious. Some material may be inappropriate for pre-teenagers.

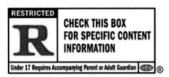

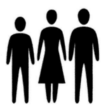

Contains some adult material. Parents are urged to learn more about the film before taking their young children with them.

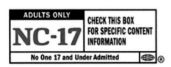

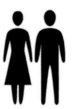

Clearly adult. Children are not admitted.

TABLE 7.3
Video and Computer Games Ratings

RATING CATEGORIES

EVERYONE
Content is generally suitable for all ages. May contain minimal cartoon, fantasy or mild violence and/or infrequent use of mild language.

EVERYONE 10+
Content is generally suitable for ages 10 and up. May contain more cartoon, fantasy or mild violence, mild language and/or minimal suggestive themes.

TEEN
Content is generally suitable for ages 13 and up. May contain violence, suggestive themes, crude humor, minimal blood, simulated gambling and/or infrequent use of strong language.

MATURE
Content is generally suitable for ages 17 and up. May contain intense violence, blood and gore, sexual content and/or strong language.

ADULTS ONLY
Content suitable only for adults ages 18 and up. May include prolonged scenes of intense violence, graphic sexual content and/or gambling with real currency.

RATING PENDING
Not yet assigned a final ESRB rating. Appears only in advertising, marketing and promotional materials related to a physical (e.g., boxed) video game that is expected to carry an ESRB rating, and should be replaced by a game's rating once it has been assigned.

NOTE: Rating Category assignments can also be based upon a game or app's minimum age requirement.

received an E (Everyone) or E10 + rating, 21% a T (Teen: 13 and up), and 11% an M (Mature: 17 years and up). (There is also an AO or Adults Only rating, but this is very seldom used.) Of the top 20 best-selling games (by units sold), 10 were rated M in 2016, including the latest entries in the *Call of Duty* and *Grand Theft Auto* series. Top-selling E-rated titles include sports series (e.g., *Madden NFL 17, FIFA 17*) and Pokemon variations.

Music/recordings
In 1985, the trade organization Recording Industry Association of America (RIAA) reached an agreement with the National Parent Teacher Association and

TABLE 7.3

CONTENT DESCRIPTORS

- **Alcohol Reference** - Reference to and/or images of alcoholic beverages
- **Animated Blood** - Discolored and/or unrealistic depictions of blood
- **Blood** - Depictions of blood
- **Blood and Gore** - Depictions of blood or the mutilation of body parts
- **Cartoon Violence** - Violent actions involving cartoon-like situations and characters. May include violence where a character is unharmed after the action has been inflicted
- **Comic Mischief** - Depictions or dialogue involving slapstick or suggestive humor
- **Crude Humor** - Depictions or dialogue involving vulgar antics, including "bathroom" humor
- **Drug Reference** - Reference to and/or images of illegal drugs
- **Fantasy Violence** - Violent actions of a fantasy nature, involving human or non-human characters in situations easily distinguishable from real life
- **Intense Violence** - Graphic and realistic-looking depictions of physical conflict. May involve extreme and/or realistic blood, gore, weapons and depictions of human injury and death
- **Language** - Mild to moderate use of profanity
- **Lyrics** - Mild references to profanity, sexuality, violence, alcohol or drug use in music
- **Mature Humor** - Depictions or dialogue involving "adult" humor, including sexual references
- **Nudity** - Graphic or prolonged depictions of nudity
- **Partial Nudity** - Brief and/or mild depictions of nudity
- **Real Gambling** - Player can gamble, including betting or wagering real cash or currency
- **Sexual Content** - Non-explicit depictions of sexual behavior, possibly including partial nudity
- **Sexual Themes** - References to sex or sexuality
- **Sexual Violence** - Depictions of rape or other violent sexual acts
- **Simulated Gambling** - Player can gamble without betting or wagering real cash or currency
- **Strong Language** - Explicit and/or frequent use of profanity
- **Strong Lyrics** - Explicit and/or frequent references to profanity, sex, violence, alcohol or drug use in music
- **Strong Sexual Content** - Explicit and/or frequent depictions of sexual behavior, possibly including nudity
- **Suggestive Themes** - Mild provocative references or materials
- **Tobacco Reference** - Reference to and/or images of tobacco products
- **Use of Alcohol** - The consumption of alcoholic beverages
- **Use of Drugs** - The consumption or use of illegal drugs
- **Use of Tobacco** - The consumption of tobacco products
- **Violence** - Scenes involving aggressive conflict. May contain bloodless dismemberment
- **Violent References** - References to violent acts

NOTE: Content Descriptors are applied relative to the Rating Category assigned and are not intended to be a complete listing of content. When a Content Descriptor is preceded by the term "Mild" it is intended to convey low frequency, intensity or severity.

TABLE 7.4
Music Industry Rating Logo

```
PARENTAL
ADVISORY
EXPLICIT CONTENT
```

The Parental Advisory is a notice to consumers that recordings identified by this logo may contain strong language or depictions of violence, sex, or substance abuse. Parental discretion is advised.

Parents Music Resource Center to identify potentially objectionable content (profanity or depictions of violence and sex) in music releases. There are no age-based guidelines, just a simple logo marking mature content. According to the RIAA, the Parent Advisory Label or "PAL Mark" is "a voluntary initiative for record companies and artists, permitting them greater freedom of expression while also giving them the opportunity to help parents and families make informed consumption decisions." The PAL Mark is "typically applied prominently" to packaging "if strong language or depictions of violence, sex or substance abuse are present in a recorded work."[51] In other words, music labeling is a self-regulatory process; individual record companies and their artists decide whether to add the label (Table 7.4).

Rating Systems Summary and Discussion
While the rating systems provide parents with useful information, all ratings are subjectively assigned by board members whose training and expertise are unknown, using instruments and methods that are not publicly available. Greater transparency in the process and greater involvement of child development experts (especially those with children who play such games) might reassure parents.

In an effort to be comprehensive, systems may become so complex as to confuse parents and therefore go unused. (For example, when should parents be concerned about "comic mischief" or "violent references": two of the many video game content descriptors?) Simplicity might be preferable, focused on descriptors in areas of concern to parents such as violence, sex, nudity, strong language, and drug use. A review of systems used in other countries may be helpful; for example, the multination European PEGI game ratings system[52] includes age-based ratings and seven simple icons for concerns such as bad language, fear (material that might scare young children), and discrimination

(content that depicts or refers to cruelty to or harassment of groups of people based on race, religion, ability, sexual preference, etc.).

The Federal Trade Commission has raised concerns about the marketing of violence to youth, and published a series of reports from 2000 to 2009.[53] These reports included results of "undercover shopper" sting operations, to see if children aged 13–16 years were able to purchase or view mature-content media. A follow-up 2013 survey[54] found that 24% were able to buy a ticket for an R-rated movie, 30% could purchase an R-rated film on DVD, 47% bought an explicit-content-labeled music CD, and 13% acquired an M-rated video game—considerable improvement in enforcement over earlier surveys. Young adolescents with game consoles and computers in their bedrooms tend to spend more hours with games in general and violent content in particular[55]; where practical, parents may wish to keep technology in areas of the home more subject to casual monitoring.

Another issue is "ratings creep," or stretching of the boundaries of acceptability in various rating categories. This has been particularly apparent in the MPAA rating system for the PG and PG-13 categories. Content analyses of films rated PG-13 from 1988, 1997, and 2006 show a trend toward increased violent content (but not sexual content) in the PG-13 category.[56] What was once R content now passes for PG-13, which concerns parents but benefits the movie industry, since it broadens the film's potential audience.

CARA sponsors a Web site, www.filmratings.com, that allows parents to search for a movie by name and get brief information on its rating (e.g., "Star Wars: The Last Jedi" is "rated PG-13 for sequences of sci-fi action and violence"). For those who want additional information, there are Web sites that have no connection to the motion picture industry and provide the user with extensive detail about a given movie, such as http://www.kidsfirst.org, www.kids-in-mind.com, and www.parentpreviews.com. Common Sense Media (www.commonsensemedia.org) also provides "family friendly" ratings based on developmental criteria from respected experts.

Monitoring and Blocking Devices

Many thoughtful parents struggle on a daily basis with how to monitor the media their children consume. In addition to limiting rental or purchase of materials, technologies are available to help parents block some media content, or restrict and control time spent with media. The speed at which technology advances, as well as the adeptness of its makers and hackers, has been daunting. The burden is unfortunately on parents, as the message from regulators essentially is that the rate at which technology develops far surpasses the rate at which laws and governmental monitoring can take place.

Fortunately, there are now a variety of options that parents can research and deploy, some of which are free and widely available. An extensive listing of devices, apps, and services for managing electronic media use and content access is pointless; such a list would be immediately obsolete. Here, we provide background on the types of options available and the thinking behind them, along with select examples and resources. When choosing methods for managing technology use, look for advice that is tailored to children's ages and likely activities (including texting, apps, video games, and favorite Web or TV series).

For televisions, the V-chip allows parents to use a "parental lock code" as a password to activate or change V-chip settings. Programs can be blocked by age category or content label. For example, a parent could block all programs rated TV-14, but if the family's primary concern is violence, the block can be specific to TV-14-V shows. The V-chip can also be set to block unedited movies on premium cable channels via the MPAA film rating system. Unfortunately, the V-chip is not seen as user-friendly; parents find it difficult to locate and complicated to program, especially given their often-limited understanding of the ratings system. Also, some parents feel that they can adequately supervise children's viewing without the V-chip.[57]

Parental controls are also built into cable set-top boxes; companies may offer to install blocking equipment for households without set-top boxes. Parents may block by channel, program name, and TV/film rating, and even hide "adult" titles from program listings. Information is available at the cable industry's Web site[58] and at individual cable company Web sites.

Game play devices, including consoles (such as Xbox and Playstation brands) and handhelds, have parental controls that can prevent playing of games based on rating (for example, all M-rated games). Some controls may limit play time, block in-game purchases, or restrict Internet access.[59] Computers, tablets, and smartphones are also potential portals of entry for material inappropriate for children. Information on securing specific tablets and phones can be found on device maker's Web sites, and at Common Sense Media.[60] Even Internet-connected toys have been cited as risks to children's privacy or security.[61,62]

The 1998 Children's Online Privacy Protection Act requires that Web site operators obtain parental consent before collecting personal information about a minor child, e.g., names, addresses, photos, and voice recordings. It allows parents to review personal information collected on their children and to revoke consent and delete the information. Web sites also cannot ask or encourage a child to submit personal information or enable a child to make such information publicly available. Information on policies, and advice for parents, teachers, and children on safe Internet use, is available from the Federal Trade Commission[63] and from Connect Safely, a Silicon valley nonprofit.[64]

A 2016 Pew Research Center survey of parents of 13- to 17-year-olds found that 39% reported using parental controls for blocking, filtering, or monitoring their child's online activities.[65] The myriad, ever-changing options include "walled garden" Web browsers for younger children and tools that limit time spent online (either total time or times of day), to reduce excessive or unsupervised Internet use. For example, in response to concerns by its own employees about their children accessing technology at earlier ages, Google created a program[66] called Family Link. This allows central management of children's access to and activities on compatible devices and apps, as well as Google searching. Parents can assess how much time is spent on various apps (such as YouTube Kids), set daily time limits on a device, see the device's current location, and even remotely lock it. Family Link requires the creation of a child Google Account, and children will be shown ads (although Google's privacy notice[67] pledges not to "serve personalized ads to your child").

There is also software that filters or blocks content by Web site address (URL), human review of Web pages, key words (such as "sex" or 'breast"), or "context sensitive" key words that avoid overzealous blocking of innocuous pages with information on "breast cancer" or "chicken breast" recipes. Some filters allow parents to override the filter for certain sites. Filtering software such as Net Nanny is controversial because filters most effective at blocking adult materials (found on hundreds of millions out of the tens of billions of indexed Web pages) overblock and prevent access to innocuous sites.[68] Studies have found that such software may somewhat reduce exposure (unwanted or sought) to online sexual materials.[69] However, no technology can replace parental monitoring or discussions with children of how to handle the inevitable exposure to inappropriate or upsetting material.

Most parents, according to the Pew Research Center survey, focus on monitoring rather than restricting teen Internet access—for example, checking what Web sites their children visit (61%) or their social media profiles (60%). It is also important for parents to recognize that they need not say yes to every device. For example, in response to concerns about younger children's access to inappropriate content and media overengagement, a movement called "Wait Until 8th" advocates delaying children's smartphone ownership until at least the eighth grade.[70] They encourage agreements among groups of families to delay their children's smartphone use, and advise those wanting to keep in touch to provide children instead with a basic phone or two-way calling watch that simply makes calls and sends texts.

CONCLUSIONS

Media literacy is a young field, evolving over the last 2 decades in response to growing concern about how mass media affect children and the potential for media-based emotional, social, and financial manipulation. This chapter has outlined an approach for clinicians and parents which is highly individualized and family based. Differing definitions, perspectives, and methodologies add to the challenge of translating existing media research into advice parents can act upon. The availability, content and interactivity of media are evolving so quickly that research done even a few years ago may offer little guidance.

For example, there is a body of research focused on reducing "screen time" at the family or school level. The goal is typically to decrease sedentary behavior or reduce obesity. Results are mixed, but useful recommendations include setting goals for screen time, using parental controls to limit TV or computer time, and trying an occasional "TV turnoff" week.[71-73] Excessive time sitting and consuming passive media is indeed a concern, but it is only one aspect of children's media use today. A focus on media content choices, the context of media use, and motivations for use may be more fruitful than a focus on hours of consumption.

Potential positives of media also deserve equal time. For example, interactive games may help children and adolescents make friends, discover new interests, express their creativity by creating or modifying content, regulate difficult emotions through play or even engage in physical activity. In multiplayer games, they can experiment with different identities through the roles they choose to play and gain experience in leading and cooperating.[74]

We need to know more about ways that the dose of media, context of media use, and children's temperament, experiences, and relationships might mediate any positive or negative effects. We can, however, draw some comfort from the knowledge that children are influenced overwhelmingly by the values and behavior of their parents (and how they are treated by others, especially caregivers and teachers). Children are in general resilient with an amazing capacity to adapt to the world. Parents, as they do for many areas of the child's life, must assess their own values and experiences, listen to various experts, and then guide the child toward productive autonomy. This includes parents becoming more conscious of their own media use, especially during family time, and setting a reasonable example.

On a societal level, concerns about media's influence—especially on violence and social isolation—can be mitigated by addressing issues known to affect children's healthy development, such as day care, educational opportunities, after-school activities, adequate healthcare, access to mental health services, and protection from violence in the home. Efforts to give parents and families more time together and to provide high-quality care for children when parents are absent are the positive supports that will help children and families cope with rapid cultural change.

ACKNOWLEDGMENTS

This chapter is an updated and revised version of Media Literacy for Clinicians and Parents by V. Susan Villani, Cheryl K. Olson, and Michael Jellinek (2005). We gratefully acknowledge the previous contributions of Drs Villani and Jellinek.

REFERENCES

1. David-Ferdon CF, Haileyesus T, Liu Y, Simon TR, Kresnow M. Nonfatal assaults among persons aged 10—24 years—United States, 2001—2015. *CDC Morb Mortal Wkly Rep.* 2018;67(5):141—145.

2. Wartella EA, Jennings N. Children and computers: new technology, old concerns. *Future Child*. 2000;10(2):31–43.

3. Thoman E, Jolls T. Media literacy - a national priority for a changing world. *Am Behav Sci*. 2004;48(1):18–29.

4. McClure ER, Chentsova-Dutton YE, Barr RF, Holochwost SJ, Parrott WG. "Facetime doesn't count": video chat as an exception to media restrictions for infants and toddlers. *Int J Child-Computer Interact*. 2015;6:1–6.

5. AAP Council on Communications and Media. Media and young minds (policy statement). *Pediatrics*. 2016;138(5):1–6.

6. Certain LK, Kahn RS. Prevalence, correlates and trajectory of television viewing among infants and toddlers. *Pediatrics*. 2002;109(4):634–642.

7. Lapierre MA, Piotrowski JT, Linebarger DL. Background television in the homes of US children. *Pediatrics*. 2012;130(5):839–846.

8. Barr R. Memory constraints on infant learning from picture books, television, and touchscreens. *Child Dev Perspect*. 2013;7(4):205–210.

9. Strouse GA, Ganea PA. Toddlers' word learning and transfer from electronic and print books. *J Exp Child Psychol*. 2017;156:129–142.

10. Anderson DA, Pempeck TA. Television and very young children. *Am Behav Sci*. 2005;48(5):505–522.

11. Radesky JS, Schumacher J, Zuckerman B. Mobile and interactive media use by young children: the good, the bad, and the unknown. *Pediatrics*. 2015;135(1).

12. Wood JM, Duke NK. Inside "Reading Rainbow": a spectrum of strategies for promoting literacy. *Lang Arts*. 1997;74(2):95–106.

13. Wright JC, Huston AC, Murphy KC, et al. The relations of early television viewing to school readiness and vocabulary of children from low-income families: the Early Window Project. *Child Dev*. 2001;72(5):1347–1366.

14. Valkenburg PM. Media and youth consumerism. *J Adolesc Health*. 2000;27S:52–56.

15. te Velde SJ, van Nassau F, Uijtdewilligen L, et al. Energy balance-related behaviours associated with overweight and obesity in preschool children: a systematic review of prospective studies. *Obes Rev*. 2012;13(suppl 1):56–74.

16. Dennison BA, Erb TA, Jenkins PL. Television viewing and television in bedroom associated with overweight risk among low-income preschool children. *Pediatrics*. 2002;109:1028–1035.

17. Li X, Atkins MS. Early childhood computer experience and cognitive and motor development. *Pediatrics*. 2004;113(6):1715–1722.

18. Meersand P. Early latency and the impact of the digital world: exploring the effect of technological games on evolving ego capacities, superego development, and peer relationships. *Psychoanal Study Child*. 2017;70(1):117–129.

19. Verenikina I, Kervin L, Rivera M, Lidbetter A. Digital play: exploring young children's perspectives on applications designed for preschoolers. *Glob Stud Child*. 2016;6(4):1–12.

20. Cantor J. Studying children's emotion reactions to mass media. In: Dervin B, Grossberg L, O'Keefe B, Wartella E, eds. *Rethinking Communication, Vol 2: Paradigm Exemplars*. Newbury Park, CA: Sage; 1989.

21. Cantor J, Omdahl BL. Effects of fictional media depictions of realistic threats on children's emotion responses, expectations, worries, and liking for related activities. *Commun Monogr*. 1991;58:384–401.

22. Rideout VJ, Foehr UG, Roberts DF. *Generation M2: Media in the Lives of 8- to 18-Year Olds*. Kaiser Family Foundation Report; 2010. Available at: https://www.kff.org/other/report/generation-m2-media-in-the-lives-of-8-to-18-year-olds/.

23. Thomas A, Chess S, Birch HG. *Temperament and Behavior Disorders in Children*. New York: New York University Press; 1968.

24. Arriaga P, Esteves F, Carneiro P, Monteiro MB. Violent computer games and their effects on state hostility and physiological arousal. *Aggress Behav*. 2006;32:146–158.

25. Ferguson CJ, Olson CK, Kutner LA, Warner DE. Violent video games, catharsis seeking, bullying and delinquency: a multivariate analysis of effects. *Crime Delinquency*. 2014;60(5):764–784.

26. Federal Interagency Forum on Child and Family Statistics. *America's Children: Key National Indicators of Well-Being*; 2017. http://childstats.gov.

27. Matsa KE. *Fewer Americans Rely on TV News; what Type They Watch Varies by Who They Are*. Pew Research Website; January 5, 2018. http://www.pewresearch.org/fact-tank/2018/01/05/fewer-americans-rely-on-tv-news-what-type-they-watch-varies-by-who-they-are/.

28. Kaiser Family Foundation. *Survey Snapshot: Teens, Sex and TV*. Pub #3229; 2002. Available at: www.kff.org.

29. Singer DG, Singer JL. Developing critical viewing skills and media literacy in children. *Ann Am Acad Polit Soc Sci*. 1998;557:164–179.

30. Kaiser Family Foundation. *Key Facts: Media Literacy*. Publication #3383. Fall 2003.

31. Shellenbarger S. Most students don't know when news is fake, Stanford study finds. *Wall Str J*; November 22, 2016. https://www.wsj.com/articles/most-students-dont-know-when-news-is-fake-stanford-study-finds-1479752576.

32. Stanford History Education Group. Evaluating Information: The Cornerstone of Civic Online Reasoning. Available at: https://stacks.stanford.edu/file/druid:fv751yt5934/SHEG%20Evaluating%20Information%20Online.pdf.

33. Edgerly S, Thorson K, Thorson E, Vraga EK, Bode L. Do parents still model news consumption? Socializing news use among adolescents in a multi-device world. *New Media Soc*. 2018;4:1263–1281. https://doi.org/10.1177/1461444816688451.

34. Jones LM, Mitchell KJ, Finkelhor D. Trends in youth internet victimization: findings from three youth internet safety surveys 2000-2010. *J Adolesc Health*. 2012;50:179–186.

35. Federal Trade Commission. *Kids and Computer Security*; 2011. https://www.consumer.ftc.gov/articles/0017-kids-and-computer-security.

36. Peter J, Valkenburg PM. Adolescents and pornography: a review of 20 years of research. *J Sex Res.* 2016;53:509−531.

37. Häggström-Nordin E, Borneskog C, Eriksson M, Tydén T. Sexual behaviour and contraceptive use among Swedish high school students in two cities: comparisons between genders, study pro- grammes, and over time. *Eur J Contracept Reprod Health Care.* 2011;16(1):36−46.

38. Cowan G, Campbell RR. Rape causal attitudes among adolescents. *J Sex Res.* 1995;32(2):145−153.

39. Steinberg L, Monahan KC. Adolescent's exposure to sexy media does not hasten the initiation of sexual intercourse. *Dev Psychol.* 2011;47(2):562−576.

40. Collins RL, Strasburger VC, Brown JD, et al. Sexual media and childhood well-being and health. *Pediatrics.* 2017;140(suppl 2):S162−S166.

41. Braun-Courville DK, Rojas M. Exposure to sexually explicit web sites and adolescent sexual attitudes and behaviors. *J Adolesc Health.* 2009;45:156−162.

42. Durkin K. Videogames and young people with developmental disorders. *Rev Gen Psychol.* 2010;14(2):122−140.

43. Dogruel L, Joeckel S. Video game rating systems in the US and Europe: comparing their outcomes. *Int Commun Gaz.* 2013;75(7):672−692.

44. Rideout V. *Parents, Children & Media.* Kaiser Family Foundation; 2007. https://files.eric.ed.gov/fulltext/ED542901.pdf.

45. Gabrielli J, Traore A, Stoolmiller M, Bergamini E, Sargent JD. Industry television ratings for violence, sex, and substance use. *Pediatrics.* 2016;138(3):e20160487.

46. Federal Trade Commission. *Marketing Violent Entertainment to Children: A Review of Self-regulation and Industry Practices in Motion Picture, Music Recording & Electronic Game Industries.* Washington, DC; 2000.

47. Understanding the Film Ratings. Motion Picture Association of America Website. www.mpaa.org/film-ratings/.

48. Price J, Palsson C, Gentile D. What matters in movie ratings? Cross-country differences in how content influences mature movie ratings. *J Child Media.* 2014;3:240−252.

49. About the Ratings Process. ESRB Website. http://www.esrb.org/ratings/faq.aspx#14.

50. Entertainment Software Association. Essential Facts About the Computer and Video Game Industry: 2017 Sales, Demographic, and Usage Data. Available at: http://www.theesa.com/wp-content/uploads/2017/04/EF2017_Final-Digital.pdf.

51. Parental Advisory Label. Recording Industry Association of America Website. https://www.riaa.com/resources-learning/parental-advisory-label/.

52. Pan European Game Information. https://www.pegi.info.

53. Federal Trade Commission Report to Congress. *Marketing Violent Entertainment to Children: A Sixth Follow-up Review of Industry Practices in the Motion Picture, Music Recording & Electronic Game Industries.* Washington DC; 2009.

54. Federal Trade Commission. *FTC Undercover Shopper Survey on Entertainment Ratings Enforcement Finds Compliance Highest Among Video Game Sellers and Movie Theaters.* FTC Press Release; March 25, 2013. https://www.ftc.gov/news-events/press-releases/2013/03/ftc-undercover-shopper-survey-entertainment-ratings-enforcement.

55. Olson CK, Kutner LA, Warner DE, et al. Factors correlated with violent video game use by adolescent boys and girls. *J Adolesc Health.* 2007;41:77−83.

56. Leone R, Barowski L. MPAA ratings creep: a longitudinal analysis of the PG-13 rating category in US movies. *J Child Media.* 2011;5(1):53−68.

57. Jordan A. *Parents' Use of the V-Chip to Supervise Children's Television Use.* Annenberg Public Policy Center, University of Pennsylvania; 2003.

58. NTCA Foundation-The Internet & Television Association. TV Parental Controls. https://www.controlwithcable.org/tv-parental-controls-2/.

59. Entertainment Software Rating Board. Parent Resoures Center: Setting Controls. https://www.esrb.org/about/settingcontrols.aspx.

60. Common Sense Media. *Everything You Need to Know about Parental Controls*; July 14, 2016. https://www.commonsensemedia.org/blog/everything-you-need-to-know-about-parental-controls.

61. Federal Bureau of Investigation. *Consumer Notice: Internet-connected Toys Could Present Privacy and Contact Concerns for Children.* FBI public service annoucement; July 17, 2017. https://www.ic3.gov/media/2017/170717.aspx.

62. Silfversten E. *A Smart Toy Could Have Personal Details for Life, Not Just for Christmas.* RAND Blog; December 23, 2017. https://www.rand.org/blog/2017/12/a-smart-toy-could-have-personal-details-for-life-not.html.

63. Federal Trade Commission. *Protecting Your Child's Privacy Online*; July 2013. https://www.consumer.ftc.gov/articles/0031-protecting-your-childs-privacy-online.

64. Connect Safely. Safety Tips and Advice. http://www.connectsafely.org/safety-tips-advice/.

65. Anderson M. *Parents, Teens and Digital Monitoring.* Pew Research Center Report; January 2016. Available at: http://www.pewinternet.org/2016/01/07/parents-teens-and-digital-monitoring/.

66. Nazerian T. *Need to Go on a 'tech Diet'? Current Ways to Fight Your Device Addiction.* EdSurge Website; 9, 2018. https://www.edsurge.com/news/2018-02-09-need-to-go-on-a-tech-diet-current-ways-to-fight-your-device-addiction.

67. https://families.google.com/familylink/privacy/notice/.

68. Stark PB. The effectiveness of Internet content filters. *A J Law Policy Inf Soc.* 2008;4(2):411−429.

69. Ybarra ML, Finkelhor D, Mitchell KJ, Wolak J. Associations between blocking, monitoring, and filtering software on the home computer and youth-reported unwanted exposure to sexual material online. *Child Abuse Neglect.* 2009;33:857−869.

70. Wait Until 8th Website. https://www.waituntil8th.org/.
71. Wahi G, Parkin PC, Beyene J, Uleryk EM, Birken CS. Effectiveness of interventions aimed at reducing screen time in children: a systematic review and meta-analysis of randomized controlled trials. *Arch Pediatr Adolesc Med.* 2011; 165(11):979–986.
72. Altenburg TM, Kist-van Holthe J, Chinapaw M. Effectiveness of intervention strategies exclusively targeting reductions in children's sedentary time: a systematic review of the literature. *Int J Behav Nutr Phys Activity.* 2016;13:65.
73. Schmidt ME, Haines J, O'Brien A, et al. Systematic review of effective strategies for reducing screen time among young children. *Obesity.* 2012;20:1338–1354.
74. Olson CK. Children's motivations for video game play in the context of normal development. *Rev Gen Psychol.* 2010;14:180–187.

CHAPTER 8

Functional Assessment of Social Media in Child and Adolescent Psychiatry

CAROLY PATAKI, MD • JEFF Q. BOSTIC, MD, EdD • KARA TABOR-FUMARK, MD • MICHAEL FELDMEIER, MD • ROXY SZEFTEL, MD • STEVE SCHLOZMAN, MD • ERIC PIACENTINI, BS

KEY POINTS

- Social media promotes social connectedness in youth
- Functional assessment of social media can identify risks and benefits for youth
- Social media promotes resilience and wellbeing
- High social media use is associated with psychological distress

INTRODUCTION

Young people in every generation personify current trends in social communication in contemporary culture. Millennials, (Generation-Y), those born between 1977 and 1995, our social media pioneers, represent the first cohort to embrace social media as an integral part of daily life. Millennials, now "the parents" and Generation-Z (Gen-Z) utilize social media in surprisingly similar ways, seamlessly "multi-tasking" with various devices, throughout the day and into the night.[1,2]

Youth today represent Gen-Z, those born between 1996 and 2009, social and digital media "natives,"[1] who are effortlessly fluent with social media platforms including Facebook, Texting, Snapchat, Instagram, YouTube, and Twitter,[1] as well as with digital media such as live video gaming.[1] For today's youth, social media is no longer primarily for "entertainment," but instead it is embedded in their daily lifestyle.[1] These youth are experts in the ongoing ebb and flow of engagement and interaction with peers, friends, admirers, and family, generating an ever-expanding set of social connections at many levels and geographic distances. The explosion of social and digital media in the past 2 decades has catapulted today's youth into a whirlwind of multifaceted social engagement with continuous repartee.

Social and digital media pervade the daily lives of youth. The impacts of social media on mood and behavior, positive and negative, affirming and disparaging, have profound and far-reaching influences on the development of today's youth. Growing up with devices ever present to communicate with "virtual friends" and in "virtual realities" has dramatically altered the way that youth engage with each other, and their parents. The net effect of this shift, with one's physical presence now eclipsed by an endless supply of novel virtual "others" is yet to be fully investigated and understood. A "functional assessment" of social and digital media can provide a window into youths' inner world and illuminate their level of social connectedness through social media, as well as enhance an understanding of their cognitive and emotional development.

SOCIAL MEDIA PLATFORMS POPULAR WITH YOUTH

The proliferation of social media has provided numerous opportunities for youth to interact spontaneously with peers and to share thoughts and reactions instantaneously, using a variety of unique social networking sites. Described below are some of the more familiar and popular social media platforms frequently used by youth:

Facebook: A social media platform founded in 2004 by Mark Zuckerberg and peers, which connects users with friends, family, acquaintances, and businesses and enables connections to friends of friends. Facebook allows users to post messages, pictures, and videos to Facebook friends and Facebook groups, whose members can share, "like," "dislike," and comment. Facebook offers a complex "timeline" of autobiographical events and updates that can be posted and viewed. The platform currently has around 1.6 billion active users.[3]

YouTube: A video-sharing platform founded in 2005 that allows users to make and upload a personal video on almost anything, from instructions on how to set up a printer, for example, to stand-up- comic videos. Users can view, rate, and share videos. One billion active users watch YouTube videos each month.[3]

Twitter: Started in 2006; a social network that allows users to tweet up to 140-character messages to their followers and to retweet the tweets of others, enabling followers to view tweets of other users whom they are not following.[3]

Instagram: Launched in 2010; this photo-sharing application enables users to take photos, apply filters to their images, and share the photos instantly. The app is targeted toward mobile social sharing and has currently gained more than 700 million users.[4]

Snapchat: Launched in 2011 is an app that allows users to send and receive time-sensitive photos and videos known as "snaps," which "disappear" from the recipient's screen once the brief time limit expires (images and videos still remain on the Snapchat server).[3]

The integration of digital and social media into the lives of children and teens is a worldwide phenomenon (where the devices and Internet are available). A school-based survey of 404,523 11- to 15-year-olds from 30 European and North American regions,[5] in collaboration with data from a World Health Organization survey,[6] found a trend for increased use of social media to predict greater ease in personal interactions with friends of the opposite sex.[5] In contrast to the typical belief of some that adolescent social media may be associated with social isolation, the authors of the school-based study conclude it can instead be helpful to youth in initiating in-person connections with peers.[5]

However, given the vast reach of social media used by youth, from engaging with friends, to "meeting" strangers online, to seeking infinite and constant stimulation, parameters are needed for youth to maintain safe and healthy use of it. The benefits and risks of social media in assisting youth to fine-tune social skills and increase social connections are becoming evident.[7] Converging evidence from genetic, behavioral, and neuroimaging studies shows bidirectional influences between social connectedness and healthy brain development during adolescence.[7] Risks and potentially negative influences of social media may be exerted on mood and behavior, especially in vulnerable youth. Overall, social media offers a unique opportunity to expand adolescent social connections and engagement and promotes resilience and well-being.[7] Identifying the optimal forms of social media and degree of use for a given youth can be approached through a functional assessment of the benefits and risks for that youth.

THE EVOLUTION OF SOCIAL MEDIA

Until the early 2000s, more traditional forms of media predominated such as television (TV), telephone, music via compact discs, TV music videos, radio, magazines, newspapers, and movies. Traditional media, lacking the "live" interaction that is social media's draw, is noticeably less appealing to today's youth. A generation ago, it seemed alarming that US high school students were spending more hours per day watching television than they spent in school.[8] A survey almost 20 years ago concluded that youth, from elementary school through high school spend 6–8 hours per day immersed in media.[9] Despite the high level of media usage among youth at that time, few long-term studies monitored the effect of technology on the quality of their lives.

An increasing array of social and digital platforms comprise the media diets of children and adolescents, while TV viewing has decreased significantly in preschoolers and to a lesser degree in school-age children.[10,11] A study in 2015[12] found that 96% of US preschool-age children from a low-income pediatric clinic had access to a mobile device and 75% reported that they owned one. 92.2% of children as young as 1–2 years of age in this study[12] had already used a mobile device. The American Academy of Pediatrics recently published a policy statement (Council on Communications and Media) and a technical report[11] based on a comprehensive review of the literature on the benefits and risks of social and digital media in youth. A very brief summary of their findings is provided below.

SOCIAL MEDIA IN EARLY CHILDHOOD

Very early in life, children are now regularly exposed to social and digital media by parents. Very young children, 2 years and younger, appear to benefit most from digital media such as videos, interactive touch screens, and touch screen games, when adult caregivers are part of the interaction.[11,13] There is some evidence that in very young children, building a "relationship" with a screen character may promote learning in the short-term.[11,14] Current consensus indicates that social media use in young toddlers is most effective when it is engaged in jointly with an adult.[11]

SOCIAL MEDIA IN SCHOOL-AGED CHILDREN

The data are both limited and mixed regarding the benefits and risks of high levels of social media use in school-aged children. Limitations of existing studies include small numbers of subjects, variable methodologies, and varied targets and outcome measures used, leading to questions about how closely these studies can be generalized to a population of school-aged children in the United States.[7,11,15] One of the interesting findings, however, is that social media "multitasking," assumed to be typically adolescent preoccupation, is also frequent in school-aged children,[11] who use it while playing with peers or doing homework. Among the benefits of social media use in this age group are increased exposure to new ideas, new social contacts, and learning about diversity through social media exposures. Risks of social media use, particularly evident in youth with extensive use, include the long daily sedentary periods contributing to obesity, diminished in-person peer interactions, and negative effects on sleep.[11] Use of social media has been associated with elevated risk of impaired impulse control, poor self-regulation, and poor mental flexibility.[15]

SOCIAL MEDIA IN ADOLESCENTS

Social connectedness of adolescents to peers, friends, family, teammates etc. through a multitude of social media and in-person experiences is critical to emotional and psychological well-being and optimal neurobiological brain development.[7] Adolescence, however, is also a developmental period of risk taking, evolving social judgment, and the emergence of many psychiatric disorders. Social media in adolescence may lead to health and safety risks, especially in vulnerable teens with emerging psychiatric illness, depression, and/or poor impulse control. As an example, the dangerous and seemingly ubiquitous habit of texting while driving can lead to devastating consequences. Social media use in adolescents presents specific challenges with respect to individuation and sense of self-worth and identity. First, the entire gamut of "cyber criticism" to cyberbullying can have significant and long-term impacts on mood, sense of self-esteem, and depressive ideation. The "metrics" of social media can also alter how youth evaluate their "status" and identity. For example, reactions to posts from friends on Facebook, including how many "Likes" they receive for a post, or negative responses may validate their self-perception, or lead to feelings of rejection and dejection.[16]

DIGITAL MEDIA PLATFORMS POPULAR WITH YOUTH: SOCIAL VIDEO GAMES

Many children and adolescents are hesitant to express emotional or sensitive information but are quite willing to converse about themselves regarding an activity they are motivated by and highly interested in—video games. Given the pervasive use of video games by today's youth, experts recommend a broader perspective on video games, with clinicians balancing benefits against potential risks and negative effects of problematic video gaming.[17] Video game playing is typically a daily activity and preoccupation for many youth, so clinician literacy about gaming provides a valuable opportunity to better understand the importance of gaming among youth. Acceptance of daily video game use as "typical," facilitates a dialog with young patients. The Video Game Initial Questionnaire (VG-IQ)[18] (see Appendix 8.1) takes a broad view of the social context of the video game diet of today's youth and elicits information about favorite video games, habits while playing, how social an activity it is, and what impacts it has on the rest of the youth's life.

Video game play serves as not only an individualized experience but has also evolved to facilitate social interaction on a number of levels. Seventy-two percent of 13- to 17-year-olds play video games on a computer, game console, or portable device, with 84% of boys and 59% of girls playing regularly.[19] Through this modality, children and teens "meet" new people to play with online, form relationships with online players, and may strengthen existing friendships. Communication usually takes place over a microphone chat or through typed text. Young people can also view other players who broadcast themselves playing over several media channels including YouTube, Twitch, and Facebook. Young video gamers can also communicate through message boards and walls with other spectators in real time. A young person's ability to broadcast him-self or herself to millions of viewers with a few clicks of a button has been facilitated by intrinsic features in con-sole and computer hardware. Players can then inform potential viewers of their participation through social media outlets such as Twitter, Facebook, Instagram, or Snapchat.

SOCIAL MEDIA AND DIGITAL MEDIA EXPOSURE FOR AMERICAN YOUTH: 2017

Youth of all ages are enthusiastic participants and vora-cious consumers of assorted social media platforms and digital media. For a majority of US teens, a smartphone, nearly a bodily appendage, enables them to reach out to peers and contacts in an instant, at any time of the day or night. For US adolescents, laptops and/or iPads are also rarely far away and used daily.[19]

The PEW Research Center report[19] examined the use of technology and social media in 1060 teens aged 13−17 years.

Table 8.1[19] reveals that the vast majority of US teen-agers have and use smartphones daily. Facebook re-mains the most highly used social media networking

TABLE 8.1
Social and Digital Media Use in US Teens

Social/Digital Media Platform	All Teens	Female Teens	Male Teens
Facebook	71%	70%	72%
Facebook friends[a]	145	175	72
Instagram	52%	61%	44%
Instagram followers[a]	150	200	100
Snapchat	41%	51%	31%
Any cell phone	88%		
Smart phone	73%		
Texting (among cell owners)	91%		
Texts sent or received/day[a]	30	40	20
Twitter	33%	37%	30%
Twitter followers[a]	95	116	61
Video games (console)	80%	70%	91%
Video games (online or phone)	71%	59%	84%

[a] Median number.

site and is used by boys and girls similarly. Most teens use multiple social media sites and go online daily. About a quarter of teens are online "constantly." Female teens are more engaged in social media that favors con-versations and posting pictures, while male teens are more engaged in action-based video gaming.[19]

The data are mixed regarding the impact of social media on youth' physical and emotional health. Strong interpersonal social support systems, including those through social media can positively impact and miti-gate psychological stress.[20] Facebook users with greater numbers of Facebook friends report higher levels of perceived social support and psychological well-being.[20] On the other hand, a critical factor determining positive or negative impacts of social media on adoles-cents is how a teen or young adult feels during and after social media interactions.[20] Young adult social media users vary in their comfort level while using social media and feeling overwhelmed by it.[20] College social media users who experienced "communication over-load" reported psychological distress and diminished self-esteem.[21] "Communication overload" appears to mediate the sequelae of negative self-esteem.[21] In healthy adolescents with reasonable use of social me-dia, data suggests positive self-esteem and increased sense of social connectedness.[7]

INFLUENCE OF SOCIAL AND DIGITAL MEDIA ON YOUTH DEVELOPMENT AND BEHAVIOR
Social Media, Self-Esteem, and Peer Friendships

Studies examining social media use in adolescents and their self-esteem have found that higher use can be asso-ciated with positive or negative self-esteem.[7,20,22] Emotionally, healthy teens who use social media regularly, but not excessively, generally feel more con-nected to their peers, share parts of their lives, and derive a sense of well-being through engaging with their peers, all of which promote positive self-esteem.[22] On the other hand, teens who use social media excessively due to fear of missing out[23] have negative psychological consequences, especially in female ado-lescents. Conversely, adolescents with preexisting anxi-ety, depression, and ruminative qualities may feel internally driven toward excessive use of social media.[23]

Adolescents' self-esteem rating while using social media was found to be directly related to recent receipt of perceived positive and/or supportive feedback (associated with positive self-esteem) about their posts or profile, or negative feedback (associated with report of diminished self-esteem).[16]

Social and/or digital media can indeed be problematic when it replaces in-person peer relationships. Given the high level of stimulation derived from playing "live" video games with online peers, for example, a preference for online video game peers over in-person friends remains a risk particularly in youth with difficulties making and maintaining friends. For some children, games on iPhones, iPads, or even "live" video games serve as "virtual babysitters" impeding social interactions with peers and increasing their social isolation and peer rejection. Peer rejection, in turn, serves to further drive children to prefer gaming over real-life experiences with friends.[9]

Friendships among youth are often sparked by sharing similar music choices,[24,25] through social media or other digital platforms. Music available online is consumed more and assigned greater importance by adolescents and young adults compared to older adults.[24] Whereas choice of music in youth may enhance peer affiliation,[25] youth with lower self-esteem seem more likely to demean musical choices divergent from their own. Among adolescents, music choices may contribute to both the selection and discontinuation of friends.[25]

CASE 1

Kim was a 14-year-old male teen who had recently moved to the US from Seoul, Korea. He had entered the ninth grade without knowing anyone, and though he understood English, he struggled to speak English fluently and was hesitant to speak to peers or teachers in school. Kim felt lonely the first few weeks of school because of his lack of familiarity with US teen culture and difficulty with spoken communication. Life changed for Kim when, one day, he was placed in a group of four for a science lab; his lab partners quickly traded phone numbers and social media handles with each other. As the group maintained contact, Kim particularly enjoyed using Snapchat because he could primarily communicate with his new friends through pictures without the pressures of having to speak perfect English. This prompted him to exchange Snapchat with other peers and his social network broadened.

Social Media's Impact on Female and Male Identity and Body Image

Social media is among the dominant influences on adolescents' internalization of ideal body image. For past generations of female adolescents "appearance magazines" (such as Teen, Cosmo Girl, and Seventeen) were reported to influence their ideas of perfect body image, and for up to half of adolescent females, magazine pictures induced them to diet.[26] Early adolescent girls across many different cultural backgrounds gravitate toward comparing themselves to each other and their ideals. These comparisons are facilitated by social media platforms such as Facebook, where pictures can be easily and quickly posted to all of one's Facebook friends (and sometimes their "friends"), with prompt responses to one's evolving sexual and feminine identities.

A study of 438 young female 13- to 15-year-olds surveyed over 3 years found that both Facebook use and body image concerns increased over this interval.[27] While this may simply represent an increased focus on appearance with increasing age, increased body image concern reported at the outset, interestingly, predicted more Facebook friends prospectively, generally associated with positive self-esteem in teens.[27] On the other hand, a systematic review of the impact of social networking on body image concern and eating disorders[28] found increased social networking in adolescents to be directly related to both body image concerns and eating disordered behaviors. The correlation between increased social network use and body image concerns and eating disorder behaviors was found in male teens as well as females.[28]

Social Media's Influence on Sexual Attitudes and Behaviors

Current social media platforms contribute to adolescent notions of sexuality by providing access to a wide range of sexual information and erotica. Sexual material is easily accessible online, with the potential for live sexting, or sharing sexual photos or videos. Sexting with a stranger, for example, may at first seem harmless, arousing, and a way to interest another person; however, it may progress to unwanted overtures or actual sexual "threats" or unwanted acts of sharing photos with individuals or in more public places.

Video games, Internet chat rooms, and Web sites provide ample options for adolescents to explore sexual interests. An international survey of 11- to 15-year-olds from 30 countries in Europe and North America reported that electronic media communication led to increased ease in communicating with the opposite sex.[5] Digital media including Web-based sites and social networking sites are now being launched to provide sex education and sexual health information.[29] A recent social media–delivered sexual health intervention[30] for young adults (16- to 25-year-olds) sent to their Facebook showed increased use of condoms to prevent sexually transmitted diseases in a 2-month follow-up. The use of social media to influence sexual attitudes and sexual risk behaviors in the short-term continues to be explored.

Social Media and Aggression

Cyberbullying is a significant public health concern in youth, in some cases leading to serious mental health problems including school refusal, depression, anxiety, and even suicide.[31] Exposure to some violent material through social and digital media seems inevitable in our society, and exposure often begins in early childhood. In past generations, evidence suggested that regular viewing of violence in media among young adults was associated with an acceptance of violent solutions to conflict and desensitization and reduced tendency to feel sympathy for a victim.[32] Traditional bullying and cyberbullying have been reported to share similar psychological outcomes among youth, including suicidal ideation and suicidal behaviors.[33] The frequency of youth cyberbullying has been difficult to ascertain due to the lack of a precise definition, leading to a wide range of reported cyberbullying prevalence rates with a median of 23%.[34] The relationship between social media and cyberbullying are complex with a consensus that cyberbullying occurs mainly among youth, with marginal rates in adulthood.[31] The most commonly cited social media platforms on which cyberbullying occurs include Facebook, texting, Twitter, and rarely Instagram.[31]

CASE 2

Jessica was a 16-year-old popular junior in high school (HS) who has been dating Cliff, the pitcher of their HS baseball team, also aged 16 years, for the past 6 months. Jessica and Cliff entered into a sexual relationship early in their relationship, and Jessica would often sext Cliff revealing pictures of herself when they were apart which she thought of as "special" and fun. Recently, Jessica decided that they needed some time apart because her parents were pressuring her to spend more time studying for the SAT. Cliff was crushed by her rejection of him and texted the entire baseball team intimate pictures of her, which she had previously sent to him. The next day at school, many male students made lewd comments to her about her body. Jessica ignored their comments, but they continued to harass her for the next week. Jessica felt so humiliated and powerless that she refused to go back to school. Isolated and demoralized, Jessica began to have suicidal thoughts, which she did not act on.

Social Media's Impact on Anxiety and Depression

Given the universal use of social media use among today's US youth, research is evaluating the relationship between social media use and mood and anxiety disorders. Studies have identified both positive and negative outcomes of social media on youth. Positive outcomes associated with social media use include increased social capital, perceived social support, and life satisfaction.[35] Other potential benefits include provision of a forum for practicing socializing and empathy, particularly for introverted youth, and the ability to connect with like-minded peers, thereby bolstering self-esteem.[22] However, a trend in research of extremely high users of social media sites suggests a negative association between social media use and mental health in young adults.[36]

Multiple cross-sectional studies in the United States and internationally have concluded that high frequency social media use in young adults correlates with an increased frequency of depression, perhaps through mediating factors if not directly.[37] In one study, individuals in the highest quartile of social media site visits per week had nearly three times the odds of developing depression (adusted odds ratio 2.74, 95% confidence interval 1.86−4.04).[37] A Lebanese study conducted in the same year found that higher specific use of Facebook-related tools, such as the "like" and "add friend" buttons, was also associated with depression.[38] Higher use of social media has been associated with both depression and anxiety, including social anxiety and obsessive-compulsive disorder.[36]

Conversely, a study of how depressed adolescents use social media found both "positive use" and "negative use" of social media.[39] In this study, depressed adolescents' mood was reported to improve when they used social media "positively," that is, for entertainment, distraction, to seek social connection, or as a creative outlet.[39] However, when depressed adolescents used social media "negatively,", that is, posting negative comments, sharing risky behaviors, cyberbullying, or comparing themselves to others, they had exacerbations of depressed mood.[39]

Researchers are also examining whether the type of engagement in social media can predict the likelihood of depression and anxiety. When social media networks are used to maintain and strengthen social ties with family and close friends, the resulting social support can be beneficial.[40] Researchers compared active consumption to passive consumption of social media.

In the context of Facebook use, active consumption is defined as the interactions on the site between a user and a friend, including text exchanges, feedback such as clicking the "like" button, and photo tagging. Passive consumption is the degree to which users pay attention to the general broadcasts shared by their friends (including status updates and public conversations) without reciprocally engaging. The authors concluded that active communication had a positive effect on well-being by increasing bonding social capital.[40] This makes intuitive sense as personal messages exchanged between friends and family serve to facilitate and maintain relationships. In contrast, passive consumption of social media content was associated with a decrease in social capital and an increase in loneliness.[40] Teens are also prone to immediate "contagion" of behaviors, both positive and negative, which social media, including Facebook, Instagram, and Twitter, have empowered due to the ease of posts reaching so many "friends" and "followers" instantaneously. The advantages of this "mega" communication ability are that many creative and positive ideas and works of art, music, and writing can be easily shared. The dangers, however, include potential "contagion" or "copycat" of self-destructive and suicidal behaviors. For individuals who have had suicidal thoughts or behaviors in the past, the risks of suicide attempts may be even higher.

The directionality of the relationship between deleterious forms of social media use and depression remains unclear and supports the need for clinicians and researchers to investigate the functions that social media serves youth and young adults.

- Do depressed or socially anxious individuals turn to social media for validation? For these individuals, social media interactions may offer a less intimidating forum for social engagement than face-to-face ones.
- Does frequent social media use take the place of more valuable and emotionally healthy face-to-face interactions, creating a cycle of isolation which may contribute to thereby depression? In addition, does the feeling of "time wasted" by spending time on social media negatively influence mood?[39]
- Does exposure to unrealistic portrayals on social media give the impression that others are more beautiful, intelligent, or moral or simply living happier lives, leading to envy and depression via social comparison?[39]

The relationship between social media use and depression is likely bidirectional. Newer studies, with the capacity to directly observe and manipulate participants' social media use, will allow for more definitive conclusions.

CASE 3

Janine was a 17½-year-old teen with a history of depression, anxiety, and self-harm behaviors including recurrent cutting. Janine considers herself artistic, with a strong interest in photography, and often takes pictures. Janine is very responsive to positive feedback about her photos that she posts on Facebook and Instagram. When Janine is feeling sad or hopeless, she looks at her old posts and reads the positive comments left by friends and followers. This lifts her mood considerably. Additionally, Janine boosts her own spirits and supports her friends by commenting positive things on their posts. Janine has found consistent solace and support by being involved with social media and surrounding herself with the positivity she draws from it.

PARENTAL PERCEPTIONS

Parents appear to vary dramatically in their awareness of social media networks that their children are using and hold diverse notions of acceptable versus risky social media used by their children.

- Among parents who are Facebook users, the vast majority of parents (83%) say they're "Facebook friends" with their teenager.[19]
- 55% of parents limit the amount of time their children spends online.[19]
- 65% of parents engage in "digital grounding."[19]

CASE 4

Henry is an 11-year-old boy who has always been temperamental and prone to conflict with peers. He received a basketball role-playing video game he can play with others in person or alone. Henry enjoyed the game, and briefly played with a local peer, but then complained the peer didn't keep up, so he began playing more alone. Parents report he has been so engaged in the game that it has begun interfering with his homework and that he will "sneak" play until late into the night. When invited to a friend's sleepover, he told parents he'd rather stay home and catch up on his game.

FUNCTIONAL ASSESSMENT OF SOCIAL AND DIGITAL MEDIA IN PSYCHIATRIC EVALUATION OF YOUTH

The social media and digital media diets of our child and adolescent patients warrant careful assessment. Existing data suggest that the social media diet of youth profoundly affects their social connectedness, peer relationships, and physical and emotional health and brain development.[7,16,20–23] A useful model for the examination of the influences—positive and negative—of social and digital media on youth is exemplified by a functional assessment of social and digital media diet in their daily lives. An example of such an assessment tool is provided here to illuminate impacts of social media and identify specific functions of social media in a given youth's life.

WHAT IS A FUNCTIONAL MEDIA ASSESSMENT?

A functional assessment seeks to derive the function served by a given behavior or activity. Often used clinically with youth to understand and better predict undesirable behaviors, functional assessments typically involve the identification of the settings or context in which the behaviors occur, including the antecedents to behavior, description of the undesired behavior, and the actual consequence of that behavior.[41] For example, a high school student with academic skill deficits who shares funny YouTube videos on his phone during math class and receives negative feedback from the teacher for being disruptive may "accomplish" a diversion from academic tasks and/or attain peer status, which sustains the seemingly dysfunctional behavior. The functional assessment of social and digital media use seeks to identify the potential constructive and destructive functions that the specific media use serves so that appropriate interventions may be identified.

A youth, for example, may surf the Internet to find out health-related information and seek support in online chat rooms about sensitive issues which appear to have a positive function; however, if this behavior is excessive, it may become negative as the adolescent fails to complete school assignments, resulting in conflicts with teachers and parents. Efforts by parents or clinicians to alter undesired behaviors require attention to their "functions" in order for a reasonable solution to be found. Clinicians are faced with the often formidable task of identifying the various perceptions by adolescents, parents, and teachers regarding the behaviors in question and developing an integrated functional assessment and plan. Attention to strengths and challenges and to overall motivation surrounding maladaptive behaviors remains paramount. The paradigm among youth of gravitating toward activities yielding immediate gratification is inherent to development but may be markedly amplified for modern youth due to the immediacy of reciprocal interactions with peers on social media and its easy accessibility.

WHAT ARE THE COMPONENTS OF A FUNCTIONAL ASSESSMENT OF SOCIAL MEDIA?

The components of a functional media assessment include (1) identification of the daily social media diet, (2) antecedents the youth's social media use, (3) the social media behaviors of the youth, and (4) the consequences of their use of social media.

A systematic way to identify the social media diet and inquire about video game use is provided in Table 8.2 and Appendix 8.1, respectively.

THE SOCIAL MEDIA DIET

The specific media preferences of a youth can be ascertained by questions related to his or her daily consumption and about the context surrounding the consumption.

An assessment of the youth social and digital media diet might include the following questions to the youth and to parents or caregivers:

- What forms of social/digital media do you regularly use?
- How much time do you spend with each of your social/digital media platforms (e.g., Facebook, Instagram, Twitter, Texting on cell phone, computer video gaming, watching YouTube)?
- How much time do you spend each day (outside of school) with in-person relationships?
- Who monitors your media diet?
- What kind of social/digital media do your parents use, and how much social media do you use together?
- *How does the social media diet relate to a youth's development? Is this social media diet developmentally appropriate?*
- *Does the youth access social media that are "designed" for his or her age group?*
- *Does the youth understand the messages provided by the platform, and do the messages enhance this youth's life?*
- Given the easy accessibility to the Internet for today's youth and many social media sites, younger teens may seek out social media sites that they are

TABLE 8.2 Social Media "Diet"					
Social Media	**Setting**	**Antecedents**	**Behavior**	**Functions**	**Consequences**
Texting					
Facebook					
Instagram					
Snapchat					
Twitter					
Video games					
YouTube					
Chat rooms					

not prepared for, these interactions or feedback from strangers online can be disturbing to them.

- *How does the media diet support adolescent individuation and social connections?*
- *Does the social media diet assist youths in making helpful peer choices?*

SETTINGS

The settings of social/digital media may include comments that reveal antecedents to its use: "I play video games after school to relax and catch up with my online gaming players." "I go on Facebook to catch up with my friends intermittently from 4 p.m. to 11 p.m.," "I text my best friend when I'm really angry," or "I use a combination of Facebook, Snapchat, Instagram and texting for about 3 hours each night while I'm doing homework."

"Chat room" conversations, for example, may be social encounters that occupy hours with strangers and may expose vulnerable youth wittingly or unwittingly to planned sexual encounters that may exploit them.

Settings while engaging in social media are both revealing of a youth's level of connectedness, for example, engaging in social media mainly alone at home while others are present, and may even incur danger, for example, texting while driving or crossing the street without looking up.

ANTECEDENTS

After the settings are clarified, the circumstances leading to the use of social media can be explored, with particular attention to circumstances fueling positive interactions as well as dysfunctional/problematic use of social

media. For example, a youth may report going to play video games to block out family conflicts, when tired of schoolwork, or to sustain a romantic connection to a peer period

- When do you/your child engage with social media (times of day and hours/day)?
- What circumstances lead you/your child shifting to social media activities?
- When do you most notice that you/your child wants to engage in social media?

BEHAVIORS

Both positive and negative behaviors should be explored that are associated with social media use.

- What do you/your child most enjoy from social media?
- What happens when you engage with social media?
- Do you usually find that your mood changes, in what way?
- Do you lose track of time while you're engaged in social media?
- How do others (peers, friends, or family) describe you when you're online?
- Have any problems occurred during social media interactions (e.g., cyberbullying, feeling excluded, "hate' responses, depressed mood)?

CONSEQUENCES

The following questions may spark discussions that are useful in clarifying the consequences of social and digital media for a given youth:

- How does your/your child's social media diet impact daily life?

- How does social media affect your child's mood?
- Does social media usage incur risks for your child, such as texting while driving, or increase social isolation?
- How does social media impact your child's functioning?
  1. At school?
  2. At home?
  3. With family?
  4. With peers?

FUNCTIONS OF SOCIAL AND DIGITAL MEDIA

Once the setting, antecedents, behaviors, and consequences of social media are clarified, a clinician and child may determine the functions that these media play in the life of the youth.

Discussion of the social media use often can illuminate a youth's particular psychosocial challenges. Social media choices occur for reasons, and preoccupations often suggest desires to master particular conflicts. As functions of social media unfold, emerging themes can provide an open channel into the mind of a youth. For a clinician, learning about a youth's "favorite" social media platform, YouTube video choices, favored Web sites, and video game choices may provide insights into important aspects of the child or adolescent's inner world. Understanding how a given youth's social media diet influences his or her daily life may be helpful in eliciting mood, thought processes, and sense of self-esteem. For certain youth, a focus on their social media may elucidate important challenges around competency in social situations, body image perceptions, poor judgment, and/or difficulties with impulsivity. In other words, many of the developmental issues that are germane to children and adolescents may emerge through discussion of a social and digital media in a clinical setting.

FUNCTIONAL APPROACH TO SOCIAL AND DIGITAL MEDIA PROBLEM SOLVING

A functional assessment of social media may reveal targets for intervention. Youth are predictably influenced by the social media habits of their peers, older siblings, and parents. A functional assessment can identify antecedents and contexts that lead to unhelpful social media choices, and the consequences that youth encounter can spark therapeutic problem solving. For example, if a youth engages in a daily Internet chat with strangers and then increases chat time when a chat room "friend" is identified, risks potentially setting

up in-person meetings with strangers from the chat room. Therapeutic targets may include decreasing Internet chat and increasing opportunities in the "outside" world to develop meaningful and safe social encounters. This intervention could address potential social skill deficits that may be contributing to a predominance of Internet socializing. Adolescents who are uncomfortable disclosing personal information to adults are often more willing to discuss sensitive topics by describing how characters in a video game or avatars in an online interactive virtual "world" such as Second Life (secondlife.com)[42] might feel. The VG-IQ[18] (see Appendix 8.1) can be used to elicit information on video game functions for a given youth, its meaning to youth, and the potential problem behaviors related to it that will benefit from clinical intervention. Table 8.3 provides a functional structured approach to social media and digital media problem solving.

CLINICAL APPLICATIONS

The four case histories presented within this chapter reveal diverse clinical situations from which a functional assessment of social media can extract the functions served and consequences for each patient. Myriad functions may be identified and their consequences are elucidated. When social and digital consequences are harmful to a child or adolescent, a clinical intervention can be provided using more affirmative strategies with positive reinforcements. Table 8.4 presents a functional assessment of the social and digital media behaviors, with settings, antecedents, behaviors, functions, and consequences, using the case histories presented in this chapter.

The intervention targets for each of these cases become quite different. For Kim, his social media use has been helpful, yet also reveals needs for assistance with social relationships at his new school. Target interventions for Kim may include helping him to expand his social interactions by "practicing" in-person social interactions with his new friends, yet also "checking" with them through social media, to understand what is acceptable and appropriate. Jessica is in need of support to manage a disparaging reputation created by her peer (Cliff). Her awareness of how "viral" a picture could go/become and cannot be retracted. Interventions for her imminently will target how to cope with the harassment from male classmates about her body, and her "tarnished" image, how to identify her "real friends" and elicit their support to help her to resume school. Janine has not only found social media a positive way to "put herself out there" but has also followed what was modeled for her. For Henry, interventions will

TABLE 8.3
Functional Social and Digital Media Problem Solving Interventions

Social Media Problem (Examples)	Frequency	Severity	Skills Needed	Interventions Planned	Efficacy of Plan
1. Isolation from friends in-person					
2. Cyberbullied					
3. Playing videogames 24/7, can't wake up for school					
4. Rejection from social media "friends"					
5. Date raped after meeting a stranger through social media					
6. FOMO					
7. Feeling depressed after overstimulation on Facebook					
8. Feeling anxious after social media use					
9. Texting while driving					

FOMO, fear of missing out.

likely include utilizing videogames as a reward for do-ing schoolwork successfully, as well as a reward for engagingt meaningfully with peers. While limiting video game play, or even "removal" of it may seem helpful, the opportunities for finding/playing other games (as he becomes more independent) favor efforts now to help him "consume a healthy portion" of this part of his media diet.

CLINICIAN'S MEDIA LITERACY
The social and digital media diet affords clinicians a lens through which to focus on pertinent issues and modalities when engaging with youth. Clinicians can be more effective in their communication with and evaluation of youth by becoming literate in social and digital media and including a functional assessment of social and digital media in their psychiatric evalua-tions. The social media diet of a given youth often yields a useful gauge of sensitive issues impacting that child and provides a facile way of potentially connecting with that youth. Most youth are drawn to a range of social and digital media platforms used in "multi-tasking" style. The array of platforms yielding multiple loyalties to online friends, followers, and contacts is a virtual representation of the "developing" adolescent. Clinicians familiar with youths' social media diet are often positioned to help troubled young people

consider substituting similar, but healthier, social me-dia diet choices. The greater fluency that clinicians have with the social world of youth—for example, the staccato language of instant messaging and Twitter, the emotional impact of Facebook "friends" on mood and behavior, and the influences of the images of Insta-gram and Snapchat on friendships, the easier it is to begin a meaningful dialog with a young person.

The sheer enormity of social media exposure in youth, and its rapid fire lead a dialog about it to be both challenging and compelling. From texting, to chatting, to sharing ephemeral video images, to tweet-ing and Facebook "liking," these cumulative stimuli provide a snapshot of a youth's emotional life which can be reflected back in insightful ways. The dialog is "virtually" always well worth the effort.

FUTURE DIRECTIONS
Social media has transformed the way people commu-nicate and continues to expand and evolve at a rapid rate. Young users of "massively multiplayer online role-playing games" such as "World of Warcraft"[43] may seek newer versions with greater immersion, while other youthful users gravitate toward even easier access to social media networking by using novel devices such as Snapchat spectacles.[44] Social trends are now identi-fied rapidly through tweets from Twitter and the

TABLE 8.4
Functional Assessment of Social Media: Cases 1—4

Case	Setting	Antecedents	Behaviors	Consequences	Function(s)
Kim	Use of Text and Snapchat outside of school (<1 h/day)	Kim had felt isolated, and social media invitation allowed him to join a group of four	He texted and then widened from texting to snapchatting	He felt positively and more a part of a group; interests could be shared with others; he contributed to the group (via pictures and comments)	Social media allowed Kim, unfamiliar with American rules of social engagement and the language, to more easily communicate
Jessica	Texting with boyfriend	As they became more intimate, she shared intimate pictures through social media with Cliff	Intimate material was shared to a boyfriend, who then shared with others	Jessica stopped going to school	Her efforts to create additional intimacy or connection with Cliff initially were helpful, but then amidst a break up could be used to harm her
Janine	Instagram posting of pictures	Feels disconnected; hard to speak, but likes to express self through art/pictures	Posted pictures on Instagram	Others responded positively and she keeps their messages; she now writes positive posts for others	She was able to express herself more easily through pictures; positive posts reinforced her and modeled how to engage with language, relaxing her fears about communicating to others
Henry	Video game	He plays alone outside school for as many hours as possible	He plays alone and prefers the game to other social activities or academic efforts	His isolation has increased, his schoolwork has diminished; he is not sustaining local peer connections	The game distracts him from other less appealing activities such as school; he avoids social interactions, and he regulates his mood by focusing on the game characters which he can titrate interactions as he needs/prefers

sentiments contained within them such that the popularity of movies can be predicted in advance of their release.[45] For clinicians, the effective application of social media knowledge allows more personalized and frequent attention to a youth's emerging behavioral patterns. Text messaging interventions, social networking sites, and online Web sites are increasingly incorporated into health education with positive effects so far on sexual health among adolescents.[29,30] Social media, like other technological advancements enables and requires modifications in how clinicians assess, educate, and treat patients. For now, we seek to promote a balanced social media diet for youth and to understand the longer-term impacts of social media on their development. A functional assessment of benefits and risks with social and digital media allows clinicians to provide individualized guidance about a youth's media diet and help to prioritize and offer positive targeted interventions.

APPENDIX 8.1: VIDEOGAME QUESTIONNAIRE

Name: _____   Age: ____ Gender____ Date:____

CHECK THE TYPES OF VIDEOGAMES YOU PLAY (see examples)

- ☐ Shooting games (Call of Duty, Battlefield, Overwatch, Fortnite, Grand Theft Auto)
- ☐ Building/User created (Minecraft, Robloks)
- ☐ Action/adventure/platformer (Lego Star Wars, Sonic, Super Mario, Skylanders)
- ☐ Strategy/MOBA (Starcraft, League of Legends)
- ☐ Sports (Madden, FIFA, NBA2K, MLB2k, etc)
- ☐ Racing (Forza, Need for Speed, Mario Kart)
- ☐ Fighting/Martial Arts (Street Fighter, Mortal Kombat, Super Smash Bros., Injustice)
- ☐ Single-Player RPG/Fantasy (Elder Scrolls, Dragon Age, Pokemon)
- ☐ Mobile Games (Angry Birds, Clash of Clans, Pokemon Go)
- ☐ Open World/Sand Box Games (Exploration (Minecraft, Terraria)
- ☐ Sci-fi/Space/Futuristic (Mass Effect, Destiny)
- ☐ MMORPG (World of Warcraft)
- ☐ Horror Games (Resident Evil, Friday the 13th)
- ☐ Puzzle (Tetris, Candy Crush)
- ☐ Other game types _____

OTHER ACTIVITIES

- ☐ Anime _____
- ☐ Cartoons _____
- ☐ TV shows/Movies _____
- ☐ Fantasy/Fiction _____
- ☐ Sports _____
- ☐ Music _____
- ☐ Art _____
- ☐ Religion _____
- ☐ Clubs _____
- ☐ Other _____

FAVORITE GAMES (or other activities if you don't play video games)

1) What is the first game you played? _____

2) What is your favorite game now? _____

3) What do you like best about it? _____

FAVORITECHARACTER

1) Who is your favorite character? _____

2) What do you like best about him/her? _____

SOCIALVIDEO GAMEPLAY (check all that apply)

1) What is your favorite way to play?
☐ By myself
☐ With friends in person
☐ With friends online
☐ With family
☐ Other

2) How do you contact friends to play?
☐ I don't
☐ Text message
☐ In-game messaging
☐ Phone call
☐ Other Social Media

3) Where do you play the most?
☐ My Bed or Room
☐ Family/Living Room
☐ Other

4) How do your game skills compare to others?
☐ Much worse
☐ Worse
☐ Same
☐ Better
☐ Much better

5) How often do you have problems/conflicts playing with others?
☐ Always
☐ Frequently
☐ Rarely
☐ Never

6)Sometimes my play gets in the way of:
☐ Sleep
☐ School
☐ Homework
☐ Friends/Family

7) On social media:
☐ I I don't use social media at all
☐ I watch/follow certain games only
☐ I share my game progress/achievements
☐ I make comments/discuss games
☐ I play with multiple screens

8) Do you feel safe playing or on internet?
☐ Never
☐ Sometimes
☐ Usually
☐ Always

9) Does the internet feel more comfortable than real life?
☐ Always
☐ Usually
☐ Sometimes
☐ Never

REFERENCES

1. Grenados N. Gen Z Media Consumption: It's a Lifestyle, Not Just Entertainment. https://www.forbes.com/sites/nelsongranados/2017/06/20/gen-z-media-consumption-its-a-lifestyle-not-just-entertainment/#3f1adc6f18c9.
2. Newswire: Millennials: Technology=Social Connection. Consumer 2-26-2014. http://www.nielsen.com/us/en/insights/news/2014/millennials-technology-social-connection.html.
3. www.blog.hubspot.com/blog.
4. www.techcrunch.com.
5. Boniel-Nissim M, et al. International trends in electronic media communication among 11-to-15- year−olds in 30 countries from 2002 to 2010: association with ease of communication with friends of the opposite sex. *Eur J Public Health.* 2015;25(suppl 2):41−45.
6. Currie C, Zanotti C, Morgan A, et al., eds. *Social Determinants of Health and Well-being Among Young People. HSBC International Report from the 2009/2010 Survey. Health Policy for Children and Adolescents, Copenhagen.* Copenhagen, Denmark: WHO Regional office for Europe; 2012. No 6.
7. Lamblin M, et al. Social Connectedness, mental health and the adolescent brain. *Neurosci Biobehav Rev.* 2017;80:57−68.
8. Comstock G, Paik H. *Television and the American Child.* San Diego, CA: Academic Press; 1999.
9. Roberts D. Media and youth; access, exposure and privatization. *J Adolesc Health.* 2000;27(suppl):8−14.
10. Loprinzi PD, Davis RE. Secular trends in parent-reported television viewing among children in the United States. *Child Care Health Dev.* 2016;42:288−291.
11. Reid Chassiakos Y, Radesky J, Christakis D, Moreno MA, Cross C. AAP Council on Communications and Media. Children and adolescents and digital media. *Pediatrics.* 2016;138(5):e20162593.
12. Kabali HK, Irigoyen MM, Nunez-Davis R, et al. Exposure and use of mobile media devices by young children. *Pediatrics.* 2015;136:1044−1050.
13. Lovato SB, Waxman SR. Young children learning from touch screens: taking a wider view. *Front Psychol.* 2016;7:1078−1083.
14. Calvert SL, Richards MN, Kent CC. Personalized interactive characters for toddlers 'learning of seriation from a video presentation. *J Appl Dev Psychol.* 2014;35:148−155.
15. Nathanson AI, Alade F, Sharp ML, Rasmussen EE, Christy K. The relation between television exposure and executive function among preschoolers. *Dev Psychol.* 2014;50:1497−1506.
16. Valkenburg PM, Peter J, Schouten AP. Friend networking sites and their relationship to adolescents' well-being and social self-esteem. *CyberPsychol Behav.* 2006;9:584−590.
17. Granic I, Lobel A, Engels RC. The benefits of playing video games. *Am Psychol.* 2014;69:66−78.
18. Feldmeier M. The Video Game Initial Questionnaire (VG-IQ)-C (Child Version). 2017 (personal communication. The author gives permission for use of this questionnaire).
19. Lenart A. *PEW Research Center. Teen, Social Media and Technology Overview;* 2015. www.pewresearch.org.
20. Nabi RL, Prestin A, So J. Facebook friends with (health) benefits? Exploring social network site use and perceptions of social support, stress, and well-being. *Cyberpsychol Behav Soc Netw.* 2013;16:721−727.
21. Chen W, Lee K-H. Sharing, liking, commenting and distressed? The pathway between facebook interaction and psychological distress. *Cyberpsychol Behav Soc Netw.* 2013;16:728−734.
22. Richards D, Caldwell P, Go H. Impact of social media on the health of children and young people. *J Pediatr Child Health.* 2015;51:1152−1157.
23. Oberst U, Wegmann E, Stodt B, Brand M, Chamarro A. Negative consequences from heavy social networking in adolescents: the mediating role of fear of missing out. *J Adolesc.* 2017;55:51−60.
24. Franken A, Keijsers L, Dijkstra JK, Bogt T. Music preferences, friendship, and externalizing behaviors in early adolescence: a SIENA examination of the music marker theory using the SNARE study. *J Youth Adolesc.* 2017;46:1839−1850.
25. Selfout MHW, Branje SJT, ter Bogt TFM, Meeus WHJ. The role of music preferences in early adolescents' friendship formation and stability. *J Adolesc.* 2009;32:95−107.
26. Field AE, Cheung L, Wolf AM, et al. Exposure to the mass media and weight concerns among girls. *Pediatrics.* 1999;103:36.
27. Tiggemann M, Slater A. Facebook and body image concern in adolescent girls: a prospective study. *Int J Eat Disord.* 2017;50:80−83.
28. Holland G, Tiggemann M. A systematic review of the impact of the use of social networking sites on body image and disordered eating outcomes. *Body Image.* 2016;17:100−110.
29. Guse K, Levine MA, Martines Lira A, et al. Interventions using new digital media to improve adolescent sexual health: a systematic review. *J Adolesc Health.* 2012;51:535−543.
30. Bull SS, Levine D, Blkack AR, et al. Social media-delivered sexual health intervention A cluster randomized controlled trial. *Am J Prev Med.* 2012;43:467−474.
31. Garett R, Ford LL, Younf SD. Associations between social media and cyberbullying: a review of the literature. *mHealth.* 2016;2:46.
32. Cantor J. Media violence. *J Adolesc Health.* 2000;27(suppl):30−34.
33. Bannik R, Broeren S, van de Looij- Jansen PM, de Waart F, Raat H. Cyber and traditional bullying victimization as risk factor for mental health problems and suicidal behavior in adolescents. *PLoS One.* 2014;9(4):e94026.
34. Hamm MP, Newton AS, Chisholm A, Chulhan J, Milne A, et al. Prevalence and effect of cyberbullying on children and young people: a scoping review of social media studies. *JAMA Pediatr.* 2015;16:770−777.
35. Ellison NB, Steinfield C, Lampe C. The benefits of Facebook "friends" social capital and college students' use of online social network sites. *J Comput Commun.* 2007;12(4):1143−1168.

36. Primack B, Escobar-Viera C. Social media as it interfaces with psychosocial development and mental illness in transitional age youth. *Child Adolesc Psychiatr Clin N Am.* 2017; 26:217–233.

37. Lin LY, Sidani JE, Shensa A, et al. Association between social media use and depression among U.S. young adults. *Depress Anxiety.* 2016;33:323–331.

38. Naja WJ, Kansoun AH, Haddad RS. Prevalence of depression in medical students at the Lebanese university and exploring its correlation with Facebook relevance: a questionnaire study. *JMIR Res Protoc.* 2016;5:e96.

39. Radovic A, Gmelin T, Stein BD, Miller E. Depressed adolescents' positive and negative use of social media. *J Adolesc.* 2017;55:5–15.

40. Burke M, Marlow C, Lento T. Social network activity and social well-being. Proceeding of the 28th ACM conference on human factors in computing systems. *Atlanta.* April 10–15, 2010:1909–1912.

41. Gable RA, Quinn M, Rutherford M, et al. Addressing problem behaviors in schools: use of functional assessments and behavior intervention plans. *Prev Sch Fail.* 1998;42:106–119.

42. Second Life. www.secondlife.com.

43. 2017 (personal communication).

44. Kaplan AM, Haenlein M. Users of the world, unite! the challenges and opportunities of social media. *Bus Horizons.* 2010;53:59–68.

45. Asur S, Huberman BA. *Predicting the Future with Social Media.* March 29, 2010. arXiv:1003.5699v1 [cs.CY].

CHAPTER 9

The Use of Film, Literature, and Music in Becoming Culturally Competent in Understanding African Americans

ARDIS C. MARTIN, MD

Mass media play a vital role in the ways that people are seen. However, they often distort the ways in which racial and ethnic minorities are perceived, perpetuating a racist ideology which negatively impacts how those minorities are treated in society.

This chapter explores (1) the roles that media play in perpetuating and maintaining individual, structural, and systematic racism and its subsequent impact on racial and ethnic disparities in healthcare, (2) the role that cultural competency, cultural humility, and cultural attunement can play in decreasing these disparities, (3) how individual practitioners' implicit and explicit biases continue to negatively impact African American's access to healthcare and treatment, and (4) how film, literature, and music can be used both to counteract these images and as a method of teaching cultural competency about African Americans to help practitioners in psychiatry better treat their patients.

A decade has passed since the seminal reports by the American College of Physicians,[1] the Institute of Medicine,[2] and the Surgeon General[3] helped shed light on the existence of racial and ethnic disparities in healthcare that continue to exist today. In 2010, the American College of Physicians[4] updated its findings about the sources of racial and ethnic disparities, the importance of correcting these disparities, and their recommendations in doing so. Ethnic and racial minorities continue to receive lower-quality healthcare, have poorer access to healthcare, remain underrepresented in the health professions, and have poorer health status overall compared to their majority counterparts, even when adjustments are made for access to insurance and socioeconomic status. In addition, a clinician's lack of cultural awareness, bias, prejudice, and stereotyping, either overtly or unconsciously, continues to be a factor in the differences in the healthcare that racial and ethnic minorities receive. A study by van Ryn and Burke-Miller[5] showed that physicians tend to assess African Americans more negatively than their white counterparts with regard to their intelligence, feelings of affiliation, likelihood of risk behavior, and adherence to medical advice. In short, healthcare providers' diagnostic decisions as well as their feelings about their patients are influenced by the latter's race or ethnicity. Improving health providers' cultural awareness and sensitivity to their own biases are crucial if we are to improve minorities' access to affordable healthcare, practice culturally competent care, and increase diversity among health professionals. The psychological distress associated with the racism and discrimination that minorities deal with on a daily basis, continues to play a role in the persistence of health disparities as well.

Chao et al.[6] found that African Americans experience more discrimination than their majority counterparts. On a daily basis, African Americans may experience discrimination in many ways: in dealing with the police, in the justice system, at the workplace, when applying for a loan, when trying to obtain property, or simply while shopping and automatically being seen as suspect. This discrimination is traumatic in nature and associated with increased mental health issues. It is important for providers to be aware of this continued struggle and not present a view of a post-racial colorblind society that doesn't reflect reality for African Americans. Doing so disregards their experience and is itself discriminatory in nature.[7]

In 2012, the Institute of Medicine[8] pointed out that the lived experience of race in America has biological and health consequences—"In order to fully address these issues, systematic racism and the social and economic inequalities that exist need to be addressed in order to truly cause change and improve the health of minorities."

THE ROLE OF CULTURAL COMPETENCE

Cultural competence is defined as the ability of providers and organizations to interact effectively with people of different cultures to deliver healthcare services that meet the social, cultural, and linguistic needs of their patients.[9,10] Pedersen[11] emphasized the importance of identifying clinician awareness/attitude as essential components of cultural competence, underscoring the benefits of practitioners becoming aware of other cultures while actively assessing their own belief systems and values about different cultures. Waters and Asbill[12] highlight the importance of *cultural humility*: having an openness to explore one's own cultural perspectives and biases, generating a healthy curiosity that motivates continued exploration, self-examination, and self-awareness to learn and expand on one's understanding. Cultural competence is an ongoing pursuit that requires continual growth and study. Providers must take an active role in learning and continuing to learn.

Hoskins[13] introduces the concept of "cultural attunement," emphasizing the importance of the relationship between providers and the patients they treat. Cultural attunement involves (1) acknowledging the pain of oppression, (2) engaging in acts of humility, (3) acting with reverence, (4) engaging in mutuality, and (5) maintaining a position of "not knowing." Cultural attunement is also a lifelong process that needs to be maintained.

With regard to African Americans, "acknowledging the pain of oppression" is crucial and involves practitioners learning about such topics as slavery, the struggle for civil rights, the experience of discrimination and microaggressions, and the impact that these experiences have had on their minority-group patients. Practitioners are also encouraged to explore their own cultural background and their personal views about race and racism: to become aware of their own prejudices and stereotypes, no matter how subtle. Betancourt[14] reports how efforts by doctors to become culturally competent enhance their ability to provide higher-quality care to patients from racially and ethnically diverse groups, which in turn may alleviate the mental and health disparities that currently exist for minorities.

A NEW WAY TO TEACH: VIA FILM, LITERATURE, PHOTOGRAPHY, AND MUSIC

Film, literature, and music can effectively be used to facilitate cultural competency, cultural humility, and cultural attunement. Literature and film have long been used in medical education to help stimulate discussion on such topics as morality, empathy, and ethics. Mullin[15] described how literature can also be used to promote cultural competency by providing a powerful medium through which one can learn to recognize one's own assumptions and develop empathy, awareness, and appreciation for those who are culturally different. This is done via critical thinking and analysis of characters' feelings, struggles, achievements, and overall life experiences through the stories read (e.g., Freedom Summer, Mississippi Trial: 1955) in a less threatening and anxiety-provoking way, especially when the themes may be painful.

Alexander et al.[16] described several reasons for using movie clips in teaching: they capture the attention through words, sight, and sound, allowing the viewer to experience the subject matter more fully. They can expand awareness of diverse lifestyles of which the viewer may have little or no first-hand knowledge. They engage the humanistic side of physicians, allowing them to emotionally experience situations, leaving a longer-lasting impression. They imprint visual images in memory, stimulating the symbolic and imaginative rather than just the linguistic and rational parts of the brain. They enable physicians to draw on past experiences when faced with a similar situation in the future, providing a frame of reference for interacting with an ethnic minority patient—or at least reminding them to monitor and question their own assumptions so they don't interfere with the process of treatment. This is very important in trying to increase cultural awareness.

There are several examples in the research literature of the effectiveness of movies in medical education. Lim et al.[17] developed a curriculum using documentary films as a way of teaching cultural competency and diversity in medical training. Through selected films (e.g., The Color of Fear, Black and Blue), the participants can access more directly the emotional impact that racism, prejudice, and discrimination can have on people of color. Lim and colleagues found that through the viewing of documentary films, dialog about difficult topics like racism is more easily attained; by objectifying the topics, viewers feel safer acknowledging their feelings and discussing them more freely. Participants are better able to understand difficult topics and experience the emotional impact of them, promoting uncomfortable feelings of "self-reflection and self-revelation that are necessary to build trust and facilitate change." Film provides viewers with a vicarious affective experience, allowing them to acknowledge and process their emotions in a less-threatening environment. Thus they are better able to acknowledge when they are using biases and prejudices so that they avoid a negative outcomes in the treatment of their patients.

MUSIC'S INFLUENCE IN AFRICAN AMERICAN CULTURE

America's view of minorities has often been reflected in popular music. This has historically depicted African Americans in a negative light. The "Coon" songs[18] of the 1900s are the most prominent representations of the racist ideology that existed and which has had long-lasting effects on the way that African Americans are seen and treated in society, and by extension in medicine. These songs were sung on the radio and often in minstrel shows by white actors in blackface, portraying through song and dance the image of African Americans as shiftless, lazy, childlike, inarticulate buffoons.

Music can build both an emotional connection with and provide insight into the cultural history of African Americans. It can be used to convey the feelings and struggles of African Americans and effectively teach majority culture about the African American experience. African Americans have used a wide range of musical genres, including country and western, gospel, R&B, rap, hip-hop, reggae, and blues to tell their stories. Music has long been a source of spiritual strength, free expression, and guidance within the African American community.

Music has effectively been used to document the trials and tribulations of the African American experience from the times of slavery to the civil rights movement to the current struggles that African Americans face with continued systematic racism and violence. It has also recorded their triumphs and successes, promoting a sense of pride, identity, and the understanding that they are not alone in their struggle.

During the times of slavery, songs like "Nobody Knows the Trouble I've Seen" were used to uplift the spirit and provide relief during a time of struggle and pain.

They were also used to pass along secret messages and give guidance to those who wanted to escape from slavery through the Underground Railroad.[19] Abolitionist Harriet Tubman used the song "Wade in the Water" as a message to tell runaway slaves to exercise caution—making sure that they stayed off the trails and traveled in the water to ensure that the slave catcher's dogs lost their scent, increasing their chances of successfully escaping captivity. According to folklore, the song "Follow the Drinking Gourd" was encoded with a map and instructions for slaves to escape North.[20] These songs also provided direction for those who felt lost to the circumstances they were forced to endure, providing a voice of encouragement to resist and refusal to comply with the situations they were in. Virginia slave Nat Turner used the song "Steal Away" to alert others to come together to discuss their plans for the historic slave rebellion that occurred in August 1831.[21] Gospel music today continues to be a source of strength in the African American Church to deliver praise to God, guidance to followers, and comfort and enlightenment in difficult times. It also reinforces the great importance of religion in the community.

In secular culture, especially for African American youth, hip-hop, R&B, rap, and reggae have provided blacks with an opportunity to express their story of struggle and that of their families, their experience of racism and discrimination and, in some instances, their triumph against the odds. Many songs in hip-hop and rap express what life is like for those who live in poverty and are surrounded by violence, how it affects them and those around them, and sometimes propels them into action and protest. It expresses what it is like to be faced with prejudice and police harassment, e.g., racial profiling, police shootings,[22,23] and how people deal with these facets on a daily basis. By acknowledging the importance of music in the lives of African American youth, child and adolescent psychiatrists will be closer to understanding what issues are foremost in their patients' lives and the potential impact on their mental health.

Music has provided African Americans with another form of self-expression, encouraging them to enlist in political and social activism, and encouraging them to stand up for their rights and to protest and to take action. Music has been used to galvanize people and a nation to acknowledge and challenge the discriminatory practices of the time that continue to exist and impact African Americans today.

Nina Simone's song "Mississippi Goddam"[24] was written as a response to the murder of civil rights leader Medgar Evers in Mississippi, the bombing of four little girls at the 16th Street Baptist Church in Alabama, and the desegregation protests in Tennessee. It describes the pain caused by these situations:

Alabama's gotten me so upset

Tennessee made me lose my rest

And everybody knows about Mississippi Goddam.........

It describes the fatigue and anger about being told to wait to get your rights when often there was no intention to change:

Oh, but this whole country is full of lies,

You're all gonna die and die like flies

I don't trust you any more

You keep on saying "Go slow!"

"Go slow!" But that's just the trouble

"Do it slow", Desegregation, Do things gradually, "Do it slow"

But bring more tragedy, "Do it slow"

Why don't you see it, Why don't you feel it

I don't know, I don't know.........

And it emphasizes the need for action in order to attain equal rights:

You don't have to live next to me

Just give me my equality

Everybody knows about Mississippi

Everybody knows about Alabama

Everybody knows about Mississippi Goddam, that's it.

Billie Holiday's rendition of Abel Meeropol's poem, "Strange Fruit,"[25] expressed and brought light to the ugliness of racism, in particular the lynchings that occurred during the Jim Crow era. John Coltrane's Song "Alabama"[26] acknowledged and expressed the pain associated with the church bombing in Alabama where four little girls were killed. James Brown's song "Say it Loud, I'm Black and I'm Proud"[27] helped spread a sense of pride about being black in America, and served as a rallying cry for the Black Power and civil rights movement. Gil Scot Heron's song "The Revolution Will Not Be Televised"[28] served as a wake-up call to America to confront these important social/racial issues. Sam Cooke's song "A Change Is Gonna Come"[29] expressed his own struggles and views of ongoing racism during the civil rights movement. "Lift Every Voice and Sing"[30] was named the Negro National Anthem by the The National Association for the Advancement of Colored People (NAACP) in 1919 because of how it powerfully voiced the cry for freedom and affirmation for African Americans. The song also helped promote wide support for passing the Civil Rights Act of 1964.

More recently, Young Jeezy's song "My President"[31] expressed his pride about the election of the first African American president, Barack Obama. Jay Z's song "Minority Report"[32] was written as a response to the devastation that African American's endured in the aftermath of Hurricane Katrina, and Lauryn Hill's song "Black Rage"[33] was re-released in response to the Michael Brown killing in Ferguson, Missouri, acknowledging the increase in police violence toward African Americans.

Protest songs to popular songs such as these help practitioners better understand issues that may affect African American youth and their families. By acknowledging issues that their clients might deal with on a daily basis, they can appropriately empathize and help youths and their families more effectively. By being aware of these subtle issues in the lives of their clients, practitioners may be more sensitive to clients' needs and be better able to help them process the pain of these occurrences.

POWER OF THE WRITTEN WORD

The American people have this to learn: that where justice is denied, where poverty is enforced, where ignorance prevails, and where any one class is made to feel that society is an organized conspiracy to oppress, rob, and degrade them, neither person nor property is safe.

FREDERICK DOUGLASS

Published writings have also been used to demean and undermine the African American experience. The book *The Bell Curve*[34] by Richard Herrnstein and Charles Murray serves as an example of scientific racism[35] in which the authors purport that African Americans have lower IQs, and further claim this is predictive of their lower socioeconomic status and their supposed propensity for criminal behavior.

Literature, plays, and poetry written by African Americans can be useful in contradicting these racist views and helping practitioners obtain yet another perception of the African American experience, helping to challenge preconceived notions. African American youth may also find the process of expressing themselves through written verse, journaling, short stories, and plays to be therapeutic. Practitioners' interest in these forms of communication can help them obtain glimpses into their young patients' worlds and be more effective in treating them by being open and supportive about the content of their expression. The following works showcase, through various forms of artistic expression, the different life experiences that

African American's have experienced in America—collectively and individually.

Lorraine Hansberry's play *A Raisin in the Sun* [36] describes the struggle of a lower-class African American family as they try to overcome financial insecurity and racism while gaining acceptance and advancement in society. August Wilson's play *Fences*[37] chronicles the difficulties of race relations and economic hardship on a married couple in the 1950s and its impact on their family. Ntozake Shange's play *For Colored Girls Who Have Considered Suicide/When the Rainbow is Enuf*[38] chronicles the oppression of seven women and their experiences living in a racist and sexist society. Suzan-Lori Parks play *The Death of the Last Black Man in the Whole Entire World* [39] showcases the erasure of African Americans and their history (from slavery to modern times) from the Western World, as if these experiences had never happened.

W.E.B. Dubois's book, *The Soul of Black Folks*,[40] refers to the "color line" and "symbol of the veil" to describe the racial divide between blacks and whites, which ensures better opportunities and treatment for whites and inferior or no treatment for blacks, preventing whites from accepting blacks as Americans and impacting blacks' visions of themselves. Frederick Douglass, in his autobiography *A Narrative on the Life of Frederick Douglass, an American Slave*[41] illustrates the struggle he went through to escape from slavery and the toll it took on him, both mentally and physically. Ralph Ellison's *The Invisible Man*[42] expresses the plight of African Americans who, despite their education and intelligence, continue to struggle to be "seen" and accepted into majority society because of the color of their skin.

Among more recent works, *The New Jim Crow: Mass Incarceration in the Age of Colorblindness* by Michelle Alexander[43] examines the racial hierarchy and discrimination that still dominates American society, especially within our justice system. This has led to disproportionate numbers of African Americans being incarcerated based on racist policies and procedures. Ibram X. Kendi's *Stamped From the Beginning: The Definitive History of Racist Ideas in America*[44] describes how discrimination and racism are still active and deeply rooted in our society, a part of our national identity. *Black Stats: African Americans by the Numbers in the Twenty-First Century*[45] by Monique W. Morris, gives an account of real life experiences of African Americans in the United States with regard to discrimination and social injustice.

More personal works providing insights include Ta-Nehisi Coates's *Between the World and Me*,[46] which is a letter to his son that addresses questions about history, identity, survival, and freedom for African Americans that is yet to be achieved. *Black Man in a White Coat: A Doctor's Reflections on Race*[47] by Dr Damon Tweede is a memoir which poignantly points out the challenges a person of color faces in the medical field with regard to race, as well as the health disparities that continue in medicine. *Citizen: An American Lyric*[48] by Claudia Rankine uses essays, poetry, images, and art to examine race, identity, and what it's like to be black in America. It profiles the racial injustices that continue to exist—exposing the overt racial aggression and microaggressions[49] that African Americans have to endure on a daily basis, impairing their ability to live life freely.

These powerful themes can have many deleterious effects on the self-esteem and identity of African Americans struggling with who they are and who they want to become. It is important for practitioners to not dismiss the issues of slavery and civil rights as belonging to the past, assuming they don't affect the present-day lives of their minority clients. Although things are better with regard to overt racism, their clients may still be deeply affected by the subtler forms of discrimination and racism that still permeates our society and deserve to be taken seriously.

THE WAR OF IMAGES

Every negro boy, every negro girl born in this country until this present moment undergoes the agony of trying to find in the body politic, in the body social, outside himself or herself, some image of himself or herself which is not demeaning.

JAMES BALDWIN (1963)

American film and television have often propagated negative images of African Americans from slavery to modern times, offering their own standards of civility and beauty, often reducing blacks to caricatures—one-sided and superficial (e.g., The Uncle Tom, The Mulatto, The Pickaninny, The Jezebel). The film "Birth of a Nation" by D.W. Griffith, is infamous for its portrayal of blacks in an extremely racist manner—as subservient, ignorant, and violent. It also served as propaganda to induce fear of blacks and as an endorsement for the continued practices of slavery and of the Klu Klux Klan when it was released in 1915.[50] It became very important for African Americans to become masters of their own fate and begin crafting their own images which better represented the diversity of their people and their experiences, helping to improve their own sense of self-worth and self-esteem.

The following films—fictional and documentary—can be effective in relaying the personal views and experiences that African Americans face with regard to the racism and discrimination that they've had to endure, and which continues to be a very prominent part of their daily lives. In addition, these films can be used to help practitioners learn more about their own underlying assumptions. As with music and literature, movie clips can be used in discussion about cultural issues in psychiatry.

12 Years a Slave by John Ridley, based on a 19th century memoir[51] poignantly captures the viciousness and inhumanity of slavery through the lens of a freed man, Solomon Northrup, who is captured and returned to a life of servitude in the South. The film portrays the atrocities and indignities he had to endure. Paul Webb's film *Selma*[52] provides a glimpse of the struggle that African Americans had to face during the civil rights movement while they trying to achieve their basic civil liberties. Justin Simien's film *Dear White People*[53] uses satire to examine the way that blacks see themselves and how majority society sees them, while exposing the stereotypes and prejudices that continue to exist under the dismissive guise of living in a color blind, post-racial society.

The 2016 documentary *I am Not your Negro*,[54] by Raoul Peck and based on the writings of James Baldwin, provides a scathing view of what it was like to be black in America in the 1960s, struggling for equality while being met with hatred and violence. It has startling similarities to the struggles that African Americans still face today.

Another documentary, "Dark Girls,"[55] by D. Channsin Berry and Bill Duke, takes a hard and painful look at the concept of "colorism" and the divisions that can exist within the African American community based entirely on skin color. Through personal accounts, the documentary offers a unique opportunity to see another side of the long-term effects of slavery and racism in the lives of blacks. It delves into the world of African American self-hatred, intraracism, self-identity, and ultimately helps us examine African American views of beauty within the community.

In the documentary *13th*,[56] Spencer Averick and Ava DuVernay explore the racial inequality that still exists in the prison systems of the United States. The criminalization of African American men has its roots in slavery and has extended from Reconstruction and Jim Crow to modern day police violence and police profiling.

The documentary series "Eyes on the Prize"[57] by Henry Hampton et al. captures the real life struggle of African Americans during their pursuit for equality and justice in America during the Civil Rights Era. Lastly, the documentary "Through A Lens Darkly: Black Photographs and the Emergence of a People"[58] by Thomas Allen Harris et al. beautifully illustrates how African American photographers have used photographs to expose some of the horrors that blacks have experienced in America, as well as their humanity, improving their self-identity and sense of self-worth through images that are more accurate and positive representations.

SUMMARY

As these examples show, books, films, music, plays, and documentaries, can serve as windows into the experiences of African Americans. By adding a historical context to these experiences and acknowledging the oppression African Americans have dealt with, the practitioner is able to learn more about how these events affect the lives of their clients and their experiences in the world. Literature, songs, and movies can also help practitioners recognize their own prejudices and underlying assumptions. This is essential to delivering culturally competent and culturally attuned care, which in turn may help reduce disparities in healthcare.

As we seek to improve psychiatric care through cultural competency, the goal is to provide practitioners with the opportunity to be well informed, to challenge their beliefs, and to minimize unwarranted assumptions about the people they interact with and care for.

While it is important to learn about a minority group's experience, it is crucial to consider and acknowledge each individual's own unique experience, providing patient-centered care, acknowledging their collective as well as their individual experiences. Each African American will have a different take on his or her own experience as a member of the black race, and thus be affected and interact with the world differently. If we assume that what applies to one person in a group applies to all its members, we risk creating new harmful stereotypes and promoting discrimination which can could be further detrimental to their health.

This reminds us to assess from our patients' perspective the pertinent issues that led them to seek treatment, and not to assume that information learned about a patient's background, or an ethnicity or culture, will lead us in the right direction. The goal of using different forms of media to become culturally competent in understanding African Americans and other minorities is to challenge the negative images that have been instilled by majority society, to combat their deleterious effects by providing a visceral, enjoyable, and interesting way to learn about a group's experience in a safe and nonthreatening manner, while respecting patient individuality.

REFERENCES

1. Groman R, Ginsburg J, American College of Physicians. Racial and ethnic disparities in health care. *Ann Intern Med.* 2004;141(3):226−232.
2. Institute of Medicine. *Report Brief. Unequal Treatment: What Health Care Providers Need to Know about Racial and Ethnic Disparities in Health Care;* 2002. Available at: https://www.nap.edu/html/10260/disparities_providers.pdf.
3. Mental Health: Culture, Race, and Ethnicity. *A Supplement to Mental Health: A Report of the Surgeon General;* 2001. Available at: www.ct.gov/dmhas/lib/dmhas/publications/mhethnicity.pdf.
4. American College of Physicians. *Racial and Ethnic Disparities in Health Care* (Position Paper). Philadelphia: American College of Physicians; 2003.
5. van Ryn M, Burke-Miller JK. The effect of patient race and socio-economic status on physicians' perceptions of patients. *Soc Sci Med.* 2000;50(6):813−828.
6. Chou T, Asnaani A, Hofmann S. Perception of racial discrimination and psychopathology across three U.S. ethnic minority groups. *Cult Divers Ethn Minor Psychol.* 2012;18(1):74−81.
7. Institutional Racism and the Social Work Profession: A Call to Action. Available at: https://www.socialworkers.org/diversity/InstitutionalRacism.pdf .
8. Institute of Medicine. *How Far Have We Come in Reducing Health Disparities? Progress since 2000: Workshop Summary.* Washington: National Academies Press (US); 2012.
9. Betancourt JR, Green AR, Carrillo JE. *Cultural Competence in Health Care: Emerging Frameworks and Practical Approaches.* New York: The Commonwealth Fund; 2002.
10. Cultural Competence. *Substance Abuse and Mental Health Administration;* 2016. Available at: https://www.samhsa.gov/capt/applying-strategic-prevention/cultural-competence.
11. Pedersen PB. The making of a culturally competent counselor. *Online Read Psychol Cult.* 2002;10(3). Available at: https://doi.org/10.9707/2307-0919.1093.
12. Waters A, Asbill L. Reflections on cultural humility. *CYF News.* Aug. 2013.
13. Hoskins M. Worlds apart and lives together: developing cultural attunement. *Child Youth Care Forum.* 1999;28(2):143−150. Available at: https://www.researchgate.net/publication/.
14. Betancourt JR. Cultural competence——marginal or mainstream movement? *New Engl J Med.* 2004;351(10):953−955.
15. Mullin NL. *Using Literature to Promote Culture Competence: A Bullying Prevention Companion Bibliography, Volume II, K-12;* 2014:1−210. Available at: http://chpdp.org/wp-content/uploads/2014/11/Using-Literature-to-Promote-Cultural-Competence.pdf.
16. Alexander M, Hall MN, Pettice YJ. Cinemeducation: an innovative approach to teaching psychosocial medical care. *Fam Med.* 1994;26(7):430−433.
17. Lim RF, Diamond RJ, Chang JB, Primm AB, Lu FG. Using non-feature films to teach diversity, cultural competence, and the DSM-IV-TR outline for cultural formulation. *Acad Psychiatry.* 2008;32(4):291−298.
18. Racism and Prejudice in Music. *The Parlor Songs Academy: Lessons in America's Popular Music History;* 1999. Available at: http://parlorsongs.com/issues/1999-8/aug99feature.php.
19. National Geographic. The Underground Railroad. Available at: http://www.nationalgeographic.com/features/99/railroad/.
20. Bresler J. Follow the Drinking Gourd: A Cultural History. Available at: followthedrinkinggourd.org.
21. LaFraniere S, Lehren A. The Disproportionate Risk of Driving While Black. Available at: https://www.nytimes.com/2015/10/25/us/racial-disparity-traffic-stops-driving-black.html.
22. California Police Killings Database Reveals "Clear Racial Disparities." Available at: https://www.theguardian.com/us-news/2015/sep/07/california-police-shootings-database-racial-disparity.
23. Secrets: Signs and Symbols. Pathways to Freedom: Maryland and the Underground Railroad. Available at: http://pathways.thinkport.org/secrets/music2.cfm.
24. Allan L. *Strange Fruit [recorded by Billie Holiday]. On Lady in Autumn: The Best of the Verve Years.* [CD]. USA: Polygram Records; 1991. Song lyrics available at: http://www.songlyrics.com. - Billie Holiday.
25. Meeropol A. 1939. Strange Fruit [song]. Song by Billie Holiday. On Jazz at the Philharmonic; 1954.
26. Coltrane J [song]. Alabama. On Soundtrack - Malcolm X (Music From the Motion Picture Soundtrack); 1964.
27. Brown J, Ellis A. James Brown Orchestra [song]. Say it Loud, I'm Black and I'm Proud. On Star Time; 1968.
28. Heron GS [song]. The Revolution Will Not Be Televised. On Small Talk at 125th and Lenox; 1971.
29. Cooke S [song]. A Change Gonna Come. On Ain't That Good News; 1964.
30. Johnson JR, Johnson JW [song]. Lift Every Voice and Sing; 1905.
31. Jeezy and Nas. My President. On The Recession; 2009.
32. Jay Z, Dre Dr, Baston M [song]. Minority Report. On Kingdom Come; 2006.
33. Lauryn H. Black Rage [song]; 2012.
34. Murray C, Herrstein R. *Bell Curve: Intelligence and Class Structure in American Life.* New York: Free Press; 1996.
35. Dennis RM. Social darwinism, scientific racism, and the metaphysics of race. *J Negro Educ.* 1995;64(No. 3):243−252.
36. Hansberry L. (Playwright). A Raisin in the Sun; 1959.
37. Wilson A. (Playwright). Fences; 1985.
38. Change N. (Playwright). For Colored Girls Who Have Considered Suicide/When the Rainbow is Enough; 1976.
39. Parks SL (Playwright). The Death of the Last Black Man in the Whole Entire World [play]; 1989−1992.

40. DuBois WEB, Gibson D, Elbert M. *The Souls of Black Folk*. Penguin Books; 1996.

41. Douglass F. *Narrative of the Life of Frederick Douglass, an American Slave*. Anti-Slavery Office; 1845.

42. Ellison R. *The Invisible Man*. Modern library; 1992.

43. Alexander M. *The New Jim Crow: Mass Incarceration in the Age of Colorblindness*. New York: The New Press; 2012.

44. Kendi IX. *Stamped from the Beginning: The Definitive History of Racist Ideas in America*. New York: Nation Books; 2017.

45. Morris MW. *Black Stats: African Americans by the Numbers in the Twenty-first- Century*. New York: The New Press; 2014.

46. Coates T. *Between the World and Me*. New York: Spiegel and Grau; 2015.

47. Tweede D. *Black Man in a White Coat: A Doctor's Reflections on Race*. New York: Picador; 2016.

48. Rankine C. *Citizen: An American Lyric*. Minneapolis: Graywolf Press; 2014.

49. Owen J, Tao KW, Imel ZE, Wampold BE, Rodolfa E. Addressing racial and ethnic microaggressions in therapy. *Prof Psychol Res Pract*. 2014;45(4):283−290.

50. Griffith DW, Aitken H (Producers), Griffith DW (Director). *The Birth of a Nation* [motion picture]. Los Angeles, CA: Triangle Film Production; 1915.

51. Pitt B, Gardner D, Kleiner J, Pohlad B, McQueen S, Miclchan A, Katagas A (Producers), McQueen S (Director). *12 Years a Slave* [motion picture]. Los Angeles, CA: 20th Century Fox; 2013.

52. Colson C, Winfrey O, Gardner D, Kleiner J (Producers), DuVernay A. (Director). *Selma* [motion picture]. Los Angeles, CA: Paramount; 2014.

53. Brown E, Le A, Lebedev J, Lope A, Simien J, White L (Producers), Simien J (Director). *Dear White People* [motion picture]. Santa Monica, CA: Lionsgate; 2014.

54. Grellety R, Peck H, Peck R (Producers), Peck R (Director). *I am Not Your Negro* [motion picture]. Auburn AL: Magnolia Studios; 2016.

55. Duke B, Berry DC. *Dark Girls* [motion picture]. Utah: Doc Club; 2011.

56. Barish H, DuVernay A, Averick (Producers), DuVernay A (Director). *The 13h* [motion picture]. Netflix; 2016.

57. Vecchione J, Else J (Producers), Hampton H (Director). *Eyes on the Prize, Volume I and II* [television-DVD]. US: PBS; 1987−1990.

58. Harris TA, Bennett A, Perry D, Willis D, Steward K (Producers), Harris TA (Director). *Through a Lens Darkly: Black Photographers and the Emergence of a People*. New York: First Run Features; 2014.

CHAPTER 10

Mass Media Outreach for Child Psychiatrists

CHERYL K. OLSON, SCD • LAWRENCE A. KUTNER, PHD • EUGENE V. BERESIN, MD

In July 1899, an editorial in the *Journal of the American Medical Association* bemoaned the difficulty of "instilling correct ideas of insanity into the public mind":

"There is such an opportunity for sensationalism that newspaper reporters in particular are rarely able to keep their imagination in restraint and the average literature they produce on the subject is about as thoroughly untrustworthy as it can well be. The physician who unguardedly allows himself to be interviewed on any remarkable incident or phase of the subject [of insanity] is liable to have to repent it…"[1]

As this century-old quote shows, physicians have long been aware of the potential of mass media for public education, but also (often rightly) critical of inaccuracies and sensationalism in media reports.

This debate was been renewed, although with a politically laden twist, in the United States in 2017 with calls for a lifting of the "Goldwater Rule"—an ethics guideline dating back to the 1960s prohibiting psychiatrists and other mental health professionals from commenting publicly on the mental states of public figures. The presidential campaign of 2016 led to heated discussions about whether such a prohibition was a "gag order," contradicted a "duty to warn," or served a greater good. In 2017, the American Psychoanalytic Association sent an e-mail[2] to its members allowing them to make public statements on the mental health of President Donald Trump without violating that organization's ethical guidelines.

Child and adolescent psychiatrists may see little reason to get involved with media reporters or producers, and plenty of reasons to avoid them. There is the fear of being viewed as a self-promoting popularizer, rather than a serious clinician or researcher. There is concern about being misquoted or having statements taken out of context, to the detriment of their reputation and of the public's education. Moreover, uncertainty about the expectations, methods, and motivations of media professionals create uncomfortable feelings of confusion and lack of control.[3]

In this paper, we will suggest several reasons why psychiatrists should get involved with the media. We will demystify some of the workings of the news media, so that when a reporter calls, you can be better prepared and increase the odds of a positive outcome. We will describe ways to proactively reach out to media professionals in order to educate the public or support improved mental health policies. Finally, we will look at more sophisticated uses of media, including media campaigns.

WHY GET INVOLVED WITH THE MEDIA?

The Need to Raise Public Awareness About Mental Illness and Effective Treatment

Surveys in the United States and other countries have found that many people have little understanding of what mental illness looks like, what symptoms characterize different illnesses, and what is meant by labels such as "schizophrenia."[4] Stigmatizing myths about causality persist; for example, many members of the public believe that schizophrenia and depression are caused by "the way a person was raised" or due to "one's own bad character."[5] Misconceptions about medication are rampant, including concerns that they "turn kids into zombies" and merely put off dealing with real problems.[6]

The Need to Reduce Stigma and Other Barriers to Care

While certainly the cost of and access to services affect whether a child will receive treatment, research suggests that beliefs about mental health problems and treatment may be even greater obstacles to care.[7] These include parent knowledge about symptoms of mental illness, and parent beliefs about the seriousness of the symptoms, the need for treatment, and the likely effectiveness of mental health services. Also, parent expectations about their child's treatment predict the level of parent involvement in therapy and whether treatment is terminated prematurely.[8] Given that half of US adolescents with *severely impairing* mental disorders have never received mental health treatment,[9] removing barriers to care is a critical priority.

The Need to Counteract Media Misinformation that Contributes to Stigma

Unfortunately, a significant amount of today's health-related media content is confusing, misleading, or downright wrong. Poor reporting can, for example, lead viewers to misconstrue research results, dangerously halt medical treatment, or turn to unproven "cures."[10] Selective reporting can also reinforce myths, such as the belief that mentally ill persons are dangerous.[11] In fact, perceptions of the dangerousness and unpredictability of mentally ill people, particularly those with schizophrenia, may have increased in recent decades, despite gains in knowledge.[12,13] Reviews of press coverage in the United States, United Kingdom, Canada, and New Zealand have found that mental illness is frequently linked with violence.[14] In one US study of major newspapers' reporting of mental illness, crimes, and/or violence perpetrated by a mentally ill person was the focus of 26% of such stories and was by far the most common theme.[15] Perceptions such as these make people wary of contact with the mentally ill and may increase support for coercive or counterproductive policies.[16]

Entertainment media can also perpetuate harmful stereotypes. A review of Disney animated films[17] found a surprisingly high number of stigmatizing comments, including "crazy" thoughts, ideas, behaviors, or clothing, with the implication that these traits were irrational and inferior. Studies of television programs aimed at young children[18,19] also found frequent negative stereotypes, especially in cartoon programs; "twisted" or "nuts" characters were typically portrayed as threatening or disrespected. The authors were concerned that these shows may promote stigmatization and verbal harassment in real life.

Mental illness is a common theme in movies, including horror films. These not only present the mentally ill as scary and dangerous but can also affect the image of psychiatrists and the expectations that children and their parents have about the nature and outcome of therapy.[20]

The Need to Counterbalance Information From Special Interests

Much of the health information presented to the public is put forward by special interests, such as pharmaceutical companies. Some advertising has the potential to benefit, as when therapies widely viewed as effective for undertreated conditions are advertised.[21] But when celebrities are paid to make the rounds of talk shows to promote medications,[22] news stories are based on corporate press releases or conference abstracts,[23] and the benefits of new medications are exaggerated and risks overlooked,[24] disinterested physicians must come forward to balance the picture.

Similarly, according to the Pew Research Center <http://www.pewinternet.org/2013/11/26/part-two-sources-of-health-information/>, 80% of adults who search for health information online begin with a search engine such as Google. The listings on these search engines can be altered by corporations and other groups with financial interests through search engine optimization techniques or simply purchasing advertisements that look like noncommercial listings and are placed on the first page of the results of such searches.

THE POTENTIAL OF MASS MEDIA TO TEACH, AND COUNTERACT STIGMA

If we wish to educate the public, it's far easier to reach them through their usual channels of information—and this includes reaching out through the mass media. According to the 2014 National Science Board survey, television is still America's most popular source of current news, although the Internet surpasses it as a source of science and medical news specifically.[25]

At the same time, a growing number of health education and medical intervention programs have made use of highly targeted media—including "personalized" voice mail messages and text messages on cell phones.[26] Similarly, blogs and podcasts have essentially removed the middleman when using print and broadcast media, allowing individuals to create and distribute educational and other materials directly to larger but highly targeted audiences. While these are powerful tools and areas in which media-savvy psychiatrists may wish to become involved, their use is beyond the scope of this paper, which focuses on electronic and print mass media.

Intelligent news coverage has led to needed changes in health and research policies and legislation,[27] and television programs have repeatedly shown themselves—intentionally or accidentally—to be highly effective health and science public education tools. Even entertainment programming content has been shown to influence health-related knowledge and behaviors, such as family discussions and choices about healthcare, deciding to visit a doctor or clinic, or encouraging others to seek help.[28,29]

HOW TO WORK WITH MASS MEDIA OUTLETS

While clinicians and researchers readily acknowledge the power of mass media as public health and public education tools for mental health promotion, primary prevention, and stigma reduction, few psychiatrists receive any formal training in how to use those tools. In addition, many health professionals are concerned that attempts to work with the media may be viewed by colleagues as little more than self-aggrandizement.

To counteract these problems, we incorporated both formal and informal media training into the curriculum of the child and adolescent psychiatry training program at the Massachusetts General Hospital/McLean Hospital. These include seminars in health communication, structured practice sessions such as mock broadcast and print interviews, and opportunities to work on media-based outreach projects. Several of the points emphasized in these sessions can be readily used by experienced psychiatrists who wish to explore the use of mass media as extensions of their clinical practice or research.

There are three general types of "triggers" for contact with mass media

- **Contact by a reporter or producer about a specific story.** This is probably the most common first interaction between physicians and the press. For example, you may receive a telephone call from a journalist who is writing a news story about some local children who had been sexually abused or who is producing a television feature story on the supposed increase in autism over the past few generations.

- **Promotion of a story idea that you have developed.** This includes promotion of new clinical services or a book, interpretation of research findings for the general public or for public policy makers, or even an organized mental health-related media campaign.

- **The use of natural opportunities such as breaking national news to help guide coverage of that news and related topics.** For example, concerns and publicity over the use of antidepressant medications by children provided child psychiatrists with

opportunities to reach out to the press not only on that specific topic but also on the nature of childhood depression, the purpose and limits of these types of studies, and the predicaments of parents who are seeking help for children who have mental illnesses.

When you receive a telephone call from a reporter asking for your comments or insights into a story, your first response should be to ask a few questions of your own. (Psychiatrists who work for academic medical centers may find that their employers have a policy of channeling all such calls through a public affairs office, where the staff will do this. Even so, it's a good idea to verify some information with the reporter or producer.)

What, exactly, is the name of the publication, podcast, online news service, or broadcast program? A reporter who says he's with the *Enquirer* may mean the venerable *Cincinnati Enquirer* or the supermarket tabloid *National Enquirer*.

What, exactly, is the focus of the story? Knowing this before you start can help you structure what you say and help ensure that your statements are taken in context.

What's the deadline? Reporters who work for daily publications or news broadcasts often have only hours to put together a story. If you can't meet the reporter's deadline, simply say so.

Also recognize that reporters, radio talk show hosts, and others who may call for an interview have a wide range of experience and expertise that may color their coverage of a topic. A few have doctoral degrees in medicine, psychology, or a related subject; others haven't set foot in a science classroom since high school and may spend most of their workday reporting on fires and local politics.

No matter what their background, most journalists are simply trying to get their facts straight, put issues into perspective, and present them in a way that is interesting and attractive to their audience. The challenge for psychiatrists who present information on mental health is to help reporters achieve their goals in ways that also help us achieve ours.

This challenge is sometimes made more difficult because the priorities of the media can stand in stark contrast to the priorities of mental health professionals.[30] Let's say you're contacted by a reporter who's writing a story in response to the suicide of a local and popular high school athlete.

The reporter's focus for the story—especially if that reporter is relatively unsophisticated—may be quite different from what you might wish to get across to the public about the underlying issues. If your voice is to be heard, you need to gently guide the reporter and shape or "frame" the story; address the reporter's assumptions about the nature of the problem or issue, the causes of the problem, moral or value judgments associated with those perceived causes, and/or potential remedies for the problem.[31]

1. *Why did the child kill himself?* You should, of course, decline to answer that question. However, you can use it to segue to the larger issue. For example, you might begin your response with, "I can't comment on this specific child because I didn't know him. However, we do know that the large majority of young people who kill themselves are depressed; but their depression can look different than depression in adults."

2. *We know that most of these kids who shoot other people and themselves—like Adam Lanza, the school shooter in Newtown, CT—play a lot of violent computer games. Do you think this kid played those games? Shouldn't we just ban them?* Always correct a false premise before attempting to answer any question. Otherwise your silence acts as a tacit endorsement of the premise. "I think that you and a lot of other people are making some assumptions that aren't supported by research. Let's look at them one at a time."

3. *But this kid had everything going for him. He was smart and popular. What happened?* Again, you can use this to help shape the reporter's story by talking about the myths of depression and suicide, as well as the need for treatment. "Depression is a brain disorder. One of the things it does is give a person a distorted picture of his life. Even though other people may say he's doing well, he may feel hopeless and doomed. Both medication and talk therapy can help. The big problem is getting teenagers to go for that help."

By acknowledging the reporter's questions, correcting false premises, and segueing to relevant materials that lend insight to the story, you are helping shape it so that it is more likely to address the following important issues that might otherwise have been missed:

1. Perspective. The epidemiology of suicide and of adolescent depression.

2. Identification of children at risk. What are the symptoms of depression among adolescents? Why are these symptoms sometimes missed, even by family, friends, and teachers? How does adolescent depression present itself differently than adult depression?

3. Primary prevention. What can schools and parents do to help these children before they become

suicidal? What can be done to help prevent additional suicide attempts ("contagion") by teenagers in the community?

4. Posttrauma intervention. What can parents and teachers say to teenagers and younger children who are frightened or upset by the adolescent's suicide?

These same techniques can be used in a proactive rather than a reactive manner. Whether you're promoting the expansion of services at a community mental health center or working on a national stigma reduction initiative, you'll be much more effective if you start with a detailed plan for both strategy and implementation. Key issues the plan must address include:

- **Whom are you trying to reach with your message?** Be as specific as you can, e.g., parents of children who are making the transition to middle school. There are times when you can effectively use mass media to influence a very small but critical group of individuals, such as state legislators who are about to vote on a particular bill. The pioneering political media specialist Tony Schwartz was one of the first to use low-cost targeted radio advertising to great effect.[32]

- **What exactly is your message?** Media interviews give you only limited time or space to get your point across. Focus on between one and three clear points you'd like to make. If you find yourself thinking in vague terms ("My goal is to tell parents about childhood stress."), you need to rethink your approach.

- **What are the specific responses you want from your target audience when they receive your information?** Too often, mental health professionals focus exclusively on conveying detailed information, such as the symptoms of posttraumatic stress disorder. In many situations, other types of responses are at least as important. How should a person feel upon seeing, hearing, or reading your message? (Reassured? Empowered? Ashamed?) What specific behaviors do you want from that person? (Speak with their child or spouse about the topic? Call a clinic to set up an appointment?)

- **How will you know if your efforts are successful?** Did readers contact you for more information? Did clinical appointments increase? Was a bill passed in the legislature? Defining your criteria for success ahead of time will sometimes lead you to reexamine whether you're offering the information your target audience needs in order to give the specific responses you hope for.

Another important pitfall to avoid is what we call the education trap. It's tempting to be didactic. That is, of course, what's been demonstrated and reinforced throughout our formal schooling. But journalists are there to tell stories, not primarily to teach.

We encountered this when working recently as consultants to a major market public radio outlet that wanted to revamp its health coverage on both its broadcast and podcast operations. It was recovering from a failed, very expensive podcast that had lapsed into teaching rather than telling compelling stories that, as a side benefit, allowed the audience to learn. It was a subtle shift that had a profoundly negative affect on their audience size.

A well-told story can be far more compelling than any statistical analysis. That does not mean that you should ignore statistics; rather, they are best used to reinforce and complement the stories you tell to make your points, not as the primary tool for making your points.

While more published studies are needed, there is evidence that reaching out to reporters with accurate background information and ideas for positive stories can improve the amount and tone of mental health coverage.[33] Both predictable (e.g., the holiday season) and unpredictable (the 2017 confluence of two major hurricanes and an earthquake in North American within a few weeks) events can provide opportunities to reach out to the media on children's mental health issues. Although the window of opportunity may be brief, the key issues listed above still apply. For example, a school shooting in a different state might make reporters more interested in the issue of posttraumatic stress disorder among school-age children. Before you speak with a reporter about the topic, you should clearly define your target audience, your message, the behavioral responses you want, and your criteria for success.

If the story is based on newly published research, it's important to provide information that helps reporters put new information into context. For example, a mention in one small study that a quarter of schizophrenic patients had carried weapons during psychotic episodes led to hysterical headlines about dangerous mental patients.[34]

Be explicit about what the data mean and what they don't tell us, as well as what the practical implications might be. Try to put the data into a real world context. If your goal is to increase the recognition of depression, it's more compelling to state that every high school classroom has at least one student with undiagnosed depression—and to give examples of what untreated depression might mean for that child's future—than to recite population statistics.

Take advantage of the power of imagery—whether a video image or photograph, or images created by phrases or metaphors—to get your points across. When a person who looks like your next-door neighbor describes her struggle with schizophrenia, the visual impression she makes (so different from the iconic image of a violent, disheveled "crazy" person) may convey a stronger and more memorable message than any of her words.

WHAT OTHERS HAVE DONE TO EDUCATE THE PUBLIC ABOUT MENTAL ILLNESS

Because little is known about what works to educate the public about mental illness (and disorders of children and adolescents in particular), it's important to share information on what has been tried and what approaches seem most effective.[35]

For the past 20 years, the Carter Center in Atlanta has offered Rosalynn Carter Fellowships in Mental Health Journalism[a] to reporters and producers in a variety of media. While the focus has been on American journalists, it has helped develop similar programs in Colombia, New Zealand, Qatar, Romania, South Africa, and the United Arab Emirates. The 1-year program combines formal training in Atlanta with financial support and professional guidance from both mental health professionals and senior journalists on a media project. While most of the fellowship participants are traditional general assignment or medical reporters, a few have been mental health professionals as well as journalists. It has also published a resource guide for journalists on covering behavioral health issues[36] that could be of use to psychiatrists interested in working with the media.

The World Psychiatric Association has collected information on programs from 11 countries, including the United States, designed to educate the public and reduce stigma and discrimination related to schizophrenia and other mental illnesses. Some of these involve the distribution of media materials such as videotapes, efforts to work with reporters, critiques of poor news coverage, or awards for good reporting. (This compendium collection can be viewed or downloaded at http://www.openthedoors.com/english/01_02.html, although it is no longer being updated.) Unfortunately, these efforts tell us little about the best ways to educate the public about mental illness; there is a dearth of published information on the evaluation of educational media materials and the campaigns which use these materials. Most programs rely on

---

[a]https://www.cartercenter.org/health/mental_health/fellowships/index.html.

informal measures such as feedback from conference participants or counts of requests for materials.

A notable exception is the *Like Minds, Like Mine* campaign, which was initiated by the New Zealand Ministry of Health in 1996.[37] This research-based campaign includes strategically placed television, radio, and cinema advertisements (including nationally known and respected people who had experience with mental illness), public relations activities to support the advertising messages (including media interviews and placed articles), and more targeted locally based education and grassroots activities. National tracking surveys found high awareness of campaign messages and significant changes in attitudes and behavior. For example, 62% of those surveyed reported discussing the advertising one or more times with someone else. Most important were the reports of reduced stigma and discrimination related to family, the public, mental health services, media content, police, and housing. More information on the ongoing campaign, including the National Plan,[38] can be found at https://www.likeminds.org.nz/.

England's *Time to Change* (TTC) campaign, another promising effort to change public attitudes and reduce discriminatory behavior toward people with mental illness. *TTC*, launched in 2009 and funded (by several charities) through at least 2021, has a substantial social media component. A national survey linked awareness of *TTC* with increased odds of seeking help and comfort disclosing a mental illness.[39] Also worth noting are the public education campaigns developed by the Royal College of Psychiatrists in Great Britain, including *Defeat Depression* from 1992 to 1996[40] and Changing Minds from 1998 to 2003.[41,42] *Defeat Depression* was meant to encourage earlier treatment-seeking by educating the public and reducing stigma. *Changing Minds* broadened the effort to include anxiety, schizophrenia, dementias, alcohol, and other drug misuse, and eating disorders. In addition to encouraging the public "to stop and think about their own attitudes and behaviour in relation to mental disorders… and become more tolerant of people with mental health problems," the campaign designers sought to reduce discrimination against people who suffer from these problems. Surveys suggest that these campaigns may have contributed to encouraging small shifts in attitudes (for example, regarding perceptions of dangerousness, and whether a mentally ill person is to blame for his or her condition), but it's not clear whether discriminatory behaviors were affected. Survey data tables, campaign materials, and information on the recent Royal College of Psychiatrists campaign *Partners in Care* (addressing the needs of families caring for someone who is mentally ill) can be found at <http://www.rcpsych.ac.uk/healthadvice/partnersincarecampaign.aspx>.

SUMMARY

Working with the media can be a positive experience and a valuable complement to a clinical practice or a research program if psychiatrists overcome their discomfort and develop realistic expectations and clear goals. For clinicians, it provides opportunities to counter misinformation and stereotypes, to remove barriers to seeking diagnosis and treatment, to improve therapeutic relationships, compliance with treatment, and clinical outcomes, and to increase social and political support for families who struggle with mental illness. For researchers, it can help bring key public policy issues to the forefront and clarify confusing issues related to mental health. It is also important to network with colleagues locally and internationally to build our limited knowledge base of innovative and effective ways to use mass media for the benefit of the public's mental health.

REFERENCES

1. Reiling J, ed. *Psychiatry and Sensationalism (JAMA 100 Years Ago: July 29, 1899)*. JAMA. Vol. 282. 1999:308F (4).
2. Begley S. Psychiatry group tells members they can ignore 'Goldwater rule' and comment on Trump's mental health. *STAT*; July 25, 2017. https://www.statnews.com/2017/07/25/psychiatry-goldwater-rule-trump/.
3. Kutner L, Beresin EV. Media training for psychiatry residents. *Acad Psychiatry*. 1999;23:227−232.
4. Jorm AF. Mental health literacy: empowering the community to take action for better mental health. *Am Psychol*. 2012;67(3):231−243.
5. Pescosolido BA, Medina TR, Martin JK, Long JS. The "backbone" of stigma: identifying the global core of public prejudice associated with mental illness. *Am J Public Health*. 2013;103(5):853−860.
6. Pescosolido BA, Perry BL, Martin JK, McLeod JD, Jensen PS. Stigmatizing attitudes and beliefs about treatment and psychiatric medication for children with mental illness. *Psychiatr Serv*. 2007;58(5):613−618.
7. Owens PL, Hoagwood K, Horwitz SM, et al. Barriers to children's mental health services. *J Am Acad Child Adolesc Psychiatry*. 2002;41(6):73108.
8. Nock MK, Kazdin AE. Parent expectancies for child therapy: assessment and relation to participation in treatment. *J Child Fam Stud*. 2001;10(2):155−180.
9. Merikangas KR, He JP, Burstein ME, et al. Service utilization for lifetime mental disorders in U.S. adolescents: results of the National comorbidity Survey Adolescent supplement (NCS-A). *J Am Acad Child Adolesc Psychiatry*. 2011;50(1):32−45.

10. Shuchman M, Wilkes MS. Medical scientists and health news reporting: a case of miscommunication. *Ann Intern Med.* 1997;126(12):976–982.

11. Angermeyer MC, Matschinger H. The effect of violent attacks by schizophrenic persons on the attitude of the public towards the mentally ill. *Soc Sci Med.* 1996;43(12):1721–1728.

12. Silton NR, Flannelley KJ, Milstein G, Vaaler ML. Stigma in America: has anything changed? Impact of perceptions of mental illness and dangerousness on the desire for social distance, 1996 and 2006. *J Nerv Ment Dis.* 2011;199(6):361–366.

13. Reavley NJ, Jorm AF. Association between beliefs about the causes of mental disorders and stigmatising attitudes: results of a national survey of the Australian public. *Aust N Z J Psychiatry.* 2014;48(8):764–771.

14. Pirkis J, Francis C. *Mental Illness in the News and the Information Media: A Critical Review.* Hunter Institute of Mental Health, Mindframe National Media Initiative. Available at: http://www.mindframe-media.info.

15. Wahl OF, Wood A, Richards R. Newspaper coverage of mental illness: is it changing? *Psychiatr Rehabil Skills.* 2002;6(1):9–31.

16. Taylor PJ, Gunn J. Homicides by people with mental illness: myth and reality. *Br J Psychiatry.* 1999;174(1):9–14.

17. Lawson A, Fouts G. Mental illness in Disney animated films. *Can J Psychiatry.* 2004;49:310–314.

18. Wilson C, Nairn R, Coverdale J, Panapa A. How mental illness is portrayed in children's television: a prospective study. *Br J Psychiatry.* 2000;176:440–443.

19. Wahl O, Hanrahan E, Karl K, Lasher E, Swaye J. The depiction of mental illnesses on children's television programs. *J Commun Psychol.* 2007;35(1):121–133.

20. Butler JR, Hyler SE. Hollywood portrayals of child and adolescent mental health treatment: implications for clinical practice. *Child Adolesc Psychiatr Clin N Am.* 2005;14(3):509–522.

21. Dubois RW. Pharmaceutical promotion: don't throw the baby out with the bath water. *Health Aff;* Feb. 26 2003 (web exclusive) http://content.healthaffairs.org/cgi/content/full/hlthaff.w3.96v1/DC1.

22. Moynihan R. Celebrity selling - part two. *BMJ.* 2002;325:286.

23. Moynihan R. Making medical journalism healthier. *Lancet.* 2003;361:2097–2098.

24. Frosch DL, Grande D, Tarn DM, Kravitz RL. A decade of controversy: balancing policy with evidence in the regulation of prescription drug advertising. *Am J Public Health.* 2010;100(1):24–32.

25. National Science Board, National Science Foundation. *Science and Engineering Indicators 2016 (NSB-2016-1);* 2016 Jan. https://www.nsf.gov/statistics/2016/nsb20161/#/report/chapter-7/interest-information-sources-and-involvement.

26. Krishna S, Boren SA, Balas EA. Healthcare via cell phones: a systematic review. *Telemed e-Health.* 2009;15(3):231–240.

27. Shuchman M. Journalists as change agents in medicine and health care. *JAMA.* 2002;287(6):776.

28. Centers for Disease Control and Prevention Entertainment Education Program. Porter Novelli healthstyles survey: soap opera viewers and health information. In: *Presentation at the American Public Health Association Annual Meeting, Nov 15, 2000;* 1999. http://www.cdc.gov/communication/surveys/surv1999.htm.

29. Brodie M, Foehr U, Rideout V, et al. Communicating health information through the entertainment media. *Health Aff.* 2001;20(1):192–199.

30. Kutner L, Beresin EV. Reaching out: mass media techniques for child and adolescent psychiatrists. *J Am Acad Child Adolesc Psychiatry.* 2000;39(11):1452–1454.

31. Sieff EM. Media frames of mental illness: the potential impact of negative frames. *J Ment Health.* 2003;12(3):259–269.

32. Schwartz T. *Media: The Second God.* Garden City, NY: Anchor Press/Doubleday; 1983:97–99.

33. Stuart H. Stigma and the daily news: evaluation of a newspaper intervention. *Can J Psychiatry.* 2003;48:651–656.

34. Ferriman A. The stigma of schizophrenia (reviews: press). *BMJ.* 2000;320(7233):522 (news editor).

35. Sartorius N. Stigma: what can psychiatrists do about it? *Lancet.* 1998;352:1058–1059.

36. The Carter Center Journalism Resource Guide on Behavioral Health. Available at: https://www.cartercenter.org/resources/pdfs/health/mental_health/2015-journalism-resource-guide-on-behavioral-health.pdf.

37. Vaughan G, Hansen C. "Like Minds, Like Mine": a New Zealand project to counter the stigma and discrimination associated with mental illness. *Australas Psychiatry.* 2004;12(2):113–117.

38. New Zealand Ministry of Health. Like Minds, Like Mine National Plan 2003–2005. Wellington, NZ; September 2003.

39. Henderson C, Robinsin E, Evans-Lacko S, Thornicroft G. Relationships between anti-stigma programme awareness, disclosure comfort and intended help-seeking regarding a mental health problem. *Br J Psychiatry.* 2017. Published online in advance of print on 2017-9-21.

40. Paykel ES, Hart D, Priest RG. Changes in public attitudes to depression during the Defeat depression campaign. *Br J Psychiatry.* 1998;173(12):519–522.

41. Byrne P. Stigma of mental illness and ways of diminishing it. *Adv Psychiatr Treat.* 2000;6:65–72.

42. Crisp A, Gelder M, Goddard E, Meltzer H. Stigmatization of people with mental illnesses: a follow-up study within the changing minds campaign of the Royal College of Psychiatrists. *World Psychiatry.* 2005;4(2):106–113.

CHAPTER 11

The Use of Telepsychiatry in Caring for Youth and Families: Overcoming the Shortages in Child and Adolescent Psychiatrists

ANTHONY D. SOSSONG, MD, MS • LIORA ZHREBKER, BA •
JESSICA E. BECKER, MD • NEHA P. CHAUDHARY, MD • DAVID H. RUBIN, MD

INTRODUCTION

In recent years, the demand for child and adolescent psychiatry and other mental health services has grown. As more is understood about the early onset of psychiatric illness and as additional treatments have become available, more people who need treatment are seeking care.[1] At the same time, services have become more accessible to families through laws such as the Patient Protection and Affordable Care Act, increasing mental health service eligibility. Yet, the number of child and adolescent psychiatric providers is not nearly enough to meet the growing demand. If resources remain stable, it is estimated that by 2020, the child and adolescent workforce will barely meet only two-thirds of the demand.[1,2] Patients in rural communities are at a particular disadvantage, as child psychiatrists tend to be concentrated in urban or suburban areas and academic centers.[3] Rural populations face other barriers to mental healthcare access as well, including increased rates of poverty, delays in mental health treatment, less access to insurance coverage for mental health services, and limited transportation options.[2] Urban populations experience their own set of challenges. Access to healthcare services can be limited due to such issues as parents' work schedules, language barriers, immigration status, culture, and lack of familiarity with the healthcare system.[2,4] As high-quality videoconferencing (VC) technology becomes more affordable, there is growing interest in applying these technologies to increase healthcare accessibility and equitable delivery. The advent and regulatory acceptance of these technologies is ushering in a new potential for specialists to affect lives beyond the catchment of their traditional practice sites, while patients stand to benefit irrespective of their localities, time of day, or access to transportation.

OVERVIEW OF TELEPSYCHIATRY

The terms "*telehealth*" and "*telemedicine*" generally refer to the use of technology to deliver healthcare remotely.[1,5] The application of these terms, however, can be variable. Some organizations, such as the World Health Organization, use the terms telehealth and telemedicine interchangeably, while others refer to telehealth as a broader field and use telemedicine more narrowly.[6] The Health Resources and Services Administration defines telehealth broadly as using "electronic information and telecommunications technologies to support and promote long-distance clinical health care, patient and professional health-related education, public health, and health administration."[1]

Telehealth comprises multiple modalities, including *synchronous* (i.e., real-time) interactions between providers and patients via VC or telecommunication technology, as well as *asynchronous* interactions. Asynchronous modalities include store-and-forward technology in which a patient is recorded and the recording is reviewed later by a remote, consulting provider; video- or telephone-based consultation from a specialist healthcare provider to another healthcare provider; internet-based interventions targeted directly to patients; and delivery of care to patients using mobile technology via applications ("apps") or text messages.[5,7]

In contrast, telemedicine can be defined more specifically as the synchronous use of VC or telecommunication technology to connect a provider directly to a patient for remote diagnosis and treatment.[1] When telehealth or telemedicine is used to deliver mental healthcare, the terms *telemental health* and *telepsychiatry* are used.[1,8]

For the purposes of this chapter, we will examine telepsychiatry, a type of synchronous VC in which telecommunications-based sessions occur between a psychiatrist and patient. Telepsychiatry models of care may vary widely, and similar to traditional in-person (IP) practice, the telepsychiatrist can evaluate and treat patients directly or provide consultative services.

Telepsychiatry has found utility in nearly all aspects of evaluation and treatment encompassed by the IP encounter,[5,7] spanning many clinical locations including the outpatient, inpatient, and emergency room setting.[2,9] As the demand for child psychiatrists continues to grow without a supply of clinicians to match, telepsychiatry offers a unique avenue by which to close this gap. It holds the advantage of being able to extend care to settings in which child psychiatry care may not otherwise be accessed and allows each participating child psychiatrist to reach a larger number of patients than could otherwise be reached geographically by an individual. It also allows for flexibility to access providers beyond usual business hours, which may expand access to services for children with working parents.

Telepsychiatry has been used in several different clinical practice settings for the evaluation and treatment of youth and their families. Emergency rooms, for example, often do not have an in-house psychiatrist available for evaluations, especially at night or on weekends. In some emergency rooms, children with behavioral problems are seen and evaluated by pediatricians on an emergency basis. If a psychiatrist is available, his or her background is typically tailored to triaging adult patients and not youth. In such circumstances, a telepsychiatry consultation would allow a child psychiatrist to provide subspecialty consultation for use of medications on an urgent basis, consideration of appropriate placements and necessary levels of care, and suggestions for ambulatory clinical services for the child and family. If the child is seen by a pediatrician, additional psychiatric consultation may be available for diagnostic considerations as well. By providing these services using telepsychiatry, a single child and adolescent psychiatrist can reach to a wider catchment area at any given time.

In addition to its utility in emergency rooms, telepsychiatry can also be used in inpatient and outpatient settings. In inpatient settings, this modality is used for intake assessments, follow-up evaluations, and even family meetings. In outpatient clinics, telepsychiatry is used to colocate or embed psychiatry in primary care and specialty pediatric clinics to provide timely follow-up or consultations for youth in need of evaluations. In these settings, clinics maintain their typical duties and staffing structures while utilizing telepsychiatry where there is a shortage of onsite staff child psychiatrists. Telepsychiatry has become versatile across clinical settings, allowing for mental healthcare to be delivered both within a physician's practice, as well as in a bridging, consultative capacity until patients are able to obtain appointments in longitudinal clinics. Further, telepsychiatry may be used in any of these settings for multidisciplinary rounding and may serve teaching purposes as well as guiding the team for appropriate behavioral management or pharmacotherapy.

Telepsychiatry also expands the reach of mental healthcare beyond traditional clinical settings. Schools and childcare centers in both urban and rural areas have served as sites for telepsychiatry patients, with consultations directly to children, or to teachers, nurses, social workers, school psychologists, and administrative staff who are facing challenges with particular students.[4] There are unique advantages to using telepsychiatry in these settings, which cannot be attained through practice in traditional healthcare settings. For one, school-based programs inherently implement mental healthcare into a child and family's daily routine, which helps to minimize travel time and cost to families. Second, schools are settings in which behaviors of concern can be observed before they reach a severe level. As a result, school-based programs are a prime opportunity for preventative care, where children can be evaluated and treated before problems escalate.

TELEPSYCHIATRY VERSUS TRADITIONAL PRACTICE

As the practice of telepsychiatry becomes more widespread, studies have emerged that aim to determine its utility and efficacy in successfully managing and treating psychiatric conditions in pediatric patients. Much of the research compares telepsychiatry to traditional, IP encounters using a variety of outcome measures, including patient satisfaction and clinical outcomes, consistency and accuracy of diagnosis, and factors mediating successful implementation of a telepsychiatry program.

Effectiveness of implementation has been studied on the basis of the implementation of clinical parameters from IP evaluations in which their implementation is replicable and adaptable to the settings of telemental health.[9] A successful psychiatric evaluation is contingent upon reliability of diagnosis, as well as psychotherapeutic and psychopharmacological treatments and approaches. The replicability and efficacy of psychiatric evaluations within the telepsychiatry setting will be reviewed, based on clinical parameters and outcomes described by current literature.

As an evaluative and therapeutic service across a variety of psychiatric conditions, telepsychiatry has been found to function just as well as, if not better than, traditional psychiatric services. In a trial of 23 pediatric patients, aged 4–16 years, patients were randomized to two groups in which both groups were assessed by child psychiatrists over VC software and IP assessment, but experienced the modalities in different orders.[10] An independent, blinded psychiatrist then compared assessments of patients following the VC evaluation to those following the IP evaluation; it was found that 22 of these 23 cases (96%) were given the same diagnosis and treatment recommendations when evaluated over VC as when they were evaluated IP.[10] Reese et al.[11] similarly compared diagnostic accuracy over VC and IP evaluations, in which a sample of 21 children with diagnoses of either autism or developmental delay were assessed by clinicians in either a VC or IP modality. It was found that 83% and 86% of IP and VC assessments, respectively, matched prior diagnoses; this suggests that there was no significant difference between the assessments in the two modalities.[11]

Psychotherapy has been studied for replicability in telepsychiatry across a variety of conditions. In a randomized controlled study, 28 pediatric depression patients were placed in either VC or IP groups and underwent at least 6 (up to 8) sessions of cognitive behavioral therapy (CBT).[12] Following this intervention, both groups reported a decrease in depressive symptoms, with 82% of subjects no longer meeting depression criteria. It was additionally found that the decrease of depressive symptoms was higher in the VC group than in the IP group. A study that similarly compared VC to IP assessments explored the assessments of childhood tic disorders for pediatric participants in both VC and IP treatment.[13] A total of 20 participants were randomized to either a VC or IP group in which participants received a psychotherapeutic treatment, the Comprehensive Behavioral Intervention for Tics (CBIT). Following CBIT, it was found that there was little difference between the treatment modalities, and CBIT under both VC and IP treatment was successful in reducing the severity of tics. In a similar

randomized study exploring the effect of a CBT intervention in a sample of children with early-onset obsessive-compulsive disorder, it was found that the VC modality of treatment had better results than the IP treatment.[14]

Studies have also explored the accuracy of psychopharmacological practice in telepsychiatry compared with traditional practice. For instance, Myers et al.[15] explored the outcomes in psychopharmacological treatment of 233 patients with attention-deficit/hyperactivity disorder (ADHD), in which the patients were randomized to either a VC or IP mode of assessment and treatment. Psychiatrists were trained to prescribe medication using five ADHD algorithms of an evidence-based manual, the Texas Children's Medication Algorithm Project.[15,16] The patient treatment was supplemented by a caregiver behavioral training, which allowed the caregiver to monitor the improvement of patients following treatment. As reported by caregivers, patients in both groups improved following the treatment, although a greater improvement was observed in the VC group. At present, Myers et al.[15] is the only existing study that examines pediatric psychopharmacologic treatment through telepsychiatry.[15]

Overall, current research demonstrates that the field of telepsychiatry has potential to provide effective services where IP evaluations are not possible. This body of research demonstrates that these services benefit patients across psychiatric conditions and locations. However, there is room to continue exploring the accessibility of telepsychiatry services as it impacts populations of different socioeconomic classes, ethnicities, and geographic residencies. While a primary purpose of telepsychiatry, and telemental health in general, is to increase availability of services to those who would not otherwise access those services, the existing body of telepsychiatry research does not represent a diverse population of participants, focusing mainly on Caucasian participants of a middle socioeconomic class.[11,12,14] The Children's ADHD Telemental Health Treatment Study of 2015, for instance, is the first community-based trial exploring the effects of using VC for treatment intervention in underserved communities.[15] Future studies should specifically target underserved communities, notably rural communities who face geographic barriers and urban communities who often have concentrated underserved populations with minimal access to healthcare.[2,4]

In addition to expanding the demographic of participants targeted for studies, additional opportunities for further research include study designs with alternative interventions and larger sample sizes. While one of the studies reviewed, Myers et al.,[15] studies a sample of over 200 participants, it stands as one of the few studies with a large sample size.[15] Many of the current studies have smaller sample sizes and risk losing generalizability to the larger population.[11–13] To increase generalizability and representation of child psychiatric patients, it would be beneficial to increase the sample size. An additional factor within study design that has potential for further research is exploring interventions other than psychotherapy. At present, there is only one study that has used psychopharmacology as an intervention to determine the success of telepsychiatry in treating child mental health conditions.[15] Overall, to better represent the communities and populations who most benefit from telepsychiatry, future studies should be configured to explore interventions that have not been studied and recruit samples that represent a variety of demographics in order to show how the impact of telepsychiatry is wide-reaching.

CLINICAL CONSIDERATIONS
The Telepsychiatry Encounter

Participants in a telepsychiatry encounter are typically a patient, a parent/guardian if the patient is a minor, and a telepsychiatrist. A *telepresenter*, a medical professional or technician facilitating the patient encounter from the hospital or clinic in which the patient is participating, may also be present. Beyond the technological logistics of facilitation, onsite telepresenters also help by providing the remote telepsychiatry provider with relevant information about local culture, community resources, and other facets of local healthcare systems that contributes to a safer and more effective clinical practice.[2,17]

During a telepsychiatry encounter, the patient is brought into a designated, private room and is seated while the psychiatrist observes the patient over the video. Alternatively, the videoconference equipment is installed on a movable cart or embedded in a robot, which is either brought or remotely steered to the patient's location. The psychiatrist introduces him- or herself and conducts the interview over the screen, with or without the help of a telepresenter. Relevant records are reviewed and notes are recorded remotely, usually in electronic medical records (EMRs). If medications are needed, they are prescribed using traditional prescription guidelines through the EMR. After the encounter is complete, the physician may request to speak with the staff after the patient is dismissed from the room. Final disposition and/or treatment plans are discussed with staff directly, as would be done in a face-to-face team meeting or at the nursing station.

Webside manner, the overall etiquette surrounding each patient encounter using telepsychiatry, is similar to the "bedside manner" of an IP visit; however, there are some notable exceptions. Research has explored the factors and unique considerations that promote patient engagement in telepsychiatry. During the opening phase of an encounter, it is imperative that audio and video equipment be tested and that both the physician and patient can see and hear one another. The patient should be in the camera's field of view, so that the psychiatrist can observe facial expressions and other behaviors. It is recommended that the psychiatrist's head, shoulders, and both arms until mid-chest be in the frame of view, with 6 inches left above his or her head.[18] It is also common for the psychiatrist to pay particular attention to his or her own affect conveyance, at times accentuating expressions since nuances can be lost over video. The psychiatrist should vary his or her gaze between the camera and the screen; this allows the psychiatrist to balance their own observation of the patient with the patient perceiving eye contact and thus a sense of connection during the encounter.[19] These intentional behaviors help in establishing rapport with the patient despite the lack of physical presence and proximity.

In our clinical experience, it is common for both the psychiatrist and the patient to forget within minutes that they are interacting via a screen, especially with older adolescents and with adults. Sustaining concentration and attention with younger children can be challenging via a teleconference and often the assistance of the telepresenter or nurse in redirecting the child toward the screen is helpful. Physicians should comment on the use of technology in the session and invite the patient to comment on how the experience of a tele-based session was for him or her, in order to strengthen rapport and acknowledge the patient's experience. Currently, most randomized controlled trials have illustrated high patient satisfaction with telepsychiatry and comparability to the care provided IP.[2]

Patient Selection

While telepsychiatry has offered an avenue for easier access to mental healthcare for patients of all ages, research has particularly demonstrated the receptiveness of the pediatric population. This may be due to increased pervasiveness of social media and real-time, internet-based communication applications, which has made screen time conversations using commercial VC a typical means of communication for children and teens. In addition to this ubiquity, the perception of anonymity while using this technology may also be particularly attractive to young people.[20] Findings validate these conjectures, showing high rates of pediatric patient satisfaction with, and even preference for, VC sessions with physicians.[20] Notably, adolescent patients have expressed that telepsychiatry allows a perceived distance contributing to the patient's sense of privacy and agency; this helps them to be more open and confident with their clinicians and contributes to collaborative, joint responsibility, and decision making.[20]

Telepsychiatry has been used for youth with virtually all psychiatric conditions. While ADHD has been found to be the most commonly treated disorder, it is important to consider the impact of telepsychiatry on other patient populations as well.[2] While the benefit of telepsychiatry is clear for certain patient populations, there are others for whom aggravation of their conditions (e.g., patients with psychotic or phobic disorders) may pose a potential concern.[5] While evidence is limited, recent studies have found VC-based telepsychiatry not inferior to IP care for patients with psychotic disorders and that patients with delusions regarding television responded appropriately to telepsychiatry sessions without incorporating the sessions into their delusions.[5,21,22]

Patient Safety and Emergencies

As previously discussed, patient selection is an important part of determining appropriateness of using telepsychiatry for treatment. While a telepresenter or parent at the patient site may help facilitate a smooth interaction during a routine encounter with a pediatric patient, the uncooperative, behaviorally dysregulated, or agitated patient poses a unique challenge in the telepsychiatric encounter.[2] Given the remote nature of the clinician when practicing telepsychiatry, it is important for the psychiatrist to lay out expectations with patient families for emergency procedures and for contact between sessions.[5,22]

As with an IP encounter, the provider needs to be familiar with local services, including the closest emergency room or healthcare facility for emergency planning, and may need to respond to emergent safety concerns in real time. To ensure a timely response to psychiatric emergencies that may emerge during the session, it is imperative that the provider has knowledge of the patient's exact location during the encounter and be familiar with community resources local to the patient. In such an emergency, the provider may benefit from the assistance of a telepresenter or parent at the patient site to allow for safer monitoring of the patient while emergency services are mobilized.[3,17]

TECHNOLOGY AND SECURITY

Effective telepsychiatry requires high *bandwidth*, high monitor resolution, and consistent transmission signal strength and connectivity.[17] Further, camera quality and positioning, audio signal, room lighting, room size, and ability to capture a potentially mobile pediatric patient on camera can affect effective evaluation and treatment of a patient.[5,17] However, as technology advances, technological literacy improves among patients and providers, and as technological concerns are better addressed in the telemedical literature, technological barriers to telepsychiatry implementation have diminished.[1,20]

To maintain secure and efficient transmission of patient data, the audio and video equipment utilized in telepsychiatry encounters is set up in accordance with specific standards. For example, the generally accepted bandwidth is >386 kbits/s and the information transmission must be *encrypted*.[2]

REQUIREMENTS AND REGULATIONS

While efforts have been made toward national telemedicine licensing, at present, licensing requirements are determined by individual state medical boards. At present, a physician must be licensed in the jurisdiction of the patient's location in addition to their own.[23] However, the Federation of State Medical Boards, along with representatives from several state medical boards, helped to create the Interstate Medical Licensure Compact, which first began issuing Letters of Qualification in April 2017.[23] At present, there are 22 states that take part in this compact, which allows eligible physicians to apply for licensure in states outside of their home state that are members of the Compact.[23]

Explicit written and/or verbal consent for telepsychiatry should be obtained from pediatric patients' legal guardians or from the patient directly as regulated by local, regional, and national laws and guidelines.[23] State laws regarding the confidentiality of mental health information as well as the federal Health Insurance Portability and Accountability Act regulations must be followed, and any recording or storage of sessions should be performed only with written consent by the patient and/or patient's legal guardian.[2] The remote provider should also be versed in the mandatory reporting guidelines, civil commitment laws, age of majority, and any other ethical requirements to which the provider may be bound while providing remote care. These standards and regulations must be followed for the location at which the patient is receiving care.[2,7]

Further, the American Telemedicine Association guidelines require that practitioners comply with laws and regulations both in the provider and patient site jurisdictions.[2] At the same time, in order to protect themselves, providers must also verify that their malpractice insurance covers telemedicine practice and covers practice in the patient's jurisdiction.[2]

PAYMENT AND REIMBURSEMENT

Financial sustainability has been a barrier to implementation of telepsychiatry programs and services. While over 30 states require parity between payment from private insurance companies for telehealth and IP services, others do not have such laws.[24] As such, insurance companies, including public payers, may not always reimburse telepsychiatry services at rates equivalent to IP services.[20] Even if there is parity in service reimbursement for the practitioner, most private payers do not compensate for clinical or technical staff at the patient site, which may limit feasibility of participation at the patient site.[15] However, the Center for Medicare and Medicaid Services has established the policy of providing a care coordination fee to telemedicine patient sites at a per patient per month rate, while Medicaid coverage for telemedicine has been expanding across geographic regions and sites of service within states.[15]

Other financial constraints to consider include costs of equipment, service lines, and data transmission.[9] These often require grant funds to accommodate costs. While decreasing technology costs allows for telepsychiatry programs to be more feasible, more research is required to determine sustainable financial means to maintain these programs.[2,25]

Despite these challenges, there are ways in which telepsychiatry can be made more financially feasible. At the present, reimbursement is available for Medicare and Medicaid holders in 46 states.[26,27] The current payment model, however, is limited in scope (as it is strictly a fee-for-services model) and has not expanded to other insurance companies. An alternate payment model to explore is value-based pay, which limits over- or underuse of services and over- or underpayment accordingly; by considering the variety of patient experiences and conditions in payment, it offers a model that is potentially more economically effective and equitable.[28] Another approach to consider is exploring the financial impacts of telepsychiatry beyond the center in which services are offered and to explore the impact on a network of medical centers in a geographic area. While the center may not itself benefit from offering the

program, implementing telepsychiatric services may contribute to decreased hospitalization and reduction of transfers by other medical centers or by other departments in the institution, contributing to decreased costs overall.[2,25]

TRAINING AND EDUCATION

As telepsychiatry becomes more widely used and adopted into new and existing communities, some child and adolescent psychiatry training programs have begun elective or required clinical training in telepsychiatry.[2] As this practice modality grows, it will be imperative for all graduate medical training in psychiatry to include formal training in the use of telepsychiatry. Training should include not only a practical overview of how to use properly configured equipment, assess patients, establish rapport, and offer treatment but also education on privacy, security, safety, licensing, and other such considerations that are unique to the practice of telemedicine. With proper training and familiarity, consistency of high-quality, value-based care delivery will be ensured.

SUMMARY

Because of its ease of use, potential for cost savings, widespread availability, and growing accessibility, telepsychiatry has become an attractive option for expanding pediatric psychiatric care to larger communities. As its use becomes increasingly widespread, care must be given to understand its unique considerations, including new regulatory factors, limitations in reimbursement, and privacy requirements. If implemented and used appropriately with this knowledge, telepsychiatry can extend psychiatric care to children and adolescents who otherwise may not receive the care that they need, thereby helping to close the gap between the demand for care and the limited available child and adolescent psychiatric workforce. By increasing the geographical reach of, and convenience of access to, scarce child psychiatrists, telepsychiatry offers boundless distribution of highly specialized care to demanding populations.

GLOSSARY

Asynchronous   Not in real-time. In the context of telehealth, for example, asynchronous interactions include a patient encounter being recorded and forwarded to a telehealth provider, or the forwarding of a photograph or lab result to assist in evaluation and treatment remotely.

Bandwidth
A measure of the maximum volume of information per unit of time that can be transmitted through a given medium (e.g., an internet connection).

Encrypted
In information technology, this refers to the crucial data security measure of providing end-to-end protection when transmitting information across a public network (e.g., the open Internet), by which data are converted to an encoded form that may only be decoded by using a unique decryption key.

Resolution
A measure of video quality. Specifically, the number of pixels, or individual points of color, contained in the graphical display. This is expressed as the number of pixels on the horizontal axis by the number on the vertical axis (e.g., 1024 × 768).

Store-and-forward
Model of care in which a patient is recorded and recording is reviewed later by a remote, consulting provider.

Synchronous
In real-time.

Telehealth
The use of technology to deliver healthcare remotely. Can be used interchangeably with the term telemedicine or defined more broadly as any such remote interaction, whether synchronous or asynchronous.

Telemedicine
The use of technology to deliver healthcare remotely. Can be used interchangeably with the term telehealth or defined more narrowly to refer to remote, synchronous encounters between a patient and healthcare provider.

Telemental health
The use of technology to deliver mental healthcare remotely. Can be used interchangeably with the term telepsychiatry or defined more broadly as any such remote interaction, whether synchronous or asynchronous.

Telepresenter
Technician assisting in delivery of telehealthcare (patient-side).

Telepsychiatry
The use of technology to deliver mental healthcare remotely. Can be used interchangeably with the term telemental health or defined more narrowly to refer to remote, synchronous encounters between a patient and healthcare provider.

Webside manner
The etiquette surrounding a patient encounter using telepsychiatry, similar to bedside manner for an in-person encounter.

REFERENCES

1. Myers K, Comer JS. The case for telemental health for improving the accessibility and quality of Children's Mental Health Services. *J Child Adolesc Psychopharmacol.* 2016;26(3):186−191. https://doi.org/10.1089/cap.2015.0055.
2. Cain S, Nelson EL, Myers K. Telemental health. In: *Dulcan's Textbook of Child and Adolescent Psychiatry.* 2nd ed. American Psychiatric Association Publishing; 2015. https://doi.org/10.1176/appi.books.9781615370306.md33.
3. Thomas CR, Holzer CE. The continuing shortage of child and adolescent psychiatrists. *J Am Acad Child Adolesc Psychiatry.* 2006;45(9):1023−1031.
4. Spaulding R, Cain S, Sonnenschein K. Urban telepsychiatry: uncommon service for a common need. *Child Adolesc Psychiatr Clin N Am.* 2011;20(1):29−39. https://doi.org/10.1016/j.chc.2010.08.010.
5. Becker J. Telemental health modalities: videoconferencing, store-and-forward, web-based, and mHealth. In: Jefee-Bahloul H, Barkil-Oteo A, Augusterfer EF, eds. *Telemental Health in Resource-Limited Global Settings.* Oxford University Press; 2017:15−32.
6. Ryu S. World Health Organization Global Observatory for eHealth. Telemedicine: opportunities and developments in member states. *Observatory.* 2012;18(2):153−155. https://doi.org/10.4258/hir.2012.18.2.153.
7. Yellowlees PM, Odor A, Parish MB, Iosif A-M, Haught K, Hilty D. A feasibility study of the use of asynchronous telepsychiatry for psychiatric consultations. *Psychiatr Serv.* 2010;61(8):838−840. https://doi.org/10.1176/ps.2010.61.8.838.
8. Yellowlees P, Shore J, Roberts L. Practice guidelines for videoconferencing-based telemental health − October 2009. *Telemed J E Health.* 2010;16(10):1074−1089. https://doi.org/10.1089/tmj.2010.0148.
9. Hilty DM, Ferrer DC, Parish MB, Johnston B, Callahan EJ, Yellowlees PM. The effectiveness of telemental health: a 2013 review. *Telemed J E Health.* 2013;19(6):444−454. https://doi.org/10.1089/tmj.2013.0075.
10. Elford R, White H, Bowering R, Ghandi A, Maddiggan B, John KS. A randomized, controlled trial of child psychiatric assessments conducted using videoconferencing. *J Telemed Telecare.* 2000;6(2):73−82.
11. Reese RM, Jamison R, Wendland M, et al. Evaluating interactive videoconferencing for assessing symptoms of autism. *Telemed J E Health.* 2013;19(9):671−677.

12. Nelson E-L, Barnard M, Cain S. Treating childhood depression over videoconferencing. *Telemed J E health.* 2003;9(1): 49–55.

13. Himle MB, Freitag M, Walther M, Franklin SA, Ely L, Woods DW. A randomized pilot trial comparing videoconference versus face-to-face delivery of behavior therapy for childhood tic disorders. *Behav Res Ther.* 2012;50(9): 565–570.

14. Storch EA, Caporino NE, Morgan JR, et al. Preliminary investigation of web-camera delivered cognitive-behavioral therapy for youth with obsessive-compulsive disorder. *Psychiatry Res.* 2011;189(3):407–412.

15. Myers K, Stoep AV, Zhou C, McCarty CA, Katon W. Effectiveness of a telehealth service delivery model for treating attention-deficit/hyperactivity disorder: a community-based randomized controlled trial. *J Am Acad Child Adolesc Psychiatry.* 2015;54(4):263–274.

16. Pliszka SR, Crismon ML, Hughes CW, et al. The Texas children's medication algorithm project: revision of the algorithm for pharmacotherapy of attention-deficit/hyperactivity disorder. *J Am Acad Child Adolesc Psychiatry.* 2006; 45(6):642–657.

17. Goldstein F, Glueck D. Developing rapport and therapeutic alliance during telemental health sessions with children and adolescents. *J Child Adolesc Psychopharmacol.* 2016; 26(3):204–211. https://doi.org/10.1089/cap.2015.0022.

18. Shore JH. Telepsychiatry: videoconferencing in the delivery of psychiatric care. *Am J Psychiatry.* 2013;170(3):256–262. https://doi.org/10.1176/appi.ajp.2012.12081064.

19. Myers K, Cain S. Practice parameter for telepsychiatry with children and adolescents. *J Am Acad Child Adolesc Psychiatry.* 2008;47(12):1468–1483.

20. Boydell KM, Hodgins M, Pignatiello A, Teshima J, Edwards H, Willis D. Using technology to deliver mental health services to children and youth: a scoping review. *J Can Acad Child Adolesc Psychiatry.* 2014;23(2):87–99.

21. Sharp IR, Kobak KA, Osman DA. The use of videoconferencing with patients with psychosis: a review of the literature. *Ann Gen Psychiatry.* 2011;10(1):14. https://doi.org/10.1186/1744-859X-10-14.

22. Turvey C, Coleman M, Dennison O, et al. ATA practice guidelines for video-based online mental health services. *Telemed J E Health.* 2013;19(9):722–730. https://doi.org/10.1089/tmj.2013.9989.

23. *Interstate Medical Licensure Compact*; 2017. http://www.imlcc.org/.

24. *About Telemedicine*; 2016. https://www.americantelemed.org/about/telehealth-faqs-.

25. Hilty DM, Cobb HC, Neufeld JD, Bourgeois JA, Yellowlees PM. Telepsychiatry reduces geographic physician disparity in rural settings, but is it financially feasible because of reimbursement? *Psychiatr Clin N Am.* 2008; 31(1):85–94.

26. Myers KM, Valentine JM, Melzer SM. Feasibility, acceptability, and sustainability of telepsychiatry for children and adolescents. *Psychiatr Serv.* 2007;58(11):1493–1496.

27. Lauckner C, Whitten P. The state and sustainability of telepsychiatry programs. *J Behav Health Serv Res.* 2016;43(2): 305–318.

28. Chernew ME, Rosen AB, Fendrick AM. Value-based insurance design. *Health Aff.* 2007;26(2):195–203. https://doi.org/10.1377/hlthaff.26.2.w195.

CHAPTER 12

Your Brain on Video Games: The Neuroscience of Media

DAVID C. RETTEW, MD • ROBERT R. ALTHOFF, MD, PHD • JAMES J. HUDZIAK, MD

The amount of time people today interface with various forms of media is astounding. From watching videos, movies, and television shows to responding to social media and playing video games, media use has become woven into the fabric of everyday modern life. Its technology can bombard the senses, and its content can elicit powerful emotions. Given all this, we should certainly not be surprised that our consumption and interaction with the many forms of media can have a substantive impact on neurodevelopment.

At the same time, the brain is not simply a passive substrate to be shaped and modified by the media or any other important environmental factor. Individual variation coupled with someone's own unique experiences lead us to expect that some people may be more impacted by media than others or be more likely to use certain types of media than others. All of these potential sources of complexity are compounded with the diversity involving "media." To a developing brain, for example, an occasional viewing of *Sesame Street* might be quite different than a regular 5-hours daily diet of violent video games. In the end, it is probably as naïve of us to expect there to be a common and unifying neurobiological effect of "media" as it would be to expect a common underlying neurobiology for other important environmental factors such as parenting, peer relations, or education. Rather, what seems much more likely is a neuroscience that varies as a function of many factors related both to the media itself and the person interacting with it.

It is with this appreciation of the complexity involved that this chapter attempts to summarize what is known about the neurobiological effects of different types of media as it relates to domains that have particular clinical and public health interest. After a short discussion regarding the mechanisms through which environmental factors such as media use are known to change brain structure and function,

particular topics that have been a focus of research will be explored namely, media effects on the brain attentional networks, the link between exposure to violent media and aggression, and the emerging neuroscience literature examining the neurobiology that may be relevant for people who become "addicted" to the Internet.

GENERAL PROCESSES

Before exploring the neuroscience underlying specific brain regions and various types of media usage, it is worth considering some general mechanisms that are involved in translating qualities of one's environment to lasting alternations in brain structure and activity. While it has been long appreciated that environmental factors can have profound effects on neurodevelopment, an understanding of the precise mechanisms behind these changes has been an exciting and rapidly developing line of investigation over the past several decades.

Epigenetics and Telomeres

One of the most important processes through which environmental factors influence brain development is epigenetic modification. In general, epigenetics refers to the mechanisms through which environmental factors cause changes in levels of gene expression without altering the specific DNA sequence.[1] While there are many specific processes that could be referred to as epigenetic modifications, perhaps the most studied and widely known in behavioral science are DNA methylation, the attaching of a methyl group to promoter regions of DNA, and histone acetylation of chromatin.[2] Both of these processes can have significant effects on overall levels of gene expression independent of the actual DNA sequence within the coding region of the gene. In contrast to the actual DNA code which remains largely static over time, epigenetic processes are much more dynamic and vary according to developmental stage, tissue type, and exposure to specific types of environments.

To date, one of the most prominent areas of epigenetic research in psychiatry relates to stressful and traumatic childhood events leading to methylation and decreased expression of glucocorticoid receptors on the hippocampus which in turn can lead to dysregulation and ultimately overactivity of the hypothalamic-pituitary-adrenal axis.[3–5] A related and more uplifting story has also revealed in animal models how more positive parenting, which in mice means increased licking and grooming of pups, can lead to increased expression of these regulatory genes and protection against the negative effects of future stress.[6,7]

Epigenetic modifications in response to media exposure has yet to be investigated systematically. Theoretically, however, it hardly seems too much of a stretch to view some forms of media exposure as a form of chronic stress, especially given research that links things such as violent video games to increased levels of physiological arousal[8] as players navigate virtual kill-or-be-killed worlds. Research has demonstrated that even indirect exposure to traumatic events through the media, such as viewing coverage of the September 11 terrorist attacks, can produce some degree of posttraumatic symptoms.[9]

Another area of genetically related research that has received increased attention involves alterations in telomere length in relation to age and stressful events. Telomeres are repetitive DNA sequences found at the ends of chromosomes that serve as protective caps, similar to the plastic ends of shoelaces.[10] Telomeres are involved in the process of cell division and tend to shorten with age.[11] Research has increasingly shown that variety of adverse and stressful events can result in premature telomere shortening.[12,13] Once again, there is a scarcity of research directly looking at changes in telomere length and media exposure, although a recent study of adults did find that increased television viewing was related to shorter telomeres, controlling for some potential covariates.[14]

SPECIFIC TOPICS RELATED TO THE NEUROSCIENCE OF MEDIA

Both the brain and the media are obviously enormous topics, and while there is much that has yet to be studied and understood, there has been mounting interest about the neurobiological impacts of media use that is often inspired by specific public health

questions and concerns. One of the longstanding challenges in research regarding the neuroscience of media involves the pace at which technology and the way people use it change over time. Thirty years ago, what research there was on the media often focused on the viewing of a few television channels from a single device in the middle of the house. Video games developed from simple games of "pong" and "breakout" to the creation of entire virtual worlds with stunning imagery and elaborate plots that can now be experienced in real-time with other players across the world. The Internet gave people access to unlimited types of content with minimal barriers, especially as computers shrunk from room-sized structures to something that fits in the palm of one's hand. This moving target of what actually counts as media has created a built-in lag in behavioral and neuroscience research as scientists constantly try to catch up in their understanding of the impact of the latest technology. Yet, despite this ever evolving world of media, a number of questions have remained a priority for many years and have been steady targets of research studies, even as many of the details related to the media itself evolve. Here, we focus on the neuroscience surrounding some specific issues that each have received a fair amount of scrutiny and that potentially have important clinical and developmental implications.

SMARTPHONES, SOCIAL MEDIA, AND THE BRAIN'S ATTENTION NETWORKS

An increasing volume of research has been devoted to understanding the bidirectional influences between various forms of media and the brain's complex attentional network systems. These efforts have been stimulated by clinical research in a number of areas, including the association between excessive television and video games use and attention problems in youth,[15] the increasing public health problem related to distracted driving from mobile phones and other devices,[16] and the hypothesis that smartphones and social media may undermine an individual's ability and even motivation to maintain focus during more long-term goal-oriented tasks.

While a thorough review of how attention is mediated in the brain is beyond the scope of the chapter, a common conceptual model that is often described considers the dynamic competition between the a more "top down" attentional network that utilizes more dorsal frontoparietal areas and is responsible for giving individuals the ability to focus and concentrate on something a person chooses versus the "bottom up" and more ventrally located attentional system which helps people become alert to something in the environment that may need more immediate consideration.[17,18] From an evolutionary perspective, it is not difficult to see how both systems are important for functioning and survival, and how an imbalance in the two systems can be maladaptive. It is also evident that companies and organizations that create media platforms such as smartphones and social media are also quite aware of these different processes and use this knowledge to the advantage of their products.

As described in the recent popular book *A Deadly Wandering*, which describes the story of a young man whose texting while driving led to the deaths of two individuals and depicts the science behind our society's increasing attempts to "multitask," current smartphone technology, with its multiple alerts and interruptions to draw a person's attention to things that may or may not be important, is designed to enhance bottom-up attentional networks at the expense of an individual's ability to maintain top-down attention. Research is now beginning to suggest that it is working. Despite the widespread appeal and popularity of modern multitasking, studies continue to demonstrate that such an approach for the vast majority of people comes at a price of reduced efficiency and accuracy. The increased public health awareness related to the risks of distracted driving are based on the growing evidence that the engagement of "secondary tasks" when driving, which often involve screens and media use, can easily undermine many of the critical cognitive components required for safe driving.[16] Unfortunately, research on some of the technological advancements such as voice activated controls, which are designed to reduce levels of distracted driving, is indicating that these developments do not offer the level of cognitive workload reduction that had been originally hoped.[19]

Even in situations that have much less potential for deadly consequences, there is the question of why there remains such a compulsion to use and check smartphones so frequently despite the increased appreciation that doing so generally decreases efficiency and degrades cognitive performance. The answer, as proposed by some, may relate to basic tendencies not only involving the brain's attentional networks but also those related to fundamental drives toward social connectedness and the inherently rewarding properties of both receiving and disclosing social information.[20] A study using delay discounting procedures showed that the added value of receiving social information via text immediately versus later is similar to that for

monetary rewards.[21] As mentioned, these principles related to attentional processes and desires for social contact have been well utilized by smartphones and social media software, which by some have been called perfect "brain hijack machine(s) (p. 146)."[22]

NEUROBIOLOGICAL EFFECTS OF TELEVISION AND VIDEO GAMES

When it comes to "older" media such as television viewing and video games, which more and more is experienced on smartphones rather than on stand-alone television sets and consoles, there is abundant data documenting the association between increased viewing, especially of noneducational programming, and higher levels of attention problems and ADHD-type symptoms.[23–25] One theory behind these associations found between media exposure and later cognitive problems involves brain overstimulation. Experimental studies in animals suggest that audiovisual overstimulation does lead to later cognitive problems[26] and may do so through its effects on the number and density of neuronal synapses during periods of rapid brain growth.[27] Some experts have also suggested that excessive media use alters a brain's arousal set point such that less audiovisually stimulating content that might be found, for example, in a typical school classroom seems increasingly dull as children become more accustomed to the many "bells and whistles" encountered in television programming and video games.[25]

A similar mechanism has been proposed to explain the link between media usage prior to bedtime, sleep problems, and daytime sleepiness.[28] In particular, it has been suggested that media such as self-luminous tablets can suppress melatonin secretion and thus interfere with normal sleep-wake cycles. An experimental study did indeed find in a transitional-age sample that viewing a tablet for 1 and 2 h did result in a measurable reduction in melatonin.[29] This effect may be more pronounced in early- to mid-adolescence compared to later in development.[30] Some of these problems may be ameliorated through dimming the brightness of the screen as much as possible.

Somewhat complicating this picture on the association between screens and alertness, however, are studies that suggest that some online and screen-based content may actually be a *treatment* for conditions such as ADHD. One recent study showed a modest improvement in some attentional tasks in children with ADHD who participated in a series of computer-based exercises designed to help subjects become better at suppressing distractions.[31] Other computerized programs try to improve cognition through the training of individuals to attend to progressively more subtle cues.[32] While it could be argued that these are custom-made applications outside of mainstream media, there are also studies of youth and young adults reporting positive associations between regular video game use and improved visuospatial cognition,[33] processing speed,[34] and improved attention skills,[35] with some also showing improvements in short-term memory,[36] and even some elements of executive functioning.[37]

Neuroimaging studies have revealed associations between video game playing and reduced gray matter in the hippocampus,[38] although the opposite has also been found.[39] This finding has been interpreted generally as being cautionary given the role of the hippocampus not only in memory but a number of other functions as well such as regulation of the stress response.[40] There are also many studies showing links between reduced hippocampal size and a number of psychiatric and cognitive disorders including PTSD, depression, and Alzheimer's disease.[41–43] Some newer studies, however, suggest a more complex association with differential responses to video games in the plasticity of the hippocampus dependent on a person's particular learning style[44] and the type of video game being played.[45] Together, these studies illustrate how responsive the brain can be to environmental factors such as video games, with the specific reaction often highly dependent on many other qualities of both the game and the user.

VIOLENT MEDIA EFFECTS ON THE BRAIN

Another domain that has received a great deal of attention relates to more violent imagery in television, video games, and online. At this point, there is general consensus based on a large number of both experimental and naturalistic studies that exposure to violent media, including the playing of video games, does indeed increase levels of child aggression while decreasing prosocial emotions such as empathy.[46] The magnitude of this association has been criticized as being overstated due to publication bias,[33,47] and experts and politicians alike continue to debate this important topic today.[48]

In addition to some of the mixed hippocampal findings discussed earlier, high usage of video games has been associated with reduced activity in the dorsolateral prefrontal cortex and diminished performance on executive functioning tasks.[17,49] The concern that violent video games may desensitize youth from the typical emotional response to violence may be mediated through changes in frontoparietal networks that link emotional and attentional processing.[17] One study demonstrated decreased prefontal cortex activation and less connectivity between the dorsolateral prefrontal cortex and dorsal anterior cingulate gyrus in adolescents during a modified Stroop task after subjects played a violent versus a nonviolent video game.[50] Another recent experimental study in which subjects played violent or nonviolent versions of the same video game demonstrated that playing the violent version changed functional brain activity with reduced connectivity in several functional networks including the default mode network and those related to sensory-motor functioning and reward processing.[51]

While the public message often implies that exposure to violent media increases everyone's propensity to act aggressively, there is some research evidence suggesting this that the link may be especially present among those who are more prone to violence in the first place. A recent study compared behavioral, physiological, and brain activity (via positron-emission tomography scan) changes related watching violent media between a group of young men who had a history of aggression versus controls.[52] The authors found differential responses related to brain activation, behavior, and blood pressure between the two groups, with those higher in trait aggression showing higher metabolism in regions of the default mode network and lower metabolism in the orbital frontal gyrus, among other changes. Physiologically, more aggressive subjects had decreases in their systolic blood pressure when seeing violent images compared to nonaggressive subjects who showed the opposite. These findings compliment research on personality traits suggesting that individuals who tend to be higher on neuroticism and lower on agreeableness and conscientiousness tend to be most vulnerable to the effects of violent video games.[53] Research studies have unfortunately too often missed this important aspect of individual factors such as a person's baseline level of aggression as a potential moderating factor in this ongoing debate over exposure to violent media as a risk factor for future aggression.

MEDIA ADDICTION AND INTERNET GAMING DISORDER

Currently, the only defined psychiatric disorder directly related to media use is Internet Gaming Disorder (IGD), an entity listed not as an official disorder but a condition for further study in the Diagnostic and

Statistical Manual of Mental Disorders, Fifth Edition (DSM-5).[54] It describes individuals who spend excessive amounts of time playing Internet-based games to a degree that results in a loss of interest in other activities, negative consequences related to overall functioning, and an inability to stop. Estimates about the prevalence rate among adolescents and young adults range widely between 0.5% and 6%.[55,56] This condition arose as the DSM-5 Substance Disorder Workgroup was charged with the categorization of nonsubstance or "behavioral" addiction behaviors such gambling, sex, exercise, and media use.

A number of studies to date have shown abnormalities in gray and white matter among adolescents with online gaming addiction. Regions include the prefrontal cortex, parahippocampal gyrus, left precuneus, middle cingulate cortex, and middle and inferior temporal cortex.[57-59] Reduced functional connectivity between cortical and striatal regions has also been documented.[60] These regions are involved in functions such as reward processing, error monitoring, and decision making, among others.[55] While these documented brain changes among individuals who meet criteria for IGD are often interpreted as representing the lingering effects of the heavy Internet use itself, questions remain as to the degree that the alternations may also be related to the underlying predisposition toward these behaviors, such as the trait of impulsivity and attention problems.[61,62] Large prospective studies such as the landmark Adolescent Brain Cognitive Development study, a multicenter study that will follow youth over long periods of time, are needed to help distinguish between these hypotheses.[63]

An ongoing debate within both the scientific community and the public relates to the degree to which IGD and other nonsubstance-related addictions should be conceptualized along the same lines of addictions to various substances such as opiates or alcohol. While this is a challenging task in the absence of a verified biosignature for bona fide physiological addictions, neuroscience research has been called upon to examine the question of whether any brain changes associated with IGD resemble the changes associated with more classic addictive disorders. A recent study found that individuals with IGD had larger volumes in the amygdala, hippocampus, and right percuneus compared to controls and stronger functional connectivity between the hippocampus/amygdala area and the left ventromedial prefrontal cortex compared to those in alcohol use disorder.[64] They concluded overall that there were substantial differences in the brain changes associated with IGD versus alcohol use disorder that may be related to

the more specific toxic effects of the substance being used. A recent study using electroencephalography also found different neurophysiological patterns between adult males with IGD and alcohol use disorder.[65] At the same time, functional MRI studies that look at the brain response to Internet gaming cues show activation in areas related to reward processing similar to that seen in both other types of substance disorders and cues to other pleasurable activities.[66-68] While much remains to be learned, the available evidence to date suggests that there are definable differences in brain volume, activity, and connectivity related to IGB that bear some, but certainly not complete, resemblance to those found with other types of addictive behavior.

CONCLUSIONS

Forces that affect thoughts, emotions, and behavior must necessarily affect the brain. As expected, our increasing consumption of ever more realistic and interactive media result in substantive and enduring changes in brain structure and activity which are mediated through processes such as epigenetic modification. Smartphones and social media take full advantage of our brain's predisposition to alert us to novel stimuli and may be contributing to a shifting of the balance between different types of attention networks. The link between high media usage and attention problems may be related to the ability of television and video games to reset the bar with regard to a child's arousal and attentional set point. Further, research suggests that the association between particularly violent media and aggressive behavior may be related to alterations in the functional connectivity between cortical and subcortical regions, particularly among those with existing predispositions for aggressive behavior. These data provide evidence that media use, particularly in youth, has the potential to modify the brain in ways that may not be optimal for overall development, and reaffirms the need to proceed cautiously as our society moves steadily forward in embracing even more screens and technology into our daily life.

At the same time, it is also evident that both the behavioral and neurobiological data regarding the impact of media is, as it is in many other areas, often inconsistent and incomplete. Furthermore, interpretation of the many of the neuroscience findings as being positive or negative remain ambiguous in many cases. With the behavioral data indicating that media use can be both part of the problem and part of the solution, it appears equally likely that universal conclusions about media use and an overall positive or negative impact on the brain are also misguided. To reflect the complexity and richness of both the media and the brain, research that seeks to improve the understanding of *how much* of *which type* of media impacting *different areas* of neurodevelopment among *particular types* of children is needed to provide practical data that can inform the guidance that clinicians and child development experts give to patients and the general public.

REFERENCES

1. Bhat V, Joober R, Sengupta SM. How environmental factors can get under the skin: epigenetics in attention-deficit/hyperactivity disorder. *J Am Acad Child Adolesc Psychiatry.* 2017;56(4):278–280.
2. McEwen BS. Allostasis and the epigenetics of brain and body health over the life course: the brain on stress. *JAMA Psychiatry.* 2017;74(6):551–552.
3. McGowan PO, Sasaki A, D'Alessio AC, et al. Epigenetic regulation of the glucocorticoid receptor in human brain associates with childhood abuse. *Nat Neurosci.* 2009;12(3):342–348.
4. Weder N, Zhang H, Jensen K, et al. Child abuse, depression, and methylation in genes involved with stress, neural plasticity, and brain circuitry. *J Am Acad Child Adolesc Psychiatry.* 2014;53(4):417–424.e415.
5. van der Knaap LJ, Riese H, Hudziak JJ, et al. Glucocorticoid receptor gene (NR3C1) methylation following stressful events between birth and adolescence. The TRAILS study. *Transl Psychiatry.* 2014;4:e381.
6. Weaver IC, Cervoni N, Champagne FA, et al. Epigenetic programming by maternal behavior. *Nat Neurosci.* 2004;7(8):847–854.
7. Kaffman A, Meaney MJ. Neurodevelopmental sequelae of postnatal maternal care in rodents: clinical and research implications of molecular insights. *J Child Psychol Psychiatry.* 2007;48(3–4):224–244.
8. Anderson CA, Shibuya A, Ihori N, et al. Violent video game effects on aggression, empathy, and prosocial behavior in eastern and western countries: a meta-analytic review. *Psychol Bull.* 2010;136(2):151–173.
9. Gil-Rivas V, Silver RC, Holman EA, McIntosh DN, Poulin M. Parental response and adolescent adjustment to the September 11, 2001 terrorist attacks. *J Trauma Stress.* 2007;20(6):1063–1068.
10. Blackburn E, Epel E. *The Telomere Effect: A Revolutionary Approach to Living Younger, Healthier, Longer.* New York: Hachette Book Group; 2017.
11. Marioni RE, Harris SE, Shah S, et al. The epigenetic clock and telomere length are independently associated with chronological age and mortality. *Int J Epidemiol.* 2016;45(2):424–432.
12. Shalev I, Moffitt TE, Sugden K, et al. Exposure to violence during childhood is associated with telomere erosion from 5 to 10 years of age: a longitudinal study. *Mol Psychiatry.* 2013;18(5):576–581.
13. Mitchell C, McLanahan S, Schneper L, Garfinkel I, Brooks-Gunn J, Notterman D. Father loss and child telomere length. *Pediatrics.* 2017;140(2).
14. Xue HM, Liu QQ, Tian G, Quan LM, Zhao Y, Cheng G. Television watching and telomere length among adults in Southwest China. *Am J Public Health.* 2017;107(9):1425–1432.
15. Nikkelen SW, Valkenburg PM, Huizinga M, Bushman BJ. Media use and ADHD-related behaviors in children and adolescents: a meta-analysis. *Dev Psychol.* 2014;50(9):2228–2241.
16. Strayer DL, Fisher DL. SPIDER: a framework for understanding driver distraction. *Hum Factors.* 2016;58(1):5–12.
17. Palaus M, Marron EM, Viejo-Sobera R, Redolar-Ripoll D. Neural basis of video gaming: a systematic review. *Front Hum Neurosci.* 2017;11:248.
18. Vossel S, Geng JJ, Fink GR. Dorsal and ventral attention systems: distinct neural circuits but collaborative roles. *Neuroscientist.* 2014;20(2):150–159.
19. Strayer DL, Cooper JM, Turrill J, Coleman JR, Hopman RJ. Talking to your car can drive you to distraction. *Cogn Res Princ Implic.* 2016;1(1):16.
20. Tamir DI, Mitchell JP. Disclosing information about the self is intrinsically rewarding. *Proc Natl Acad Sci USA.* 2012;109(21):8038–8043.
21. Atchley P, Warden AC. The need of young adults to text now: using delay discounting to assess informational choice. *J Appl Res Mem Cogn.* 2012;1:229–234.
22. Richtel M. *A Deadly Wandering: A Mystery, a Landmark Investigation, and the Astonishing Science of Attention in the Digital Age.* New York: HarperCollins; 2014.
23. Zimmerman FJ, Christakis DA. Children's television viewing and cognitive outcomes: a longitudinal analysis of national data. *Arch Pediatr Adolesc Med.* 2005;159(7):619–625.
24. Strasburger VC, Jordan AB, Donnerstein E. Health effects of media on children and adolescents. *Pediatrics.* 2010;125(4):756–767.
25. Christakis DA, Zimmerman FJ, DiGiuseppe DL, McCarty CA. Early television exposure and subsequent attentional problems in children. *Pediatrics.* 2004;113(4):708–713.
26. Christakis DA, Ramirez JS, Ramirez JM. Overstimulation of newborn mice leads to behavioral differences and deficits in cognitive performance. *Sci Rep.* 2012;2:546.
27. Wallace CS, Kilman VL, Withers GS, Greenough WT. Increases in dendritic length in occipital cortex after 4 days of differential housing in weanling rats. *Behav Neural Biol.* 1992;58(1):64–68.
28. Carter B, Rees P, Hale L, Bhattacharjee D, Paradkar MS. Association between portable screen-based media device access or use and sleep outcomes: a systematic review and meta-analysis. *JAMA Pediatr.* 2016;170(12):1202–1208.
29. Wood B, Rea MS, Plitnick B, Figueiro MG. Light level and duration of exposure determine the impact of self-luminous tablets on melatonin suppression. *Appl Ergon.* 2013;44(2):237–240.

30. Crowley SJ, Cain SW, Burns AC, Acebo C, Carskadon MA. Increased sensitivity of the circadian system to light in early/mid-puberty. *J Clin Endocrinol Metab*. 2015; 100(11):4067–4073.

31. Mishra J, Sagar R, Joseph AA, Gazzaley A, Merzenich MM. Training sensory signal-to-noise resolution in children with ADHD in a global mental health setting. *Transl Psychiatry*. 2016;6:e781.

32. Stevens C, Fanning J, Coch D, Sanders L, Neville H. Neural mechanisms of selective auditory attention are enhanced by computerized training: electrophysiological evidence from language-impaired and typically developing children. *Brain Res*. 2008;1205:55–69.

33. Ferguson CJ. The good, the bad and the ugly: a meta-analytic review of positive and negative effects of violent video games. *Psychiatr Q*. 2007;78(4):309–316.

34. Dye MW, Green CS, Bavelier D. Increasing speed of processing with action video games. *Curr Dir Psychol Sci*. 2009;18(6):321–326.

35. Dye MW, Green CS, Bavelier D. The development of attention skills in action video game players. *Neuropsychologia*. 2009;47(8–9):1780–1789.

36. Blacker KJ, Curby KM. Enhanced visual short-term memory in action video game players. *Atten Percept Psychophs*. 2013;75:1128–1136.

37. Green CS, Sugarman MA, Medford K, Klobusicky E, Daphne B. The effect of action video game experience on task-switching. *Comput Hum Behav*. 2012;28(3):984–994.

38. West GL, Drisdelle BL, Konishi K, Jackson J, Jolicoeur P, Bohbot VD. Habitual action video game playing is associated with caudate nucleus-dependent navigational strategies. *Proc Biol Sci*. 2015;282(1808):20142952.

39. Kuhn S, Gleich T, Lorenz RC, Lindenberger U, Gallinat J. Playing Super Mario induces structural brain plasticity: gray matter changes resulting from training with a commercial video game. *Mol Psychiatry*. 2014;19(2):265–271.

40. McEwen BS, Eiland L, Hunter RG, Miller MM. Stress and anxiety: structural plasticity and epigenetic regulation as a consequence of stress. *Neuropharmacology*. 2012;62(1): 3–12.

41. Apostolova LG, Dutton RA, Dinov ID, et al. Conversion of mild cognitive impairment to Alzheimer disease predicted by hippocampal atrophy maps. *Arch Neurol*. 2006;63(5): 693–699.

42. Amico F, Meisenzahl E, Koutsouleris N, Reiser M, Moller HJ, Frodl T. Structural MRI correlates for vulnerability and resilience to major depressive disorder. *J Psychiatry Neurosci*. 2011;36(1):15–22.

43. O'Doherty DCM, Tickell A, Ryder W, et al. Frontal and subcortical grey matter reductions in PTSD. *Psychiatry Res*. 2017;266:1–9.

44. West GL, Konishi K, Diarra M, et al. Impact of video games on plasticity of the hippocampus. *Mol Psychiatry*. 2017. Advance online publication, 8 August 2017; https://doi.org/10.1038/mp.2017.155.

45. West GL, Konishi K, Bohbot VD. Video games and hippocampus-dependent learning. *Curr Dir Psychol Sci*. 2017;26(2):152–158.

46. Media ATFoV. *Technical Report on the Review of the Violent Video Game Literature*. American Psychological Association; 2015.

47. Hilgard J, Engelhart CR, Rouder JN. Overstated evidence for short-term effects of violent games on affect and behavior: a reanalysis of Anderson et al. (2010). *Psychol Bull*. 2017;143(7):757–774.

48. Kepes S, Bushman BJ, Anderson CA. Violent video game effects remain a societal concern: reply to Hilgard, Engelhardt, and Rouder (2017). *Psychol Bull*. 2017; 143(7):775–782.

49. Hummer TA, Wang Y, Kronenberger WG, et al. Short-term violent video game play by adolescents alters prefrontal activity during cognitive inhibition. *Media Psychol*. 2010; 13:136–154.

50. Wang Y, Mathews VP, Kalnin AJ, et al. Short term exposure to a violent video game induces changes in frontolimbic circuitry in adolescents. *Brain Imaging Behav*. 2009;3: 38–50.

51. Zvyagintsev M, Klasen M, Weber R, et al. Violence-related content in video game may lead to functional connectivity changes in brain networks as revealed by fMRI-ICA in young men. *Neuroscience*. 2016;320: 247–258.

52. Alia-Klein N, Wang GJ, Preston-Campbell RN, et al. Reactions to media violence: it's in the brain of the beholder. *PLoS One*. 2014;9(9):e107260.

53. Markey PM, Markey CN. Vulnerability to violent video games: a review and integration of personality research. *Rev Gen Psychol*. 2010;14(2):82–91.

54. Association AP. *Diagnostic and Statistical Manual of Mental Disorders*. 5th ed. Arlington, VA: American Psychiatric Publishing; 2013.

55. Petry NM, Rehbein F, Ko CH, O'Brien CP. Internet gaming disorder in the DSM-5. *Curr Psychiatry Rep*. 2015; 17(9):72.

56. Rehbein F, Kliem S, Baier D, Mossle T, Petry NM. Prevalence of Internet gaming disorder in German adolescents: diagnostic contribution of the nine DSM-5 criteria in a state-wide representative sample. *Addiction*. 2015;110(5): 842–851.

57. Yuan K, Cheng P, Dong T, et al. Cortical thickness abnormalities in late adolescence with online gaming addiction. *PLoS One*. 2013;8(1):e53055.

58. Yuan K, Jin C, Cheng P, et al. Amplitude of low frequency fluctuation abnormalities in adolescents with online gaming addiction. *PLoS One*. 2013;8(11):e78708.

59. Hong SB, Kim JW, Choi EJ, et al. Reduced orbitofrontal cortical thickness in male adolescents with internet addiction. *Behav Brain Funct*. 2013;9:11.

60. Hong SB, Zalesky A, Cocchi L, et al. Decreased functional brain connectivity in adolescents with internet addiction. *PLoS One*. 2013;8(2):e57831.

61. Lee D, Namkoong K, Lee J, Jung YC. Abnormal gray matter volume and impulsivity in young adults with Internet gaming disorder. *Addict Biol*. 2017. Advance online publication, 8 September 2017; https://doi.org/10.1111/adb.12552.

62. Swing EL, Gentile DA, Anderson CA, Walsh DA. Television and video game exposure and the development of attention problems. *Pediatrics*. 2010;126(2):214−221.

63. Abuse NIoD. *Longitudinal Study of Adolescent Brain and Cognitive Development (ABCD Study)*. 2017. https://www.drugabuse.gov/related-topics/adolescent-brain/longitudinal-study-adolescent-brain-cognitive-development-abcd-studyNation.

64. Yoon EJ, Choi JS, Kim H, et al. Altered hippocampal volume and functional connectivity in males with Internet gaming disorder comparing to those with alcohol use disorder. *Sci Rep*. 2017;7(1):5744.

65. Park SM, Lee JY, Kim YJ, et al. Neural connectivity in Internet gaming disorder and alcohol use disorder: a resting-state EEG coherence study. *Sci Rep*. 2017;7(1):1333.

66. Ko CH, Liu GC, Yen JY, Chen CY, Yen CF, Chen CS. Brain correlates of craving for online gaming under cue exposure in subjects with Internet gaming addiction and in remitted subjects. *Addict Biol*. 2013;18(3):559−569.

67. Ko CH, Liu GC, Yen JY, Yen CF, Chen CS, Lin WC. The brain activations for both cue-induced gaming urge and smoking craving among subjects comorbid with Internet gaming addiction and nicotine dependence. *J Psychiatr Res*. 2013;47(4):486−493.

68. Sun Y, Ying H, Seetohul RM, et al. Brain fMRI study of crave induced by cue pictures in online game addicts (male adolescents). *Behav Brain Res*. 2012;233(2):563−576.

CHAPTER 13

The Role of Media in Promoting and Destigmatizing Mental Illness in Youth

CHERYL K. OLSON, SCD[a] • LAWRENCE A. KUTNER, PHD[a,b]

The mass shooting at Marjorie Stoneman Douglas High School in Parkland, Florida, in February 2018 revealed some of the underlying biases many people—including policymakers—have when it comes to the nature of mental illness. The murders were allegedly carried out by a teenager who had a long history of documented psychiatric and behavioral problems, including depression, attention-deficit hyperactivity disorder, and autism. (As of this writing, he has yet to be adjudicated.)

Dana Loesch, a spokesperson for the National Rifle Association, referred to the alleged shooter as an "insane monster," "nuts," and a "madman."[1] President Donald Trump used Twitter, the medium favored by him as well as by many adolescents, to refer to the young man as "a savage sicko."[2] A few days later, while addressing a national gathering of state governors at the White House, he added, "You know, in the old days we had mental institutions. We had a lot of them. And you could nab somebody like this, because they … knew something was off."[3]

After more than a century of growing enlightenment about the causes and consequences of mental illness, we appear to be seeing a revival of the long-held stigmas against it. These biases not only affect public perception and policy, they contribute to people's reluctance and delay in seeing effective help.

STIGMA: CAUSES AND EFFECTS

Why does stigma matter? First, stereotypes and prejudices affect whether a person with mental illness will be socially accepted or avoided and shunned by potential friends, neighbors, employers, or landlords. Second,

acceptance of these stereotypes by persons with a mental illness affects their behavior, e.g., not applying to a desired school, club, or job due to assumptions of low competence or likely failure. Third, an individual motivated to avoid a mental illness label may fail to seek out treatment or discontinue it early. Corrigan and colleagues[4] refer to these three types of stigma as public stigma, self-stigma, and label avoidance.

Stigma can result from outside-the-norm behaviors associated with mental illness symptoms and from cultural meanings attached to mental illness labels. Multiple studies[5] over time have found that labels matter, whether applied to adults or children, even when controlling for stigma associated with the socially disapproved behaviors arising from mental disorders.

A qualitative study[6] of 56 Midwestern teens who had been treated for mental disorders found that stigma affected multiple spheres of their lives. Teens described divergent stigmatizing reactions from close and extended family members: from hypervigilance and overreacting to daily problems, to accusations of being manipulative and "making up" the disorder, to being viewed as permanently damaged ("like 'you're just gonna be a screw-up your whole life' kind of thing") or even being dangerous to siblings. Several teens who reported no negative changes attributed this to having relatives with existing mental health or substance abuse problems, which made such issues more familiar and acceptable to the family.

About two-thirds reported stigma from peers, including losing friends after disclosing problems or experiencing symptoms. Thirteen (23%) found understanding and support from peers who'd faced similar problems. Eight (14%) reported rifts with friends triggered by their friends' parents: "they don't want them [their children] to pick up what I've got." A few reported friends being newly cautious or fearful, "afraid I'll go off on them."

[a]Independent consultant.
[b]Dr. Kutner is a member of the board of advisors to the Rosalynn Carter Fellowship for Mental Health Journalism at the Carter Center in Atlanta.

Ten students (18%) reported receiving extra support from school staff. They spoke appreciatively of teachers reaching out to ensure they kept up academically and willingness to be flexible. Sixteen students (29%) spoke of being stigmatized and blamed by some staff, including lowered academic expectations, being kept in less-challenging courses, not being called on in class, or treated as likely to cause problems.

How Does Stigma Differ for the Young?

As Mukolo and colleagues[7] note, there is a large body of research on stigma and adult mental illness, but comparatively few studies focus on children and youth. They speculate that on the one hand, children have less power and status than adults, so their deviant behavior may be less tolerated. On the other hand, young children may be less stigmatized as they are generally perceived due to age to be less responsible for their way of being (i.e., parents receive the blame and stigma); older children and adolescents might be seen as somewhat more culpable. Because it typically falls to parents to seek help for a mentally ill child, any "stigma by association" affecting family members may influence care-seeking.

In focus group interviews with 122 relatives of patients with schizophrenia in Germany (primarily parents of adult children with the disorder), Angermeyer and colleagues[8] focused on what they termed "courtesy stigma," or stigma applied to someone related through the social structure to a stigmatized individual. Participants described contact with mental health professionals as their primary stigmatizing experience. They reported feeling that their knowledge and experience were not valued; they were excluded or treated as a burden or irritant; and their worries and fears were disregarded or minimized. Parents (especially mothers) of adults with schizophrenia spoke of facing accusations of "wrong or bad upbringing of their children," including blame from grandparents, siblings of the ill child, and from friends who believe the illness had family origins. This left parents feeling ashamed, guilty, and helpless.

In her review of lessons from stigma research, Pescosolido[5] notes that public surveys suggest greater tolerance toward children and teens with mental health problems as compared to adults, with the exception of depression. Youth depression was seen as unlikely to improve without treatment, predisposing toward violence, and rooted in child-rearing (suggesting blame assigned to parents).

More research is needed with parents of children and adolescents to understand how this stigma by association might affect family well-being and interactions with the healthcare system.

Peer Perceptions

Negative attitudes toward people with mental illness start young and persist. A study of 577 elementary-school children found stigma and desire for social distance already present; when 34 kindergarten-age students still in the school district were followed up 8 years later, their attitudes had not changed.[9] A vignette-based survey of 303 California teens[10] found that stigma was greater when they viewed peers with mental illness as responsible for their illness or as dangerous. Perceived responsibility for one's illness evoked less pity (and desire to help) and more anger. Peers seen as dangerous were feared and avoided.

HOW STIGMA AFFECTS HELP-SEEKING

Given that normal adolescent development involves heightened sensitivity to identity concerns and peer opinions, we might expect that teens would be particularly sensitive to stigma. Clement and colleagues[11] reviewed 144 qualitative and quantitative studies of how stigma affects help-seeking. Based on the limited youth data available, they conclude that stigma may be an even-greater deterrent for young people, who tend to be acutely sensitive to dissonance between their preferred self-identity and social identity, and the stereotypes of mental illness. (Research on school-age youth is particularly needed.)

Teen boys may be especially affected by stigma. For example, a study of 274 diverse eighth graders[12] found that more boys (40%) than girls (24%) agreed that "seeing a counselor for emotional problems makes people think you are weird or different"; boys were also more likely than girls to say they were not willing to use mental health services (38%–23%). Higher perceived stigma and perceived parental disapproval appeared to account for most of the gender difference in willingness to use mental health services. The authors suggest that addressing negative views of mental illness and its treatment among youth could minimize gender disparities in service use and reduce the influence of stigma as a barrier to treatment later in life.

Parent attitudes, including feeling blamed for problems, are also a factor. Reardon and colleagues[13] reviewed 44 qualitative and quantitative studies addressing barriers perceived by parents to accessing psychological treatment for children and adolescents. Although it is far from the only barrier (others include cost concerns, trust and confidence in professionals, and a lack of knowledge of illnesses and available help), the authors single out the "frequency with which parents across studies reported the detrimental impact of perceived negative attitudes of others (as well as personal discomfort surrounding mental health) on help seeking" (p. 644).

Stigma From Healthcare and Mental Health Providers

Unfortunately, people with mental illness often encounter more stigma when seeking medical or psychological care. Henderson et al.[14] reviewed international surveys of healthcare and mental healthcare providers exploring stigmatizing attitudes. The authors note that removing stigma-related barriers to healthcare is particularly important given the reduced life expectancy faced by people with severe mental illness (20 years for men, 15 for women) in high-income nations. For example, surveys suggest that physicians may take physical symptoms of disease less seriously in patients who have a history of depression. If they view patients with schizophrenia as unlikely to adhere to treatment, it affects decisions to prescribe or refill medications and refer to specialists.

A Canadian survey[15] found that nurses and physicians often share stigmatizing beliefs found among the general public, including associating mental illness with violence, unpredictability, and weakness of character.

A large survey[16] of Swiss German psychiatric facilities found that, compared to both a general population sample and other mental health professionals, psychiatrists held more negative stereotypes about people with mental illnesses. Perhaps this reflects disproportionate contact with severely or chronically ill individuals. The review of surveys by Henderson et al. found increasing optimism about recovery and less stigmatization among psychiatrists, other physicians, and nurses who have more years of experience.

SOURCES OF STIGMA IN THE MEDIA

In a British qualitative study of 46 adolescents' perceptions of mental illness, participants who were asked about their first exposure to or sources of ideas about mental illness often mentioned media sources, including cartoons, films, and news coverage of "criminals." However, they also acknowledged that these portrayals were likely stereotypes that may differ from real life.[17]

Media content helps us develop our concepts or "mental frames" of mental illness[18] that shape how we define and talk about a problem, how we diagnose its cause, what moral judgments we make about the problem and causes, and what remedies we find appropriate.

Stigma in Movies

Butler and Hyler[19] shared anecdotes of adolescent patients' expectations about interactions with psychiatrists and psychiatric hospitalization as shaped by horror films such as *Nightmare on Elm Street 3: Dream Warriors*, where heavily drugged "zombie"-like patients are hospitalized indefinitely by all-powerful doctors. They quote one patient's recollection of films with "everyone getting handfuls of medication or shots from big metal syringes with huge needles" (p. 512). They note that most members of the public have far more experience with media depictions of psychiatrists than with the real thing. Films also influence views of what constitutes mental illness and what symptoms are serious enough to demand treatment. Mundane conditions such as attention deficit disorder are seldom depicted; dramatic psychopathologic conditions receive aggressive and often involuntary intervention.

"Because he/she is crazy!" appears to be an easy, lazy, time-tested way for writers to justify character behavior and propel a scary tale. Goodwin[20] notes that the "psycho killer" of cinema stereotype (e.g., *Psycho* and *Halloween*) bears no relation to any Diagnostic and Statistical Manual of Mental Disorders diagnostic categories, and links mental illness in general to dangerousness and otherness, i.e., being less than human. He reviewed 55 films[21] made between 2000 and 2012, chosen based on a literature search and using keywords (such as mental/psychiatric hospital, psychosis) in the Internet Movie Database. Consistent with earlier reviews of mental illness portrayal in films, "homicidal maniac" was the most common stock portrayal of mental illness, appearing in 79% of the 33 films that featured psychosis.

Stigma on Television

Diefenbach and West[22] analyzed 84 h (1 week) of 2003 prime-time broadcast television programming. Comparing the actions of mentally disordered television characters to statistics on real-world behavior, they found the fictional characters far outstripped real-world counterparts in violence, with 11 such characters (37% of that week's TV population of persons with mental disorders) committing 38 violent offenses. An accompanying telephone survey of 419 random respondents found that 58% believed television affects people's attitudes about mental illness (though 65% disagreed that their own attitudes were so affected) and that heavy viewers of television were more likely to agree that neighborhood-based mental health services endanger local residents.

Parrott and Parrott[23] reviewed mental illness in popular TV crime dramas (not designed for youth, but watched by many) such as *NCIS* and *Criminal Minds*. Of 983 rated characters, 5% (52) were labeled as having a mental illness, including alcohol/drug addiction (12), schizophrenia (5), and unspecified (8). Others received diagnoses that don't exist, such as "extreme Internet addiction" or very rare ones (Capgras syndrome). In line with established media stereotypes, half of the "mentally ill" characters committed acts of violence (vs. one in five nonlabeled characters) and 46% became victims of violence. Unsurprisingly, 42% showed poor grooming or hygiene, and 44% voiced delusional thoughts. One-third were unemployed (vs. 6% of other characters); none were police officers or detectives. The authors note future research might look at effects of exposure to characters who defy negative stereotypes, such as the lead character on the TNT series *Perception*, a neuropsychiatrist with a history of schizophrenia.

Media for Young Children

Content made for children is far from free of stigmatizing stereotypes. Lawson and Fouts[24] reviewed verbal and written references to mental illness in animated Disney Company feature films from 1937 to 2001. These films are often watched by children numerous times and across generations. They found that 85% of films included references to characters with mental illness, and 21% of all principal characters were so labeled (including Belle's father, Maurice, in *Beauty and the Beast*; Jafar in *Aladdin*; and Mrs Jumbo in *Dumbo*). Such labels are used to denigrate and create social distance from characters, making them objects of fear or derisive fun. Maurice is hauled away in a "lunacy wagon." Hyenas in *The Lion King* laugh hysterically, roll their eyes, and gnaw their own legs.

Wahl and colleagues[25] looked at 49 G- and PG-rated children's films released in 2000–01, of which 12 included characters with a mental illness. Most were identified through comments by others: as crazy, psycho, nuts, or "a few meals short of a picnic." In eight, the characters behaved aggressively, often eliciting fearful responses, but none of those was provided with treatment. Of characters who did receive mental health treatment, in only one case was it depicted as helpful. An additional 21 of the films reviewed contained references to mental illness, including remarks meant as derogatory such as "the coaches need a shrink" or "you're certifiable."

A 2000 review by Wilson et al.[26] of children's programs aired in New Zealand (cartoon and live-action) found repeated colloquial, disrespectful references to mental illness (e.g., words like crazy, mad, wacko, nuts, freak; motions to the head or eye-rolling), with 59 of 128 episodes including at least one such reference.

The bulk were in cartoons, most of which were US-made, such as *Tiny Toon Adventures* and *Pinky and the Brain*. In some cases, the connotations of "crazy" or "mad" were spontaneous, unpredictable fun; in others, unreasonable or unacceptable behavior; overall, a loss of control was implied. (Six characters were consistently labeled as mentally ill: three comic ones and three villains.) The authors expressed concern that children would learn to view these terms and gestures as acceptable and even funny and might use them (or condone their use) to bully or harass others.

A 2007 study by Wahl and others[27] reviewed 269 h of children's TV programs (primarily on Nickelodeon, PBS, WB, and the Cartoon Network; programs included *Yu-Gi-Oh* and *Fairly OddParents*). They found 46% of programs included slang terms about mental illness, most often used to disparage people or ideas. The relatively few characters (21) labeled as mentally ill were most commonly male; two-thirds showed unpredictable aggressive or violent behavior toward others. Others treated those characters with fear and/or disrespect, including derisive slang (crackpot, nuts). On the positive side, half were shown as well-groomed, and a third described as intelligent. Few received treatment, and just one was depicted as being helped by it.

Additional studies are needed to understand whether recent children's programs have more varied or improved portrayals and whether other media sources aimed at children (such as YouTube channels) may differ.

Stigma and Video Games

Writing on the popular gaming Web site Kotaku, neuroscientist Ian Mahar[28] drew attention to horror video games that use mental illness to add "backstory" and motivation to a character's behavior, typically a villain. He notes that the "crazed killer" and "horrific insane asylum" tropes in games such as *Manhunt 2* (denounced by the National Alliance on Mental Illness), *Arkham Asylum*, and *Outlast* perpetuate negative stereotypes in ways that go beyond what's needed to convey whatever intent their designers had. He calls not for censorship, but for consideration of the effect games may have on society.

Shapiro and Rotter[29] looked at portrayals of mental illness in the 50 annual top-selling video game titles from 2011 to 2013, using wiki Web pages and YouTube videos of gameplay. Two-thirds of the 42 characters identified fit the "homicidal maniac" stereotype, exhibiting violent behaviors that are described as due at least in part to mental illness. Less frequent stereotypes included "dysfunctional invalids" (with disordered behavior, thoughts, or speech hindering or endangering a protagonist), "paranoid conspiracy theorists" played for laughs, comic eccentrics, and depressed "afflicted victims."

Stigma in News Reports

News coverage of mass shootings has repeatedly connected violence and mental illness. McGinty and colleagues[30] reviewed a random sample of stories about serious mental illness (SMI) and gun violence from 1997 to 2012, drawn from 14 national and regional news sources. They found that dangerous *people* (17%) were mentioned far more often in stories than dangerous *weapons* (9%) as causes of gun violence, and that these proportions increased to 33% and 25%, respectively, in the 2 weeks following a mass shooting. Nearly 70% of news coverage of SMI and gun violence was event-focused. Mentions of dangerous people with SMI as a cause of gun violence were significantly correlated with mentions of policy proposals to restricting that population's access to guns, but not with other gun policy proposals.

A previous related study[31] exposed an online panel (N = 1797) to one of three news story conditions (or a control) about (1) a mass shooting by a person with a SMI, (2) that plus a proposal for gun restrictions on that population, or (3) instead a proposal to ban large-capacity magazines. Compared to the control group, exposure to any of the three story versions increased negative attitudes toward people with SMI, with respondents being less willing to work closely with or live near such a person. Exposure to content about limiting access to guns for people with SMI did not increase support for such policies (by contrast, exposure to content about restricting large-capacity magazines did increase support for that); however, this may be due to a ceiling effect, given a baseline support of 70% for such restrictions on people with SMI. These two studies suggest that such high volume of coverage could make the public more likely to view persons with mental illness as dangerous. Given that many well-publicized mass shootings in the United States were undertaken by adolescents or young adults (e.g., Nikolas Cruz, Adam Lanza, Seung-Hui Cho, Eric Harris, and Dylan Klebold), risk perceptions for this age group may be disproportionately affected.

A study of newspaper coverage of mental illness[32] that compared stories about youth versus adults found that child- and adolescent-focused stories were more often features, with more context about causes and treatment, as well as mental health system critiques or social trends. There was more emphasis on dangerousness and use of stigmatizing terms in the adult-focused stories.

How might exposure to such news coverage affect youth? Morgan and Jorm[33] attempted to address this by interviewing a random sample of 3746 Australian youth aged 12–25 years in 2006 about their recall of news stories about mental illness. Of the minority that recalled and could describe such a story, most focused on crime or violence, failures of the mental health system, or a well-known person disclosing a mental illness. Crime story recall was linked to greater reluctance to disclose a mental health issue, while famous-person stories were linked to perceiving mental disorders as a sickness rather than a weakness. None had any bearing on willingness to seek help.

MEDIA INTERVENTIONS THAT MAY REDUCE STIGMA

In an article about unintended consequences of anti-stigma campaigns, Corrigan[4] describes two ways that antistigma efforts have been framed. The "normalcy" frame attempts to reduce stigma by framing mental illness and its treatment as analogous to that of other health conditions. He notes Australia's *beyondblue* campaign as an example of this frame.

By contrast, a "solidarity" frame involves a form of pride in identifying as someone overcoming challenges and demonstrating resilience against stigma. He draws comparisons to the gay rights movement, stating that "coming out" has generally led to improved mental and physical health for that population and that keeping secrets does the inverse. Identifying with one's mental illness may be linked with lower self-esteem and pessimism; however, he asserts, doing so while rejecting stigma improves self-regard, hope, and social functioning. The solidarity approach involves strengthening people with mental illness through connections to peers and enlisting majority support for those who are "out" with their stigmatized identity: "I am in solidarity with people in recovery." One example from the United States of such a program is "No Kidding? Me, Too!"[34]

Media content promoting normalcy and solidarity views may both ultimately have a role in reducing stigma, depending on the goal. For example, a normalcy approach might reduce barriers to initial help-seeking and solidarity might improve self-assertion and self-care. A note of caution: the solidarity analogies Corrigan uses—gay pride and Irish-American ethnic pride—reference inherently healthy states of being stigmatized in certain times and places; misplaced pride in being anorectic, for example, with social media peer encouragement, has led to worsening health.[35] It also puts all mental disorders—from mild and time-limited to severe and chronic; from those due to traumatic events to those with primarily genetic origins—on the same plane. A person with mild depression, posttraumatic stress disorder, or marital difficulties could be deterred from seeing a psychiatrist or psychologist if they feel required to adopt a "mentally ill" identity and be out and proud with it.

The National Academies of Sciences published a comprehensive review of evidence[36] from campaigns to reduce stigma against people with mental and substance use disorders. Their evidence from large-scale campaigns, such as Canada's Opening Minds campaign[37] suggests some disillusion with top-down mass media campaigns broadly targeting populations and covering all mental disorders. More efforts now favor campaigns targeted to specific illnesses and to subgroups such as youth or healthcare providers. Many antistigma programs also prioritize in-person contact over media messages and seek to partner universities with community or grassroots groups to share program and evaluation expertise.

In their review of evidence for interventions to reduce stigma and discrimination, Thornicroft et al.[38] note that young people are underrepresented in such research (i.e., only 3.7% of participants in stigma studies) and that studies are needed to better understand what works with subgroups and what platforms, such as social media, might be best suited to reach them.

Social Media and Internet Interventions

Naslund et al.[39] note surveys showing that young adults with mental illness report using social media to feel less alone or more connected and that they gain a sense of relief knowing others share their experiences and challenges. They also highlight the need to watch for unintended harms from social media, such as the risks of relying on peers for advice that may be unreliable, and the potential for unrealistic expectations or confusion about one's own illness created by others' shared experiences.

Burns et al.[40] described Australia's Reach Out online mental health campaign for youth and their parents, created in 1998 to take advantage of the growing reach of the Internet to reduce stigma, promote mental health, and encourage help seeking. Reach Out was designed as a multicomponent initiative, including youth involvement programs and social marketing campaigns. Its Web site included five elements: fact sheets created with experts and young people; an online community forum with trained and staff-supervised peer moderators; links with social networking sites

such as Facebook; on-demand podcasts on mental health topics; and Reach Out Central, an online interactive game (described below).

A 2008 online survey of 1006 Reach Out users found that 87% were repeat visitors (a quarter used the site weekly) and 40% had been using it for more than a year. The site was highly rated for trustworthiness and providing a sense of support; 81% said they would tell a friend about Reach Out. Notably, 59% reported that they had spoken to a mental health professional about their difficulties after visiting Reach Out and 19% intended to do so. Reach Out has achieved remarkable longevity. As of March 2018, the Reach Out Web site[41] notes that 132,000 people in Australia access it every month.

Betton et al.[42] point to social media as low-barrier ways to educate, connect, and advocate for change. One example of challenging stigma is a 2013 protest against a UK supermarket chain's offering of a "mental patient" Halloween costume. Comments on Twitter spread, sparked mainstream news reports the following day, and led to that retailer (and others) withdrawing the costume, apologizing, and making a donation to the "Time to Change" antistigma campaign. The authors note the role of social media in larger antistigma campaigns, such as the Twitter #SmashtheStigma hashtag used to denote the posting of stories of hope and recovery for Australia's *beyondblue* depression and anxiety initiative, and the Stigma Watch media-monitoring Facebook page for New Zealand's ongoing "Like Minds, Like Mine" campaign.[43]

Australia's continuing national *beyondblue* campaign, established in 2000, features a youth Web site for ages 12–25 years, at https://www.youthbeyondblue.com. The site links to "healthy families" (https://healthyfamilies.beyondblue.org.au) content for parents and guardians, with checklists and information on child and adult mental health, online forums, and links to assistance. A 2011 telephone survey[44] of 3021 Australians aged 15–25 years found that about 70% were aware of *beyondblue*. That awareness was associated with better recognition of disorders and with beliefs about how to respond appropriately to symptoms in friends or family members (termed "first aid skills") that were more closely aligned with advice from health professionals.

Beyondblue's 2014–15 annual report's section on youth[45] refers to *beyondblue* survey data showing that nearly 80% of youth don't get help for anxiety or depression due to stigma. This inspired the launch in May 2015 of a half-dozen *beyondblue* animated video shorts[46] (less than 30-s each) called *Brains Can Have a*

Mind of Their Own. Aimed at youth aged 13–18 years, the videos feature a "pesky" animated brain meant to personify symptoms of depression and anxiety. The idea is to use humor to overcome concerns about stigma, providing a sense that "it's not me, it's my brain being weird." According to the annual report, the six videos led to a doubling in Web traffic in June 2015 from that of June 2014, and one in four visitors (~23,500) completed a Brain Quiz self-assessment that advises whether to seek help.

Livingston and colleagues[47] described a Canadian brief intervention called In One Voice, which used social media—the Facebook and Twitter pages for the Vancouver Canucks professional hockey team—to publicize a 2-min public service announcement featuring a player from that team and a youth-focused educational Web site, mindcheck.ca. Online samples (ages 13–25 years) of British Columbia residents were surveyed at baseline (T1), 2 months (T2), and 1 year following launch (T3). The proportion aware of the campaign grew from 24.5% at T2 to 48.6% at T3, and elevated Web site activity was sustained at T3. Small but significant reductions in personal stigma and social distance were found from T1 to T3 (but not at T2). However, respondents' self-ratings of the ability to help others with mental health issues or to seek information did not improve.

As part of a literature review on how people experiencing psychotic disorders, including schizophrenia, use the Internet, Villani and Kovess-Masfety[48] note some of the advantages the Internet offers to this population, which suffers particularly from stigma and self-stigma. For those who are socially impaired, social contact and support can be found, at no cost and across geographic boundaries, without potentially anxiety-provoking or stigmatizing face-to-face contact. They can also make use of multimodal expression (sound, image, and text) in idiosyncratic ways that may suit their need for emotional expression.

A pilot study in Israel[49] comparing Internet use of 143 individuals with psychotic disorders to that of two control groups (those with other disorders and volunteers) found that almost 80% of the former sought to create social connections online. Although severity of illness was a factor, the authors found that the Internet did offer distinct social benefits to these participants. Many were able to make meaningful online connections that turned into offline friendships and romances, similar to control participants.

Berry and colleagues[50] highlighted the benefits of the Twitter social media platform for discussing mental health problems, providing support and combatting stigma. They used the novel strategy of creating a

hashtag, #WhyWeTweetMH, explicitly labeled as a research tool, and asking mental health charities and advocates to help circulate it from September to November 2015. The tweet containing the hashtag linked to helplines and was monitored to ensure no offensive or bullying material was attached. (None was.)

An analysis of the 132 original tweets from 90 users (primarily from the United Kingdom and United States) revealed four broad motivations for tweeting. First was to provide a sense of community, connecting with others ("I am with friends even when I am unable to go out") or sending/receiving support or information. Second, people used Twitter to counter stigma and raise awareness, often using emotional terms such as "combat," "struggle," and "battle." This category received the most retweets and "likes."

Third, Twitter was perceived as a safe place for self-expression, to share honest experiences, or feel heard (as opposed to Facebook, which one commenter described as the "sparkly sunny version of people" vs. Twitter's "authentic version."). This includes airing complaints about experiences with mental health services. Finally, tweeting about mental health gave some an empowering or escapist way to cope with daily challenges of life with mental illness. This includes humor and joking—as one wrote, to "interrupt my irrational and obsessive thoughts—it does work." It also includes observing patterns in one's tweets as self-care; said one user, who apparently turned to Twitter after finding blogging too difficult, "my Twitter timeline performs as a sort of mood monitor for myself and those who personally know me."

Video Games to Counter Stigma

Because of their interactive nature and opportunity for in-depth storylines, video games have the potential to teach about and build empathy for the mentally ill. One well-known example is *Depression Quest* (available at http://www.depressionquest.com), a text-based 2013 interactive game about managing daily life as a person suffering from depression. Developer Zoe Quinn and writer Patrick Lindsey had experience with depression. In a *New Yorker* article,[51] they describe their goal as not to speak for all who suffer from depression but to communicate aspects of their experiences ("what it's like to be in that headspace"), introduce basic concepts, encourage conversation, and build understanding.

A recent commercially produced game called *The Town of Light*[52] (for PC, PlayStation 4, Xbox One, and Nintendo Switch) offers a subversive take on the horror genre, drawing on historical accounts of an actual Italian 1930s asylum to tell a story of inhumane treatment of the mentally ill. Documentary content about the asylum accompanies a deluxe edition of the game for the Nintendo Switch.[53]

Researchers have also created and evaluated games explicitly designed to reduce mental illness stigma. Cangas and colleagues recently described the design and evaluation of Stigma-Stop,[54] a game developed in Spain with the Unity3D game engine for multiplatform use. The game features characters who have depression, schizophrenia, bipolar disorder, and panic disorder/agoraphobia. Players select, locate, and "visit" one of the four characters, interact with them, and choose among responses they consider most appropriate in particular situations. If an "incorrect" option is chosen, an explanation appears, along with a recommended alternative. After the interaction, the player sees a short form with information about the disorder; more information about the character's illness and what led to it is also available. There are also four "minigames" (e.g., trivia, matching) that build knowledge about mental disorders. The pre-/postevaluation, with groups of high school students visiting the University of Almería, found significant reductions in stigma (dangerousness and stereotypes) compared to students who played a control game. The authors refer to a Web site to download the free game (registration required) in English and Spanish at http://stigmastop.net.

Australia's Reach Out program (described above) initially featured an online game called Reach Out Central.[55] Using principles of cognitive behavioral therapy, the game helped players identify and practice coping with stresses of everyday life to enhance resilience and protective factors. From a first-person perspective as a character new to town, players figured out how to settle in, navigate, and make friends—interacting with other characters, who often had their own detailed back stories and plotlines. Features included a coach/narrator, available to mentor or help the player on demand, and a mood meter (on view during play) that changed as players engaged with or avoided conversations, homework, sleep, and other activities. Mood then influenced interactions; for example, low mood impeded forming friendships; physical activities and avoiding drugs promoted progress.

A quasi-experimental evaluation of youth who played Reach Out Central found improvements on all measures for female participants, including mental health literacy, stigma, and willingness to seek help. Participants were disproportionately female, and results proved disappointing or inconclusive for male subjects. Exposure to gameplay was lower than planned, due to unexpected player difficulty with downloading new scenarios/environments, and comments indicating that most players did not find the storylines complex or interesting enough to replay them and explore the effects of alternative responses.

The game appears to be no longer available on the Reach Out Web site; a site search reveals a ReachOut Orb game for iPad or desktop use, designed to promote positive thoughts and build resilience. The site also connects visitors to a wide variety of mobile apps and tools (https://au.reachout.com/tools-and-apps) to help young people cope with low moods and anxiety, monitor their health behaviors, track a friend who may be having problems, or meditate.

Using Movies Against Stigma

Theriot[56] described a half-semester seminar for first-year students at the University of Tennessee with the deliberately attention-grabbing title of "Maniacs and Psycho Killers: Myths and Realities of Mental Illness in Pop Culture." Films shown included *The Cabinet of Dr. Caligari* (1920), *Psycho* (1960), clips from widely recognized horror films such as *Halloween* and *Friday the 13th*, and documentaries such as *Bellevue: Inside Out* (2001). Students discuss and read about concepts such as the nature of mental illness and how it is diagnosed, stigma, and how social values shape opinions and treatment. Pre/post attendee surveys using validated stigma instruments (e.g., Attribution Questionnaire–Short Form) found positive changes in attitudes, driven by changed perceptions regarding dangerousness, fear, and segregation.

An alternative and complementary approach would be to use movies that actively challenge misconceptions and stigma, such as *Canvas, Ordinary People, A Beautiful Mind, Benny & Joon, Patch Adams,* and others.

Acknowledging Media as Part of Therapy

Mental health professionals should consider asking young patients if they've seen movie, television, or video game depictions of psychiatrists, especially any interacting with children.[19] Open discussion of fears and expectations created (and hopes raised) by such depictions may help patients better engage with treatment. Media depictions of positive therapeutic relationships (such as *Ordinary People* or *Good Will Hunting*) may be helpful to patients, but they may include unrealistic situations or boundary violations that need acknowledgment.

Using Media to Reduce Stigma Among Health Professionals

Knaak[15] described promising results from a Canadian program, Understanding Stigma, designed to change misperceptions and behaviors among health professionals. Drawing on previous research showing the effectiveness of social contact and personal testimonies, which help healthcare providers see the person behind the illness, it also teaches and models what providers can say and do when working with patients who have mental illnesses. The model is especially promising in that it takes practical constraints on training into account. First, it is designed as 60- or 90-min workshop (with optional booster sessions). Second, it provides a variety of "social contact" and behavior modeling via a DVD featuring perspectives on mental illness from those affected themselves, family members, and providers who work with such patients. A single in-person speaker with lived experience also shares his/her story, including positive and stigmatizing experiences with providers. Another use of media: as they enter the workshop site, participants see a continuous-loop slideshow of famous people who have a mental illness, immediately challenging stereotypes.

A pooled analysis of six studies and over a 1000 matched pre/post surveys (using the validated Opening Minds Scale for Health Providers) found that the Understanding Stigma program led to significant improvement in all three subscales: negative attitudes, willingness to disclose/seek help for a mental illness, and preference for social distance. A free online version of the workshop is hosted on the Centre for Addiction and Mental Health Web site, www.camh.ca.

The Mental Health Program of the Carter Center in Atlanta has taken a different approach to reducing stigma by educating journalists and supporting their forays into covering mental health issues, including youth-focused topics. The Rosalynn Carter Fellowships in Mental Health Journalism[57] has supported journalists in the United States as well as several other countries (e.g., Colombia, New Zealand, Romania, Qatar, South Africa, United Arab Emirates) on in-depth, multimedia reporting on local and national mental health stories, with a goal of improving the coverage of such topics well beyond the period of each fellow's financial support.

Journalists in the program undergo on-site training in mental health and stigma-related issues at the Carter Center and get access to guidance, when requested, by other journalists and mental health professionals as they complete their projects. Non-US countries receive local administrative support, such as leadership by representatives of a university or communications-related nongovernmental organization, with a goal of developing and funding their own self-supporting programs that meet those countries' specific needs.

SUMMARY

The stigma associated with mental illness is manifold and complex, overt and subtle. It affects public policy and funding, other people's perceptions of mental illness, and the self-perceptions of those who have a mental illness. Both new and traditional media play roles in defining and reinforcing this stigma. However, there is evidence that those same media can be used as tools to reduce stigma and its broad effects.

Much of the research in this area has been conducted on adults, yet we see that children's perceptions of mental illness and the people who have it are formed at early ages, not only through direct contact but also with media portrayals of its presentation and consequences, especially the misportrayal of dangerousness. There are tremendous opportunities for both traditional and new media to play significant roles in reducing stigma and encouraging those who have mental illness to seek effective treatment.

REFERENCES

1. https://www.cnn.com/2018/02/22/politics/cnn-town-hall-full-video-transcript/index.html.
2. https://twitter.com/realDonaldTrump?ref_src=twsrc%5Egoogle%7Ctwcamp%5Eserp%7Ctwgr%5Eauthor.
3. https://www.politico.com/story/2018/02/26/trump-mental-institutions-424689.
4. Corrigan PW. Lessons learned from unintended consequences about erasing the stigma of mental illness. *World Psychiatry*. 2016;15:67−73.
5. Pescosolido B. The public stigma of mental illness: what do we think; what do we know; what can we prove? *J Health Soc Behav*. 2013;54(1):1−21.
6. Moses T. Being treated differently: stigma experiences with family, peers, and school staff among adolescents with mental health disorders. *Soc Sci Med*. 2010;70:985−993.
7. Mukolo A, Heflinger CA, Wallston KA. The stigma of childhood mental disorders: a conceptual framework. *J Am Acad Child Adolesc Psychiatry*. 2010;49(2):92−103.
8. Angermeyer MC, Schulze B, Dietrich S. Courtesy stigma: a focus group study of relatives of schizophrenia patients. *Soc Psychiatry Psychiatr Epidemiol*. 2003;38:593−602.
9. Weiss MF. Children's attitudes toward the mentally ill: an eight-year longitudinal followup. *Psychol Rep*. 1994;74(1):51−56.
10. Corrigan PW, Lurie BD, Goldman HH, et al. How adolescents perceive the stigma of mental illness and alcohol abuse. *Psychiatr Serv*. 2005;56(5):544−550.
11. Clement S, Schauman O, Graham T, et al. What is the impact of mental health-related stigma on help-seeking? A systematic review of quantitative and qualitative studies. *Psychol Med*. 2015;45(1):11−27.
12. Chandra A, Minkovitz CS. Stigma starts early: gender differences in teen willingness to use mental health services. *J Adolesc Health*. 2006;38:754.e1−754.e8.

13. Reardon T, Harvey K, Baranowska M, et al. What do parents perceive are the barriers and facilitators to accessing psychological treatment for mental health problems in children and adolescents ? A systematic review of qualitative and quantitative studies. *Eur J Child Adolesc Psychiatry*. 2017;26:623–647.

14. Henderson C, Noblett J, Parke H, et al. Mental health-related stigma in health care and mental health-care settings. *Lancet Psychiatry*. 2014;1:467–482.

15. Knaak S, Szeto A, Kassam A, et al. Understanding stigma: a pooled analysis of a national program aimed at health care providers to reduce stigma towards patients with a mental illness. *J Ment Health Addict Nurs*. 2017;1(1): e19–e29.

16. Nordt C, Rössler W, Lauber C. Attitudes of mental health professionals toward people with schizophrenia and major depression. *Schizophr Bull*. 2006;32(4):709–714.

17. Chisholm K, Patterson P, Greenfield S, Turner E, Birchwood M. Adolescent construction of mental illness: implication for engagement and treatment. *Early Interv Psychiatry*; 2016. Epub ahead of print. Available at: https://research.birmingham.ac.uk/portal/files/28131712/Archiving_Version_Adolescent_construction_of_mental_illness.pdf.

18. Sieff EM. Media frames of mental illnesses: the potential impact of negative frames. *J Ment Health*. 2003;12(3): 259–269.

19. Butler JR, Hyler SE. Hollywood portrayals of child and adolescent mental health treatment: implications for clinical practice. *Child Adolesc Psychiatr Clin N Am*. 2005;14: 509–522.

20. Goodwin J. The horror of stigma: psychosis and mental health care environments in twenty-first-century horror film (part I). *Perspect Psychiatr Care*. 2014;50(3):201–209.

21. Goodwin J. The horror of stigma: psychosis and mental health care environments in twenty-first-century horror film (part II). *Perspect Psychiatr Care*. 2014;50(4):224–234.

22. Diefenbach DL, West MD. Television and attitudes toward mental health issues: cultivation analysis and the third-person effect. *J Community Psychol*. 2007;35(2):181–195.

23. Parrott S, Parrott CT. Law & disorder: the portrayal of mental illness in U.S. crime dramas. *J Broadcast Electron Media*. 2015;59(4):640–657.

24. Lawson A, Fouts G. Mental illness in Disney animated films. *Can J Psychiatry*. 2004;49(5):310–314.

25. Wahl O, Wood A, Zaveri P, Drapalski A, Mann B. Mental illness depiction in children's films. *J Community Psychol*. 2003;31(6):553–560.

26. Wilson C, Nairn R, Coverdale J, Panapa A. How mental illness is portrayed in children's television: a prospective study. *Br J Psychiatry*. 2000;176:440–443.

27. Wahl O, Hanrahan E, Kari K, Lasher E, Swaye J. The depiction of mental illness in children's television programs. *J Community Psychol*. 2007;35(1):121–133.

28. Mahar I. *Nobody Wins When Horror Games Stigmatize Mental Illness*. Kotaku Website; July 26, 2013. https://kotaku.com/nobody-wins-when-horror-games-stigmatize-mental-illness-912462538.

29. Shapiro S, Rotter M. Graphic depictions: portrayals of mental illness in video games. *J Forensic Sci*. 2016;61(6): 1592–1595.

30. McGinty EE, Webster DW, Jarlenski M, Barry CL. News media framing of serious mental illness and gun violence in the United States, 1997–2012. *Am J Public Health*. 2014; 104(3):406–413.

31. McGinty EE, Webster DW, Barry CL. Effects of news media messages about mass shootings on attitudes toward persons with serious mental illness and public support for gun control policies. *Am J Psychiatry*. 2013;170(5): 494–501.

32. Slopen NB, Watson AC, Gracia G, Corrigan PW. Age analysis of newspaper coverage of mental illness. *J Health Commun*. 2007;12(1):3–15.

33. Morgan AJ, Jorm AF. Recall of news stories about mental illness by Australian youth: associations with help-seeking attitudes and stigma. *Aust N Z J Psychiatry*. 2009; 43(9):866–872.

34. NKM2.org.

35. Haas SM, Irr ME, Jennings NA, Wagner LM. Communicating thin: a grounded model of Online Negative Enabling Support Groups in the pro-anorexia movement. *New Media Soc*. 2010;13(1):40–57.

36. National Academies of Sciences, Engineering, and Medicine. *Ending Discrimination against People with Mental and Substance Use Disorders: The Evidence for Stigma Change*. Washington, DC: The National Academies Press; 2016. https://doi.org/10.17226/23442.

37. Stuart H, Chen SP, Christie R, et al. Opening minds in Canada: background and rationale. *Can J Psychiatry*. 2014; 59(suppl 1):S8–S12.

38. Thornicroft G, Mehta N, Clement S, et al. Evidence for effective interventions to reduce mental-health-related stigma and discrimination. *Lancet*. 2016;387:1123–1132.

39. Naslund JA, Aschbrenner KA, Marsch LA, Bartels SJ. The future of mental health care: peer-to-peer support and social media. *Epidemiol Psychiatr Sci*. 2016;25(2):113–122.

40. Burns JM, Durkin LA, Nicholas J. Mental health of young people in the United States: what role can the Internet play in reducing stigma and promoting help seeking? *J Adolesc Health*. 2009;45:95–97.

41. About us. ReachOut.com. https://about.au.reachout.com.

42. Betton V, Borschmann R, Docherty M, et al. The role of social media in reducing stigma and discrimination. *Br J Psychiatry*. 2015;206:443–444.

43. Thornicroft C, Wyllie A, Thornicroft G, Mehta N. Impact of the "Like Minds, Like Mine" anti-stigma and discrimination campaign in New Zealand on anticipated and experienced discrimination. *Aust N Z J Psychiatry*. 2014;48(4): 360–370.

44. Yap MB, Reavley NJ, Jorm AF. Associations between awareness of *beyondblue* and mental health literacy in Australian youth: results from a national survey. *Aust N Z J Psychiatry*. 2012;46(6):541–552.

45. Young people. Beyondblue annual report 2014–2015. Available at: http://resources.beyondblue.org.au/prism/file?token=BL/1645_A.

46. https://www.youthbeyondblue.com/.
47. Livingston JD, Cianfrone M, Korf-Uzan K, Coniglio C. Another time point, a different story: one year effects of a social media intervention on the attitudes of young people towards mental health issues. *Soc Psychiatry Psychiatr Epidemiol.* 2014;49(6):985–990.
48. Villani M, Kovess-Masfety V. How do people experiencing schizophrenia spectrum disorders or other psychotic disorders use the Internet to get information on their mental health? Literature review and recommendations. *JMIR Ment Health.* 2017;4(1):e1.
49. Spinzy Y, Nitzan U, Becker G, Bloch Y, Fennig S. Does the Internet offer social opportunities for individuals with schizophrenia? A cross-sectional pilot study. *Psychiatry Res.* 2012;198(2):319–320.
50. Berry N, Lobban F, Belousov M, Emsley R, Nenadic G, Bucci S. #WhyWeTweetMH: understanding why people use Twitter to discuss mental health problems. *J Med Internet Res.* 2017;19(4):e107.
51. Parkin S. Zoe Quinn's depression quest. *New Yorker;* September 9, 2014. https://www.newyorker.com/tech/elements/zoe-quinns-depression-quest.
52. Hoggins T. The Town of Light is a gruelling but worthy exploration of a wretched era in mental therapy. *Telegraph (Rev);* March 18, 2016. https://www.telegraph.co.uk/gaming/what-to-play/the-town-of-light-review/.
53. Craddock R. *The Town of Light: Deluxe Edition Is Coming Exclusively to Nintendo Switch This Spring: An Exploration of Mental Health.* Nintendo Life; February 1, 2018. http://www.nintendolife.com/news/2018/02/the_town_of_light_deluxe_edition_is_coming_exclusively_to_nintendo_switch_this_spring.
54. Cangas AJ, Navarro N, Parra JMA, et al. Stigma-Stop: a serious game against the stigma toward mental health in educational settings. *Front Psychol.* 2017;8. Article 1385.
55. Shandley K, Austin D, Klein B, Kyrios M. An evaluation of 'Reach Out Central': an online gaming program for supporting the mental health of young people. *Health Educ Res.* 2010;25(4):563–574.
56. Theriot MT. Using popular media to reduce new college students' mental illness stigma. *Soc Work Ment Health.* 2013;11:118–140.
57. https://www.cartercenter.org/health/mental_health/fellowships/index.html.

CHAPTER 14

Media's Role in Mitigating Culturally Competent Understanding of Latino Youth

MARIA JOSE LISOTTO, MD • LISA FORTUNA, MD • PAULINA POWELL • RANNA PAREKH, MD, MPH

INTRODUCTION

The Hispanic/Latino community is expected to reach 28.6% of the US population (119 million) by 2060,[1] making it the nation's largest and youngest racial and ethnic group. Unfortunately, this is and continues to be one of the most misunderstood and stereotyped communities in the United States. In this chapter, we will use "Latino" and "Hispanic" interchangeably, but distinguishing both terms remains important when understanding this community. The term "Hispanic" refers to a common language and describes those whose ancestry comes from Spain or Spanish-speaking countries. "Latino" refers to geography, specifically to individuals with Latin America origin. According to the 2010 Census "Hispanic or Latino" refers to a person of Cuban, Mexican, Puerto Rican, South or Central American, or other Spanish culture or origin regardless of race.[2]

Even though Latino population grew more than 43% from 2000 to 2010, the rate of Latino depiction in the media stayed stagnant or grew only slightly, at times proportionally declining.[2] Since mass media shapes "knowledge and beliefs of the majority about minority groups and, in turn, influence minority responses to the majority,"[3] and given the fact that children and adolescents utilize media to understand the world and connect with others, it is not surprising that the lack of Latino media representation and, at times, media's depiction of Latinos would play such a significant role in shaping their view of minorities in general.

Providers are greatly influenced by media representation of minorities, leading in some cases to stereotyping, unconscious bias, racial prejudice, and even discrimination.[4] In other cases, especially when providers are educated in a model centered in cultural humility, the media can inform and enrich the care they provide since it stimulates reflection on their own cultural background and promotes self-analysis of the care provided to minority youth.

In this chapter, we will review the impact of racial and ethnic healthcare disparities in Latinos, emphasizing how more accurate depictions of Latino youth in the media, can enhance understanding of the cultural nuances within Latino subgroups, as well as inform provider's care centered in a model of cultural humility. We will illustrate media's representation of Latinos throughout the last decade, identifying media's role in fostering development for Latino youth, while helping decrease stigma associated with mental illness in Latino groups.

Impact of Racial/Ethnic Biases on Healthcare Disparities and Child Development—Can Media Affect Provision of Care Among Latinos?

As noted in the Institute of Medicine (IOM) seminal report *Unequal Treatment*, racial and ethnic minorities tend to receive lower quality of healthcare than nonminorities, even after controlling for access-related factors.[4] The same report defines *discrimination in healthcare* as "differences in care that result from biases and prejudice, stereotyping, and uncertainty in communication and clinical decision-making."[4] The reasons for healthcare disparities are complex but may reflect socioeconomic differences, environmental degradation, differences in health-related risk factors, and access to care, and both direct and indirect consequences of discrimination.[5]

Latinos face inequities in terms of education, socioeconomic status, and access to care, and such inequities are often exacerbated by language barriers. The differences are so striking that in their report, the IOM states that Hispanic Americans "face greater barriers than any other racial and ethnic group in the U.S."[4]

The IOM identified healthcare provider bias, stereotyping, and clinical uncertainty as factors that may contribute to healthcare disparities.[4] Contemporary racial bias and discrimination can be subtle, unconscious, and imperceptible; unconscious bias can be observed even when there is no intention to discriminate.[6,7] Research shows that unconscious or implicit biases can lead to differential patient treatment based on race, gender, weight, age, language, income, sexual orientation, disability, and insurance status.[4]

The US Surgeon General report found mental health services, more so than other health and medical services, to be "plagued by disparities in the availability of and access to its services" and that "these disparities are viewed readily through the lenses of racial and cultural diversity, age, and gender."[8] As providers caring for a diverse and multicultural population, we must remain cognizant of the influence that media can have on the creation and perpetuation of racial stereotypes and of media's effect on children's development. Providers must also examine their own cognitive and affective processes that can predispose them to stereotyping, since during medical decision making, implicit social attitudes and stereotypes stored in memory may be retrieved automatically without awareness, unintentionally influencing medical care.[4]

Stereotypes not only affect providers' delivery of healthcare but may also be detrimental to academic performance and impact self-image, social development, and overall well-being in youth. There is evidence showing that stigma and cultural stereotypes can have a negative impact on student's academic performance.[9] Stereotype-threat theory posits that stigmatized group members may underperform in diagnostic tests of ability through concerns about confirming to a negative societal stereotype.[10] Stereotype-threat studies have shown that this extra pressure can undermine the targeted groups' (immigrants, minorities) academic performance[11] and even lead to behaviors that directly undermine health, such as adoption of unhealthy eating behaviors and subsequent weight gain.[12] Targeted groups are often stereotyped both in educational and professional settings, experiencing a fear of underperforming in the context of either subtle or blatant discriminatory cues.[13] However, evidence shows that when the stereotype-threat environment is reduced, members of negatively stereotyped groups can in fact outperform nonstereotyped groups.[14] Reducing the negative influence of stereotype threat could decrease the cognitive performance achievement gap leading to better educational achievements.[15]

Therefore, increasing visibility and representation of successful role models for minorities can help decrease the pernicious effects of stereotype threat.[16,17] Ethnic identification not only plays a role in stereotype threat but also seems to buffer negative effects elicited by societal devaluation and rejection of immigrants.[18,19] Subsequently, increasing nonstereotypical Hispanic representation in the media might lead to somewhat of a ripple effect, leading to improvement in individuals' academic and professional performance, while also promoting positive self-image and emotional development in youth.

The Role of Cultural Humility in Training—Education Is Bliss When Treating Latinos

Cross-cultural skills among providers play an important role in preventing poor patient outcomes and unfulfilling interactions within clinical settings.[20] Understanding concepts such as cultural competence and cultural humility will be key when examining the impact of biases when providing psychiatric care.

Cultural competence is the ability to interact effectively with people of different cultures. Cultural competent care is meant to improve the psychiatric treatment of immigrant and minorities, identified as "others."[23] Clinical programs based on cultural competence focus on caring for ethnic/racial minorities and their practices, with the purpose of breaking down cultural barriers to quality healthcare. Culturally competent care includes appreciating the "other person's" culture and perception of illness but does not encourage reflection on the provider's background,[24] missing the opportunity for the provider's own cultural experiences to inform and enrich patient care. Cultural humility, on the other hand, is the "ability to maintain an interpersonal stance that is other-oriented (or open to the other) in relation to aspects of cultural identity that are most important to the [person]"[21] and a "more suitable goal in multicultural medical education."[22] Cultural humility is a "lifelong process of self-reflection and self-critique whereby the individual not only learns about another's culture, but one starts with an examination of her/his own beliefs and cultural identities."[22]

Latino subgroups understand medical and psychiatric illnesses differently depending on the subgroups' place of origin; their history, patterns, and effects of immigration; and even the subgroup's conceptualization of Latino youth growing up as a minority in the

United States. Cultural humility training can therefore help counteract the effects of stereotyping that often occur even within the context of cultural competence training. Providers' understanding of the patients' sociocultural background and ability to empathize with that patient's lived experiences, which will likely include experiences of discrimination possibly affecting willingness to trust providers and adhere to treatment, is more important than scientific competence. For example, a patient may have a spiritual explanation for the etiology of a mental health symptom, and if he or she senses that the provider dismisses this explanation, this can close off trust.

Youth are also influenced by the media that represents them. Research suggests that schools are a powerful tool to socially and culturally influence students' beliefs, often shared with mainstream population.[25] Mass media influences how youth view and understand society and can even shape youth's social behaviors, personal beliefs, and identities.[26] Teachers could utilize media as an educational tool promoting students' critical analysis of the content of TV shows and films, helping them identify and process stereotyping and implicit bias. Clinicians can utilize media to critically examine their own biases and educate themselves on media's portrayal of minority youth. There are multiple movies and TV shows where Latinos are overrepresented as selling or consuming drugs: Training Day, Traffic, Breaking Bad, and Ozark are just some examples. Both teachers and clinicians should be aware of media's portrayal of minorities and the ability to exacerbate and perpetuate stereotypes, at times even affecting their own interactions with young minorities. Therefore, both should be well trained in appreciating the subtle bias or misrepresentations while also identifying accurate portrayal of Latinos in the media.

In sum, as clinicians striving to practice and promote cultural humility, we must work toward developing cross-cultural curricula integrated into the education of future healthcare providers, with practical and case-simulated media-based training.

How Does Media Represent Young Latinos? Teaching Practitioners Through Music, Films, TV, Social Media, and Literature

Media (radio, movies, music, news, magazines, books, photos) can be used as a powerful instructional tool to teach general concepts about child development and how these concepts apply to Latino youth. Entertainment media and news reports can carry more weight than other forms of public communication. Since racial stereotypes are reproduced and disseminated through mass media,[27] the limited and stereotypical-based

stories about Latinos skews viewer's perception of the US society.[28] Historically, Latinos have either been excluded from most American media or portrayed exclusively through decades-old stereotypes. While Latinos comprise about 15% population of the United States, stories about Latinos constitute less than 1% of news media coverage with most of these stories featuring Latinos as lawbreakers[28] or portraying Latinos in a distorted, stereotypic fashion as shown in examples below.

IMAGES ARE WORTH A THOUSAND WORDS
Films

Movies offer a wide variety of images of Latino youth and their families. Some reinforce cultural stereotypes while others explore themes of acculturation. Acculturation is a process through which a person or group from one culture comes to adopt practices and values of another culture. Other themes include intercultural conflicts within the family and identity development as a young minority living in the United States. We offer some examples that focus on acculturation as follows:

"Happy Feet," an Academy Award winner animated movie stars "Mumble," a penguin who was born looking different from other penguins in his environment. He has blue eyes, a high-pitched voice, and tap dances instead of singing. Mumble befriends "Adelie penguins," who identify themselves as "misfits," call each other "amigos," and speak with an accent. These "misfits" do not attend school like the other penguins making them look as dropouts.

A qualitative study based on this movie was conducted to better understand how Latino/a high school students understand media messages and its implications.[26] Participants watched clips of the movie and would then attend an open group where they could critically analyze clips of the movie. In this study, Latino/a students concluded that the "misfits" in "Happy Feet" appeared to represent real-life Latinos, which could lead to perpetuation of the stereotype of Latinos as criminals and uneducated. The students also pointed out how the "misfits" appeared to all look and speak alike, possibly leading viewers to homogenize Latinos, thinking they are all alike. Participants also reported identifying with Mumble given that they too often feel "different" from other groups; reported differences included race, family structure, language, immigration status, and culture.

This study shows some of the effects media can have on Latino children and their understanding of themselves and others through media. Student participants reported that they would have likely overlooked the movie's negative portrayal of Latinos if it had not been for the teacher's encouragement to objectively analyze the movie. Educators and school leaders have the chance to utilize media to engage and educate students on the value of multicultural, diverse societies. Clinicians should be cognizant of media's tendency to depict minority stereotypes, especially given that media messages greatly affect society's understanding of minority groups and their culture. Accreditation Council for Graduate Medical Education recently revised its Institutional Requirements regarding the study of cultural competency and diversity. These Common Program Requirements for residency programs[29] can use multimedia and group processing with trained leaders to promote this learning and reducing the stereotyping of Latinos.

"Real women have curves" (2002) is the story of Ana García (America Ferrera), a first-generation Mexican American teenager, who lives with her family within the Latino community of East Los Angeles. Torn between her mainstream ambitions and her cultural heritage, Ana struggles to find a balance between her family's cultural-based expectations and her dream of pursuing a higher education. Ana receives a full scholarship for Columbia University, but her traditional Mexican parents believe she needs to stay in Los Angeles in order to get married, have children, and help provide for the family. This movie is a great example of the ambivalence that many minority teenagers and transitional-age youth experience; they must decide between fulfilling their parents' expectations (usually based on their cultural roots) versus pursuing their dreams and incorporating American values into their lives. Even though all adolescents go through a period of psychosocial crisis struggling with conflicts related to identity formation, most first and second generation Latino teenagers have an added conflict related to their minority status and acculturation level. This movie allows for exploration of some of the conflicts that minority teenagers undergo during adolescence, while they strive to find their place within American peers and culture, while struggling to stay true to their family, cultural, and ethnic backgrounds. The virtue arising after successful completion of this psychosocial stage is "fidelity"; this word encompasses the conflict within minority teenagers, as they must find a balance between maintaining family and cultural loyalty, while managing the social pressure of fitting in and belonging to a same-age American peer group. This cultural conflict within families can lead to mental health distress and in extreme cases can lead to suicidality.[30]

Television

Since the 1970s, TV shows have tried to underscore topics such as the ambivalence and difficulties of acculturation. "¿Que Pasa, USA?," the first bilingual sitcom on television, centered on a multigenerational Cuban-American family in Miami struggling to hold on to its heritage while learning how to adapt in America. Later in the 1970s came "Chico and the Man," the first TV sitcom that headlined a Mexican character, Chico Rodriguez (Freddie Prinze) as the star of a show that attempted to tackle through laughter, the never-ending divide between ones own race and culture versus mainstream American culture in our society. With his role as a young Chicano veteran with a questionable past who was unable to find work, Chico represented a combination of Latino stereotypes, the potentially dangerous element of the "bandido," with the dark-haired, heavy-accent sexy but criminal "macho" and the clownish elements of the "buffoon."[31] Ed, "The Man," was a racially prejudiced, alcoholic, White Anglo-Saxon Protestant garage owner, not willing to accept the undergoing racial changes in Los Angeles. Throughout the show, Chico is shown as the tolerant and meek Latino "not confident or intelligent enough" to respond to Ed's ethnic slurs. As early as the first episode, we are introduced to Ed's stereotypical satire with lines promoting the "job stealer/uneducated/lazy" stereotype:

> Get out of here, take your flies with you... you people got flies all around you

> Everybody knows you people are lazy, even if I did give you a job you wouldn't show up, you'd be too busy taking a siesta

The 1990s "Saved by the Bell: The College Years" articulated the complexities of diversity and identity long before the rest of Hollywood identified cultural biases. In the episode "Slater's War,"[32] A.C. Slater (Mario Lopez) interacts with Theresa, the leader of the Chicano student organization, who encourages his curiosity to discover Slater's Chicano Mexican roots and his real Spanish name. Theresa also points out that one does not need to speak Spanish to be Latino, an idea that was not so obvious in the early 1990s. To this day, many still consider the "homogenous origin" stereotype to be true; they believe all Latinos share the same ethnic background, therefore Latinos must all know each other, eat spicy food, and come from Mexico, right....? As the episode progresses, Theresa pushes Slater to reflect on his heritage and stop denying his "Latino roots":

Knowing where you come from doesn't make you less of an American, it makes you more of a person… What's your real name? (…) Slater is an anglo name and you're Latino

His white and oblivious friend Zach Morris then wonders why Slater *"would even care about that,"* to which Slater replies:

Because I'm Chicano—in case you never noticed…

Slater's response shows some of the frustration felt by many minorities when they feel others do not recognize their minority status and their daily struggle to prove their identity.

As the episode progresses, Slater discovers that his father had to change his name in order to get into the military academy:

He felt he had to hide his heritage to be accepted… I don't want to do that

In a seemingly juvenile and humorous way, this episode encapsulates the difference between acculturation and assimilation, underscoring minorities' struggle to retain their native culture values and traditions, while trying to incorporate norms and behaviors from the new culture. Slater's father, as many other immigrants, had to go through the process of assimilation,[33] discarding his native culture in order to adopt American culture and become immersed and accepted into his new society.

More recently, prime-time television has tried to promote positive Latino stereotypes with shows like *"Ugly Betty"* and characters such as Dr Callie Torres (Sara Ramírez) from *"Grey's Anatomy."* Unfortunately, other shows continue to perpetuate stigmatization and Latino homogenization. Mass media tends to portray Latino male characters as muscular, dark-skinned, and aggressive men; characterizing them as criminals, drug lords, or seductive *"Latin lovers."* Latinas are equally homogenized, seen as sensual brunettes, with a curvilinear, voluptuous body, and olive skin. Strikingly, out of the limited Spanish-language TV shows on Netflix, more than 10 are drug cartel/guerrilla-related shows; Latino/a characters are almost exclusively depicted as being part of criminal organizations. Two of the most popular shows being *"Narcos"* and *"El Chapo,"* both based on the lives of drug lords, the former based on Colombian Pablo Escobar and the latter based on Mexican Joaquín "El Chapo" Guzmán.

"The George Lopez Show" is the first successful Latino comedy show with a Mexican-American lead actor since *"Chico and the Man."* Even though the show has helped increase Latino exposure in the media, it has also promoted homogenization by focusing its jokes around George's nationality as a Mexican, and by showing George interacting predominantly with Latinos, it has further fueled the misperception that Latinos only interact with Latinos.

"Ugly Betty," the most successful Latino-based program in American history, depicts Betty Suárez (America Ferrera), a 22-year-old quirky Mexican-American woman from Queens, NY, known for her braces, unusual clothing choices, sweet nature, and slight naïveté. She works at a fashion magazine in Manhattan where she is continually mocked for her lackluster physical appearance and initial lack of taste in fashion. *"Ugly Betty"* focuses on professional and physical transitions, tackling important issues in both American and Latino societies such as immigration, LGBTQ (lesbian, gay, bisexual, transgender, queer) issues, and relationships. Controversial themes like immigration are jovially introduced while underscoring and bringing into light how difficult these topics can be for many minorities. For example, Ignacio, one of the characters in the show gets deported after discovering he has been living as an illegal immigrant in the United States after having to flee his country to protect his wife from an abusive ex-husband. Ignacio's deportation and subsequent struggle to return to America culminates with him becoming a citizen, bringing hope and containment to viewers who might be undergoing similar circumstances, at least for a few hours anyway.

"Ugly Betty" has also been lauded for highlighting LGBTQ conflicts since the show provided a holding environment for Justin Suárez (Betty's nephew on the show), to explore his own sexuality with a support network beyond the nuclear family space.[34] The show exposes media's exponential improvement in the characterization portrayal of Latino women, while introducing characters that denote the multiple threats of discrimination when individual identities overlap with multiple minority classes, introducing the concept of intersectionality. This term is attributed to Kimberlé Crenshaw, JD, who in 1989 wrote "the concept of intersectionality denotes the various ways in which race and gender interact to shape the experience of many women of color."[35] Though traditionally intersectionality was applied to women, any individual can be affected by an overlapping minority status and can experience additive levels of discrimination. Professor Crenshaw goes on to conclude that "through an awareness of intersectionality, we can better acknowledge and ground the differences among us and negotiate the means by which these differences will find expression in constructing group politics."[35]

Therefore, even shows like *"Ugly Betty"* can raise awareness of the additive effects of discrimination in people with multiple minority identity status, hopefully leading to identification of policy and social mechanisms that do not account for critical cultural differences.

In *"Modern Family,"* Colombian actress Sofía Vergara's character Gloria Delgado-Pritchett, is a continuation of the "sexy spitfire" stereotype whose accent is a constant source of humor.[28] She embodies the perpetual stereotype of Latinas as "dramatic, hypersexualized women with a heavy Spanish accent." In 2013, the episode "Fulgencio" sparked great controversy due to the level of stereotyping. Gloria's mom and sister (Sonia) visit from Colombia during that episode; Sonia makes two comments that cross racial boundaries.[36]

We need more corn. Gloria, where is your garden? I will harvest some

"Where is the river?"—while Sonia is holding a laundry basket

These comments leave viewers with the idea that in Colombia, people still harvest their food in their back yard and that washing machines are still unknown to Colombians. These jokes only serve to perpetuate negative stereotyping, by portraying Sonia as the Latino "help" who serves the "white American family." The show officially calls Sonia "underprivileged," belittling her to an almost peasant-like status, while beautiful and sexy Gloria, who married the rich white American, gets to enjoy life in America. Blatant stereotypical characters in shows that reach millions of people that have no other direct exposure to Latinos only serve to further reproduce and disseminate Latino stereotypes.

Children's television shows have consistently outpaced prime time TV shows in terms of cultural sophistication and its multidimensional portrayal of Latinos. *"Sesame Street"* was a pioneer in multiculturalism showing people of different racial and ethnic backgrounds as friends and neighbors. Representations of distinct Latino cultures appears in both human and nonhuman characters (Rosita, Ovejita) with depiction of different Spanish accents, speaking to the diversity of Latin America.[37] *"Sesame Street"* depicts Latinos as proud of their roots and outwardly speak about the cultural differences and diversity within the group.[37] It focuses on geographically specific practices, portraying cultural traditions and expressions from different Latino subgroups.

"Sesame Street" paved the way for shows like *"Dora the Explorer"* debuting in the 2000s. This interactive show allows children to choose their next adventure, while it teaches Spanish to English-speaking children. *"Dora"*

(voiced by Caitlin Sanchez) is a cute 7-year-old Hispanic girl who asks questions, providing the correct answer while also validating the child's work and encouraging curiosity and perseverance.[38] Dora goes on adventures with other characters, anthropomorphic monkey *"Boots,"* talking purple backpack *"la mochila,"* and the *"singing map."* The villain fox *"Swiper,"* often steals things when Dora is not watching but she still goes out of her way to help *"Swiper,"* reflecting on positive values of altruism, generosity, and forgiveness to children. *"Dora the Explorer"* has been produced in 30 other languages and is very popular in Latin America, helping children learn English. *"Dora"* is portrayed as a bright and adventurous bilingual Latina, serving as a role model and source of connection for Latino children with a bicultural identity. However, the show does represent Latinos as monolithic, missing the opportunity to show children the heterogeneity of Latino culture.

In sum, the history and continued emergence of shows with Latino presence in television, movies, and children's literature will hopefully help counterbalance the negative stereotypes of Latinos that have continuously been portrayed in the media.

MUSIC: LATIN EXPLOSION

Music can provide insight into Latino culture and serve as a tool to connect with patients, especially adolescents. If one is from Latin America, music is a way to stay connected with one's culture; inexplicably, the same does not happen with other media such as TV characters/shows or films. To put things in perspective, Latinos listen to radio more than any other ethnic group, with 94% of Latinos older than 12 years tuning in every week.[39] Every time Latinos listen to a Spanish song, no matter what genre, artist, or country it represents, they always miss home. Society is reflected in music. Music is a key instrument for adolescents; it helps shape their identity and helps any adolescent identify with emotions, wishes, and dreams that they would otherwise have difficulty expressing. In the case of Latino youth, music not only provides an outlet for their emotions and helps them identify with their ethnic background, giving them a sense of belongingness and connectedness, but also allows for increased communication and bonding with other youth, providing cultural identification and a means for collective attachment and pride.

The complex history and evolution of Latin music goes beyond the scope of this chapter. Latin American folk and popular music comprises numerous musical styles and genres that emerged gradually within specific regions of Latin America. From very early on, the energy and creativity of Latino youth helped shape musical experiences of Americans. Between 1950 and 1960, Chicano Ritchie Valens created the rock "n" roll version of a Mexican folk song, *"La Bamba,"* the first Latino song to ever reach number 1 on Billboard.[40] Then came José Feliciano, a Puerto Rican singer, songwriter, and guitarist, best known for "Feliz Navidad" and the rendition of The Doors "Light my Fire," who won the first Latin Grammy for "Best New Artist." He was born blind due to glaucoma but was able to teach himself how to play the accordion and guitar and create bilingual music.[40] José Feliciano's life is an example of dedication and passion and his music a constant reminder of what one can achieve in America with hard work, resilience, and faith.

In 1961, Rita Moreno (portraying Anita Palacios) became the first Latina to win an Academy Award Oscar with *"West Side Story."* Unfortunately, after winning the Oscar, Rita describes not being able to find roles in movies that were not centered on stereotypical characters.[41] *"Celia Cruz"* or *"The Queen of Salsa"* was a true pioneer of Afro-Latinidad; she focused on the African elements of her identity with lyrics and costumes honoring her ethnic background by wearing flamboyant dresses, brightly colored wigs, and perilously high heels.[42] She also became an emblem of the immigrant experience after Fidel Castro barred her from returning to Cuba in 1960.[42] Celia died without being able to return to Cuba and would often speak about her longingness for her land and the hardships that immigrants go through when they must leave their country, feelings that most immigrant Latinos can relate to.

In 1980, 60% of Miami's population comprised Latinos. In that year, Gloria Estefan, lead singer for the band "Miami Sound Machine," made history with *"Conga."* The song *"Conga"* relates to the specific Cuban rhythm, but also speaks to all Latinos and their connection to music and dance:

It's the rhythm of the island, and like the sugar cane so sweet

Possibly the most powerful song for Latinos is Gloria Estefan's *"Mi Tierra"* (My Homeland), a song that touches on important issues for Latinos including immigration, separation from family, and longingness for the homeland.

La tierra donde naciste no la puedes olvidar

porque tiene tus raíces y lo que dejas atrás

(The homeland where you were born you cannot forget, because it has your roots and what you have left behind)

La tierra te duele, la tierra te da, en medio del alma, cuando tú no estás…

(The homeland hurts, the homeland gives, in the middle of the soul, when you're no longer there…)

"Selena" was the most influential US Latino "crossover" pop star of all times. She brought "Mexican Tejano" music to the masses, winning a Grammy award in 1993 and gold record in 1994 for *"Amor Prohibido"* (Forbidden Love). Her tragic death at 23 years signified an enormous loss for the music world and Latino market since she was exponentially increasing Latino presence in the media. She led the way for other bilingual artists like Ricky Martin, Jennifer Lopez, Marc Anthony, Christina Aguilera, Shakira, Pitbull, Romeo Santos, just to name a few. Latino presence in music has increased at a rate comparable with Latino growth in the United States. Some of their main achievements involve breaking barriers between Anglo-Saxon and Latin cultures, blurring the separation between Spanish and English music, while staying true to their ethnic roots. For example, in 1999 Ricky Martin became the first Latino ever to perform live in the Grammy Awards ceremony, while Shakira's song "Hips don't lie" become the best-selling single of the 2000s. In the late 1990s, a mix between hip hop, Latin, and Caribbean music gave birth to a new music genre originated in Puerto Rico: reggaeton. Puerto Rican reggaeton group *"Calle 13"* has been creating more politically engaged music as of lately, addressing issues like social justice and poverty in Latin America:

Soy, soy lo que dejaron, soy toda la sobra de lo que se robaron

(I am, I am what they left over, I am the leftover of what they stole)

un pueblo escondido en la cima, mi piel es de cuero, por eso aguanta en cualquier clima

(a town hidden at the top, my skin is made of leather, that's why it holds in any weather)

Lastly, *"Despacito"* a reggaeton-pop song, originally including Latin stars Luis Fonsi and Daddy Yankee, became the first number 1 song on Billboard's Hot 100 chart[43] after featuring Justin Bieber in the remix version. The only other Spanish-spoken song ever to reach number 1 song in Billboard was Ritchie Valens' cover *"La Bamba"* in 1987.[44] With over 3 billion views on YouTube, it has become the most-watched video in history and the most streamed song of all times.[43] *"Despacito"* is arguably the first authentic song to top the chart and cross-over to American audiences with the truest representation of what music sounds like on Spanish-language radio.[44]

In sum, music is a window into understanding Latinos. Practitioners treating Latino youth should become familiar with the style and content of the music their patients listen to since it can shed light into youngsters' inner conflicts, as well as educate clinicians on cultural and socioeconomic problems in different regions of Latin America. Places where this music can be found include the Internet on-sites like Sounds and Colors and YouTube. Listening to music like reggaeton with an open mind and curiosity can offer an opportunity for the provider to gain insights into youth culture and contemporary ideas. The latent content of the lyrics, associations, and images that each song evokes in the child or youth provides clues into the patient's conscious or unconscious psyche and a deeper understanding of the adolescent's inner struggles and overall psychological well-being.

SOCIAL MEDIA

Latinos are the group with the most presence in social media platforms,[45] and social media has become, for Latinos, a platform to creatively battle stigma and "bring voice" to Latino culture. One of the biggest social media platforms used by Latinos is YouTube. Of the top 50 single-focused YouTube channels with the most subscribers, 18% are produced by and/or feature US Latino content creators.[28] YouTube has become for Latinos a platform for bonding; videos are often shared among users who post comments and then spread them between their social network of subscribers, providing a vehicle for communication and allowing Latinos to feel connected across the globe.

Another example includes "Mitú," a social media platform created in 2012 with the objective of increasing communication between Latinos and increasing awareness of Latino culture to non-Latino communities. Mitú was initially exclusively created for YouTube, but given its successful release, the creators partnered with Snapchat to bring Mitú's voice to the Snapchat Discover stories platform, since then creating over 400 million views on Snapchat.[46] This bilingual platform contains videos, literature pieces, news, entertainment articles, cultural references, and a myriad of other media-related pieces, allowing for an increase in exposure to Latino culture. Mitú's aims to bring Latino and American cultures together, as they quote on their Twitter account (@wearmitu), "We are 200%: 100% American and 100% Latino."[47]

"Latino USA" is a newsmagazine and podcast that provides weekly insights into the lived experiences of Latino communities throughout the nation. It is the longest running Latino-focused program on US public media,[48] providing a window to the cultural, political, and social ideas that impact Latinos. Other media

platforms such as blogs, Facebook, YouTube, and Twitter can also be used as platforms to raise mental health awareness, reduce stigma, and provide information and resources for patients.

LITERATURE

Literature is one more genre that showcases elements of Latino culture and may shed light on issues relevant for youth development and provider cultural competency. Stories and narratives provide an opportunity to explore the nuances and experiences of culture, identity development, and inner psychological experiences as shared by the author and depicted by the characters he or she creates. A Latin American literature classic relating a transgenerational family history is "The House of the Spirits" (La casa de los espíritus) by Chilean writer Isabel Allende. The novel centers on the life and progeny of Clara del Valle, a clairvoyant who begins documenting her life in a journal after spending 9 years of silence following the death of her sister by poisoning. Fifty years after the book begins, her husband and granddaughter use her journals to make sense of the family history and uncover many of the secrets which have been buried throughout the years as a way of dealing with loss, betrayal, and power; the family secrets are laid bare in the search for identity while Allende describes in excruciating but powerful details some of the horrors that Chileans endured during the civil war that led to Pinochet's ascension into power.

A more contemporaneous novel that includes conflicts of identify is "Butterfly Boy: Memories of a Chicano Mariposa." In this book, Rigoberto Gonzalez tries to convey the complexities and societal shortcomings of the Latino community when it comes to homosexuality and the struggles that adolescents/young adults go through when they decide to "come out" in a society that still finds same-sex relationships taboo. The book describes the authors' personal life and experience of coming out as a first-generation child of Mexican farmworkers. This book examines complicated issues such as identity, assimilation versus acculturation, as well as the meaning that belonging to Latino culture has for immigrants and first-generation children. It also focuses on other themes like machismo and "familismo," while describing first-hand the continuous ambivalence that first-generation children feel when they are living in a country with a different language and whose culture at times contradicts their families.

Adolescents go through a complex process when they are confronted with incongruence between their families' social norms and the same age peers' norms.

For Latinos, family and community bonds are very important, while the dominant American culture is oriented mostly around individualism and personal achievements, creating conflict thus leading to stress and anxiety in many teenagers. In *"How the García Girls Lost Their Accents,"* Julia Alvarez follows a family from the Dominican Republic as they flee after their father's association with a group trying to overthrow the dictator government is discovered. The family lands in New York City, and the four sisters struggle to adjust to a different culture while retaining their Dominican heritage. This book shows the internal conflict of many immigrants, having to balance one's culture while becoming acculturated to a new society.

"Cien años de Soledad" (100 Years of Solitude) is the most translated literary work in Spanish after *"Don Quixote."*[49] This novel tells the story of the Buendía family, who move to the isolated town of Macondo, which is the mirror image of García Márquez's native town of Aracataca. This masterpiece relates Colombian history, and more broadly, Latin American history and its struggles with colonialism, civil war, labor unrest, and emergence into modernity. Through Macondo, García Márquez brilliantly reflects the current instability of many Latin American political regimens, with various dictatorships in the novel serving as a mirror image of the dictatorships found to have ruled Nicaragua, Panamá, and Cuba.[49] The tenacious matriarch of the family *"Ursula"* works devotedly to keep the family together despite its differences, personifying the stereotypical loving, matriarchal, family oriented, and religious Hispanic woman, often portrayed in the media.

Literature like other media begins to help providers develop cultural humility leading to curiosity and expanding on the understanding of culture, especially if it offers an opportunity for reflection and dialog. An appreciation for the complexity of stories is vitally important for Latino youth and providers in appreciating the cultural struggles and nuances they illuminate.

Media's Portrayal of Latino Children and Effects on Development

All immigrants undergo the process of acculturation, a dynamic and multidimensional process, during which immigrants retain aspects of their native culture while simultaneously adopting the new society's culture, foreign attitudes, norms, values, and behaviors.[31,50] Latino children, whether they were born outside or in the United states, undergo the same complex process of cultural identity formation or acculturation, allowing immigrants of all ages to survive and try to adapt to the new country and society.[51] Communication allows immigrants to become acculturated to the new social environment[52,53]; Latinos often turn to media (TV, films, news) to become acquainted with the new culture. Berg postulates that false ideas about a group can be validated by the media "and stereotypes may serve to develop norms of treatment of certain groups which, in turn, may create an unequal power structure."[54]

Since children utilize media to understand and develop higher-order thinking skills and make sense of the world,[56,57] it is not surprising that media would play a role in shaping their concepts of minority groups. The iGen and millennial generations are filled with all kinds of media and spend substantial amounts of time connected to social media, watching movies, listening to music or watching YouTube videos, blogging, e-mailing, or plainly "surfing the Web." According to a 1999 study, a child between 2 and 7 years uses media for 3.5 h a day on a typical day.[55] The time spent on each media platform is related to age, race and ethnicity, gender, household socioeconomic status, and other psychosocial factors.[55]

Research shows that implicit bias develops early in life from repeated reinforcement of social stereotypes, with implicit pro-white bias occurring as young as 3–4 years.[58] Furthermore, according to the social cognition theory, mere media exposure to stereotypical negative attributes "can unconsciously and automatically activate stereotypic associations,"[59] affecting the way one perceives and understands minorities. Since Latinos' representation in mainstream media is scarce, and when represented, they are often portrayed through stereotypes reinforcing Latino's negative attributes, children of any ethnic background might develop pervasive negative associations that could influence the future development of explicit or implicit biases against Latinos.

There is a strong relationship between acculturation and achievement of developmental milestones in Latinos. While core developmental domains are often analyzed without taking into account the individual's cultural context, we recognize that both culture and, in the last century, also media play a crucial role in the achievement of a child or adolescent's developmental milestones. The effects that stereotype-threat can have on academic/cognitive performance have been well noted above; emotional development, including self-esteem, and overall well-being have also been shown to potentially be affected by negative stereotypes. Therefore, it is not surprising that other developmental domains such as social interactions (within and between cultural groups) and personal identity/self-formation are also likely to be influenced by how the media portrays Latinos. Pervasive misrepresentations and negative stereotypes of Latinos have the potential to mitigate normal development in youth, while portrayal of successful and intelligent individuals who cherish belongingness to their culture, while simultaneously trying to adopt American culture, can in turn reinforce positive development and relate counter stereotypical information that could discourage negative cognitive associations and reinforce/foster positive development among youth.

The prevalence of mental health disorders increases during adolescence,[60] with Latino adolescents demonstrating the highest risk for depression among multiple ethnic groups;[18] Latina girls have been found to have higher rates of suicidal ideation and attempts than their African American and white counterparts on the Youth Risk Behavior Survey.[61] Latino youth commonly report episodes of perceived discrimination, and this has been associated with lower self-esteem and more depressive symptoms.[18] Since both directly and indirectly perceived discrimination can hinder self-worth, increasing vulnerability for depressive symptoms, enhancing youth's positive self-concept could help mitigate some of the negative effects of perceived discrimination. Given that minority youth with higher levels of ethnic identity exploration and resolution have reported higher levels of self-esteem,[18] it will be important for providers and educators of minority children to promote conversations that can inspire self-reflection and building skills for critically examining media depictions by youth. By increasing nonstereotypical Latino media presence, adolescents could be exposed to inspiring Latino role models who can foster their sense of belongingness and ethnic pride. Providers could then utilize media characters to engage teenagers in conversations about emotions involving their ethnic background, either by displacement or identification. This could also help ameliorate the stigma of sharing mental health symptoms by inviting a more wholistic exploration of these in the context of stories and images, which youth find easier to identity with. For example, one could explore lyrics or stories that explore emotions, distress, conflicts, and hope.

In summary, healthy development, including issues of self-esteem, are related to acculturation and cultural identity formation. To support positive development, we need to understand the effects of negative stereotypes as working against healthy emotional and social growth. In this technology-based era, the media is one of the most powerful tools to reproduce and maintain racial-ethnic, gender, and sexual identity stereotypes. Through media, we can shape children's perception by presenting an accurate representation of Latinos as a heterogeneous group, avoiding pan-ethnic stereotypes, promoting ethnic pride, and empowering the next generations of multicultural communities where diversity and inclusion are cherished.

SUMMARY

Latinos are a heterogeneous group with different levels of assimilation in the United States, varied physical characteristics, and contrasting socioeconomic and cultural backgrounds; paradoxically, their presence in mainstream media remains extremely low and slow-changing.

Children's development and mental health cannot be interpreted without considering each child's sociocultural environment, more so in the case of Latinos, who far from existing in a bubble cannot be understood without understanding their specific community and values. Practitioners trained within a model of cultural humility will be able to examine their own beliefs remaining aware of potential biases, while remaining open to others' culture and maintaining a curious stance that allows for assiduous learning and self-growth. The media plays a big role in shaping the society's perception of minorities. We must begin educating children on the risks of racial prejudice and implicit bias, increasing their awareness and exposure to media outlets that promote positive representations of minorities. Clinicians have a unique opportunity to educate themselves on Latino youth culture utilizing media as a vehicle assisting them in their journey toward providing competent and culturally sensitive clinical care, always informed from a stance of cultural humility. With this goal in mind and by promoting critical analysis of the media, while increasing exposure to positive role models for Latino youth, we can start changing old paradigms that have contributed to decades of discrimination, healthcare disparities, and racialization. In this current complex social atmosphere, with times of confusion and even contradictory ideas about diversity and inclusion, many are struggling to become culturally humble. Given the central role that media plays in the understanding and accurate portrayal of minority groups, the media has the unique opportunity to reach millions of people in a way that leads and facilitates cultural curiosity through an accurate portrayal of Latinos.

REFERENCES

1. Stepler R, Brown A. *2014, Hispanics in the United States Statistical Portrait*; 2016. http://www.pewhispanic.org/2016/04/19/statistical-portrait-of-hispanics-in-the-united-states-trends/.

2. Ennis SR, Rios-Vargas M, Albert NG. *The Hispanic Population: 2010*; 2011. https://www.census.gov/prod/cen2010/briefs/c2010br-04.pdf.

3. Faber RJ, O'Guinn TC, Meyer TP. Televised portrayals of Hispanics: a comparison of ethnic perceptions. *Int J Intercult Relat*. 1987;11(2):155–169.

4. Institute of Medicine (US) Committee on Understanding and Eliminating Racial and Ethnic Disparities in Health Care. In: Smedley BD, Stith AY, Nelson AR, eds. *Unequal Treatment: Confronting Racial and Ethnic Disparities in Health Care*. Washington (DC): National Academies Press (US); 2003. Available from: https://www.ncbi.nlm.nih.gov/books/NBK220362/.

5. Williams DR. Race, socioeconomic status, and health. The added effects of racism and discrimination. *Ann N Y Acad Sci*. 1999;896:173–188.

6. FitzGerald C, Hurst S. Implicit bias in healthcare professionals: a systematic review. *BMC Med Ethics*. 2017; 18:19.

7. Banaji MR, Greenwald AG. *Blind Spot: Hidden Biases of Good People*. Delacorte Press; 2017.

8. Office of the Surgeon General (US), Center for Mental Health Services (US), National Institute of Mental Health (US). Mental health: culture, race, and ethnicity. In: *A Supplement to Mental Health: A Report of the Surgeon General*. 2001. Rockville (MD).

9. Owens J, Massey DS. Stereotype threat and College academic performance: a latent variables approach. *Soc Sci Res*. 2011;40(1):150–166.

10. Steele CM, Aronson J. Stereotype threat and the intellectual test performance of African Americans. *J Pers Soc Psychol*. 1995;69(5):797–811.

11. Spencer SJ, Logel C, Davies PG. Stereotype threat. *Annu Rev Psychol*. 2016;67:415–437.

12. Guendelman MD, Cheryan S, Monin B. Fitting in but getting fat: identity threat and dietary choices among US immigrant groups. *Psychol Sci*. 2011;22(7):959–967.

13. McGlone MS, Aronson J, Kobrynowicz D. Stereotype threat and the gender gap in political knowledge. *Psychol Women Q*. 2006;30(4):392–398.

14. Walton GM, Spencer SJ. Latent ability: grades and test scores systematically underestimate the intellectual ability of negatively stereotyped students. *Psychol Sci*. 2009;20(9): 1132–1139.

15. Appel M, Weber S, Kronberger N. The influence of stereotype threat on immigrants: review and meta-analysis. *Front Psychol*. 2015;6:900.

16. Murphy MC, Steele CM, Gross JJ. Signaling threat: how situational cues affect women in math, science, and engineering settings. *Psychol Sci*. 2007;18(10): 879–885.

17. McIntyre RB, Lord CG, Gresky DM, Ten Eyck LL, Frye GJ, Bond CFJ. A social impact trend in the effects of role models on alleviating women's mathematics stereotype threat. *Curr Res Soc Psychol*. 2005;10(9): 116–136.

18. Umaña-Taylor AJ, Updegraff KA. Latino adolescents' mental health: exploring the interrelations among discrimination, ethnic identity, cultural orientation, self-esteem, and depressive symptoms. *J Adolesc*. 2007; 30(4):549–567.

19. Umaña-Taylor AJ, Wong JJ, Gonzales NA, Dumka LE. Ethnic identity and gender as moderators of the association between discrimination and academic adjustment among Mexican-origin adolescents. *J Adolesc*. 2012;35(4): 773–786.

20. Abraído-Lanza AF, Céspedes A, Daya S, Flórez KR, White K. Satisfaction with health care among Latinas. *J Health Care Poor Underserved*. 2011;22(2):491–505.

21. Waters A, Asbill L. *Reflections on Cultural Humility*; 2013. http://www.apa.org/pi/families/resources/newsletter/2013/08/cultural-humility.aspx.

22. Tervalon M, Murray-Garcia J. Cultural humility versus cultural competence: a critical distinction in defining physician training outcomes in multicultural education. *J Health Care Poor Underserved*. 1998;9(2):117–125.

23. Qureshi A, Collazos F, Ramos M, Casas M. Cultural competency training in psychiatry. *Eur Psychiatry*. 2008; 23(suppl 1):49–58.

24. Yeager KA, Bauer-Wu S. Cultural humility: essential foundation for clinical researchers. *Appl Nurs Res*. 2013; 26(4).

25. Gonzalez N, Moll LC, Amanti C. *Funds of Knowledge: Theorizing Practices in Households, Communities, and Classrooms*. New Jersey: Lawrence Erlbaum Associates; 2005.

26. Boske C, McCormack S. Building an understanding of the role of media literacy for Latino/a high school students. *High Sch J*. 2011;94(4):167–186.

27. Correa T. Framing Latinas: Hispanic women through the lenses of Spanish-language and English-language news media. *Journalism*. 2010;11(4):425–443.

28. Negrón-Muntaner F, Abbas C, Figueroa L, Robson S. *The Latino Media Gap: A Report on The State of Latinos in U.S Media*; 2014. https://fusiondotnet.files.wordpress.com/2015/02/latino_media_gap_report.pdf.

29. Accreditation Council for Graduate Medical Education (ACGME). *ACGME Common Program Requirements (Residency) Sections I-V Summary and Impact of Major Requirement Revisions*; 2018. http://www.acgme.org/Portals/0/PFAssets/ReviewandComment/CPR-Residency-2018-02-06-Impact.pdf.

30. Fortuna LR, Perez DJ, Canino G, Alegria M. Prevalence and correlates of lifetime suicidal ideation and attempts among Latino subgroups in the United States. *J Clin Psychiatry*. 2007;68(4):572–581. PMCID: PMC2774123.

31. Stephenson M. Development and validation of the Stephenson multigroup acculturation Scale (SMAS). *Psychol Assess.* 2000;12(1):77—88.

32. https://www.youtube.com/watch?v=ka_gdvRVxoU&t=438s.

33. Dalisay F. Media use and acculturation of new immigrants in the United States. *Commun Res Rep.* 2012;29(2): 148—160.

34. González T. A mainstream dream: Latinas/os on prime-time television. In: Montilla PM, ed. *Latinos and American Popular Culture.* Santa Barbara, CA: Praeger; 2013:13.

35. Crenshaw K. Mapping the margins: intersectionality, identity politics, and violence against women of color. *Stanf Law Rev.* 1991;43(6):1241—1299.

36. A Medium Corporation. *How "Modern" Is Modern Family?* April 2015. Retrieved from: https://medium.com/sitcom-world/how-modern-is-modern-family-42f325c2258.

37. Masi de Casanova E. Representing Latinidad in Children's television: what are the kids watching? In: Montilla PM, ed. *Latinos and American Popular Culture.* Santa Barbara, CA: Praeger; 2013:30—34.

38. Thompson NA. *Exploring Dora: The Positive and Negative of the 8-year-old Latina with a Backpack*; November 26, 2013. Retrieved from: http://www.latinpost.com/articles/4130/20131126/exploring-dora-positive-and-negative-8-year-old-latina-backpack.htm.

39. A Detailed Look at the Radio Listening Habits and Consumer Insight Among Hispanic Listeners in the U.S. The NiLP Network on Latino Issues, December 23, 2013. http://blog.rimix.com/rilatino/entrada/25003-hispanic-radio-today-2013%E2%80%8F.html.

40. Berríos Miranda M, Dudley S, Habell-Pallán M, Carroll R, Orozco D, Emmons J. American Sabor Latinos in U.S. *Pop Music*; 2017. Retrieved from: http://americansabor.org/musicians/ritchie-valens.

41. Martin L. Rita Moreno overcame Hispanic stereotypes to achieve stardom. *Miami Herald*; September 2008. Retrieved from: http://www.latinamericanstudies.org/puertorico/rita-moreno.htm.

42. Biography. (n.d.). Retrieved from: https://celiacruz.com/biography.

43. Nyren E. *'Despacito' Ties Mariah Carey's Record for Most Weeks at No. 1*; August 28, 2017. Retrieved from: http://variety.com/2017/music/news/despacito-record-mariah-carey-most-weeks-number-one-1202540973/.

44. Molanphy C. *Why America's First Spanish-Language No. 1 in Decades Is Likely to Be the Song of the Summer.* May 26, 2017. Retrieved from: http://www.slate.com/blogs/browbeat/2017/05/26/why_luis_fonsi_and_justin_bieber_s_despacito_is_no_1.html.

45. Social Media Fact Sheet. January 12, 2017. Retrieved from: http://www.pewinternet.org/fact-sheet/social-media.

46. Roshanian A. *Snapchat Discover Adds Mitu to Target Multicultural Youth*; December 14, 2016. Retrieved from: http://variety.com/2016/digital/news/mitu-snapchat-discover-1201942195/.

47. Account WA. We are mitú (@wearemitu). 2017. https://twitter.com/wearemitu.

48. Latino USA. n.d. Retrieved from: http://latinousa.org/reporter/latino-usa/.

49. SparkNotes Editors. *SparkNote on One Hundred Years of Solitude*; 2002. Retrieved from: http://www.sparknotes.com/lit/solitude/.

50. Trimble JE. Social change and acculturation. In: Chun KM, Organista PB, Marin G, eds. *Acculturation: Advances in Theory, Measurement, and Applied Research.* Washington, DC: American Psychological Association; 2003:3—13.

51. Young SL. Half and half: an (auto)ethnography of hybrid identities in a Korean american mother-daughter relationship. *J Int Intercult Commun.* 2009;2(2):139—167.

52. Kim YY. Communication patterns of foreign immigrants in the process of acculturation. *Hum Commun Res.* 1977; 4(1):66—77.

53. Wilkin HA, Katz VS, Ball-Rokeach SJ. The role of family interaction in new immigrant Latinos' civic engagement. *J Commun.* 2009;59:387—406.

54. Ramírez Berg C. Stereotyping in films in general and of the Hispanic in particular. *Howard J Commun.* 2009;2(3): 286—300.

55. Roberts DF, Foehr UG, Rideout VJ, Brodie M. *Kids & Media @ at the New Millenium*; November 1999. Retrieved from: https://kaiserfamilyfoundation.files.wordpress.com/2013/01/kids-media-the-new-millennium-report.pdf.

56. (a) Hobbs R. Literacy for the information age. In: Flood J, Heath SB, Lapp D, eds. *Handbook of Research on Teaching Literacy through the Communicative and Visual Arts.* New York, NY: Macmillan; 1997:7—14;
(b) Hooks B. *Reel to Real: Race, Sex, and Class at the Movies.* New York: Routledge; 1996.

57. Kozma RB. Learning with media. *Rev Educ Res.* 1991;61(2): 179—212.

58. Baron AS, Banaji MR. The development of implicit attitudes. Evidence of race evaluations from ages 6 and 10 and adulthood. *Psychol Sci.* 2006;17(1):53—58.

59. Devine PG. Stereotypes and prejudice: their automatic and controlled components. *J Pers Soc Psychol.* 1989;56(1):5—18.

60. Cicchetti D, Toth SL. The development of depression in children and adolescents. *Am Psychol.* 1998;53(2): 221—241.

61. Zayas LH, Lester RJ, Cabassa LJ, Fortuna LR. Why do so many Latina teens attempt suicide? A conceptual model for research. *Am J Orthopsychiatry.* 2005;75(2):275—287.

CHAPTER 15

Family Life in Television and Film: What Every Clinician Should Know

SYLVIA J. KRINSKY, MD • JOHN SARGENT, MD

THE ROLE OF FAMILIES IN TELEVISION AND FILM

The structure of the American family has been changing, and the two-parent, heterosexual, nuclear family is no longer the only acceptable family structure. Similarly, the types of families depicted on television and film have been changing and serve several different functions, which range from mirroring a version of our everyday life experiences to illustrating an idealized fantasy of family life. Fictional families that are similar to our own families can validate our experiences, whereas showing family structures that are different from our own has the potential to increase our empathy and understanding. However, television and film are embedded in a societal context and which families are represented in the mass media is decided by the dominant culture.[1,2] If we cannot find depictions of our own families, it supports an assumption that our stories do not matter.[3] Even when television and film makers consciously strive for diverse representations of family narratives, there is risk of reinforcing the internalized stereotypes perpetuated by those in power.[4] The economics of the television and film industry further complicate the debate over which types of families receive representation, as the intent of the industry is to generate profits not cultural competency.[1,2,4]

As professionals working with children and families, understanding the messages about family life embedded in popular media is useful because media can shape both parents' and children's perspectives on family life. It is important for clinicians working with families to understand that healthy families come in varied structures and to strengthen relationships and communication within the family.[5] The content of family-centered television and film can also be used to foster conversation about family life. By talking about television families and their problems, parents and children can talk about some of their own family experiences indirectly in displacement. Clips of family interactions from television and film can be used to facilitate discussion in parent education groups.[6] "Re-authoring" experiences can be used with children and parents when key elements of their experiences are absent from media.[7]

A BRIEF HISTORY OF FAMILY STRUCTURES ON TELEVISION

To understand how to most effectively use mass media representations in clinical work, let's start by examining how their depictions of family life have evolved. In a partial response to conservative social critics who blamed the death of the nuclear family on television trends toward including many different types of family structures, a study by Skill and Robinson[8] looked at the changing demographics of television families. Skill and Robinson[8] looked at 497 prime time network dramas or sitcoms where the plot focused on family life and tracked the changes in fictional family demographics over the decades. They[8] confirmed the earlier work of Moore,[9] whose smaller study of successful network prime time series over a similar time period found that when nontraditional families were present, they were frequently headed by widowed men. However, Skill and Robinson[8] expanded on Moore's work by comparing their TV family demographics to US Census data. Census data from 1960 revealed that 9% of families were headed by a single parent, most of whom were single mothers; however, on prime time network television during the 1950s, 31% of TV families were headed by single parents, more than half of whom were single fathers, like Andy Taylor on *The Andy Griffith Show*.[8] During the 1950s, single parenthood was relatively rare and typically the result of separation or divorce; however on television, single parents were most often widowed.[8] Divorced protagonists did not appear on prime time network programs until 1975 with *One Day at a Time* and *What's Happening*. In the 1980s, television single parenthood changed to include both more single mothers and more divorced single parents of either gender, and this change brought the fictional depictions of family life of the time closer to US Census data.[8] However, Skill and Robinson[8] found that even in the 1980s, single fathers remained much more common on network TV than in real life. In answer to the social critics who blamed changes on real-life family structures on the creation of their fictional counterparts, Skill and Robinson argued that changes in family structure on television lagged behind their real-life counterparts.[8,10]

Television families also differed from real life families in that they were predominantly white.[8,9] The first program centered on black family life appeared when *Julia* aired in 1968, and although black families became increasingly represented, there was minimal depiction of other racial minorities.[8] Skill and Robinson were unable to comment on whether the depictions of racial and ethnic minorities on television reinforced or refuted stereotypes as they examined only the quantity of television families of color. The study by Tukachinsky et al.[11] examined the quantity and quality of the depictions of racial/ethnic minorities on 40 of the most-viewed prime time shows from 1987 to 2009. They examined the association between positive depictions of minorities and the attitudes of non-Hispanic whites as measured on the American National Election Studies Survey. They[11] found that the prevalence of black characters peaked at 21% in the late 1980s and then remained constant at 10%–14%, which is similar to the US Census data. However, Latinos and Asian Americans were grossly underrepresented,[11] and Native Americans were practically absent.[3,11] This study also found that non-Hispanic whites' positive perceptions of blacks and Latinos were associated with the presence of positive media depictions, especially those showing higher levels of social status and lower levels of sexual objectification.[11] These results highlight the importance of media including quality depictions of people of color.

In her 2014 study, Wiscombe[12] updated the work of Skill and Robinson by examining 137 scripted family shows on network or cable television that aired for at least one full season between 2003 and 2013. The genres of shows included dramas, sitcoms, and comedies, but excluded animated series and soap operas. Of the 162 TV families in Wiscombe's sample, the heterosexual nuclear family structure remained the most commonly depicted TV family structure.[12] Single parent families were the next most commonly depicted family

structure, followed by childless families, step-families, guardians of nonbiological children, and empty-nest couples.[12] Although the largest percentage of TV families had two parents who were married, divorce continued to be common and was almost twice as common as widowhood among TV parents.[12] Single mothers were depicted more often than single fathers but not by all that much.[12] This study did not include a comparison to census data, so it is unclear how these fictional families compare to their real-world contemporaries. This study also did not examine racial or ethnic trends in fictional families.

Wiscombe[12] found that one of the biggest changes in television family structure was the inclusion of families with parents in a same-sex relationship. Previous TV family sitcoms, such as *My Two Dads* (1987–90) and *Full House* (1987–95) included parent figures of the same gender; however, their family structures reflected contrived sitcom plots rather than acceptance of sexual minority parents. The shows *Modern Family* and *The Fosters* feature gay and lesbian parents, respectively, and the show *Big Love* depicted a polygamist family. In the years since Wiscombe's study, television platforms have continued to evolve from network and cable to include Internet streaming services, and the diversity of sexual minority family structures portrayed has continued to expand.

Adults and teenagers are the target audience of prime time television shows in the studies discussed above; however, there are differences in the depictions of family in shows targeted at children. Callister et al.[13] studied a sample of 60 families on 46 different children's television shows that aired during the 2005–06 season and compared the fictional family demographics to the US Census data. They found that the racial representation of television families was similar to the census data for Caucasian, African American, Hispanic, and Asian families. However, the television families in children's programming were more likely to include two married parents and far less likely to contain single parents than the census data. Children's programming was a head of prime time television programming in racial diversity. However, children's programming remained skewed toward the two-parent nuclear family even during a time when family structures on prime time television were becoming increasingly diverse.

THE EVOLUTION OF FAMILY THERAPY THEORY

In the early stages of family therapy theory, from the 1950s to the 1980s, there was an implicit assumption that traditional heterosexual two-parent families with stereotyped gender roles was the ideal family structure and that family problems were associated with deviations from this structure. This was a false assumption, and the field of family therapy has had to evolve to create models for effectively working with families with all types of structures. Changes to the field first began with a set of critiques by feminists who challenged the expectation of stereotyped gender roles within the family. From the 1980s until the present, leaders of family therapy expanded upon theory to create approaches for working with many types of family structures, including stepfamilies, single parents, and same-sex parents. In structural family therapy, little attention was paid to the larger societal context or the racial and ethnic background of the family as the focus of treatment was for the therapist to create different interactional patterns between family members. However, family therapists eventually began understanding the impact of domestic violence and trauma in family life and began incorporating an understanding of social context into their clinical work. In the shift from structural family therapy to narrative and social constructivism, family therapy theory expanded to recognize the importance of culture and the effect of institutional racism on families of color.[14,15]

In the next sections, we will provide some examples of how divorce, single parenthood, stepfamilies, same-sex parents, and racial minorities are depicted in the media, especially on television, and we will discuss how this information informs our clinical work with children and families.

MEDIA DEPICTIONS OF FAMILIES

Divorce and Stepfamilies

Divorce is an unplanned transition in family life that always involves conflict and loss.[5] Parental separation leads to many changes to children's lives, including how often they see each parent, where they live, and sometimes even where they attend school. With parental divorce, there can also be a change in the families' socioeconomic status (often an increase in financial stress). Memorable movies that center on divorce, such as *Kramer versus Kramer* and *The War of the Roses*, frequently depict toxic high-conflict divorce. The creation of television families tends to skip the divorce process and start the series with the family in their postdivorce state, either as a single parent or stepfamily arrangement. Perhaps stories featuring the trials and tribulations of divorcing parents who learn to disagree respectfully and put their differences aside for the good of their children do not contain the drama and

conflict needed for a hit movie or TV show; however, the reduction of parental conflict is essential for children's emotional well-being.[5,16] Parents who have become stuck and polarized in power struggles have the hardest time resolving their conflicts and creating a peaceful co-parent relationship. The goal of family therapist working with divorcing families is to reduce the parental conflict and help children to have a positive relationship with both parents.[5]

Television depictions of stepfamilies in family sitcoms and dramas have been increasing but remain rare.[8,12] When stepfamilies are featured in television and film, the narratives often do not capture the realities of stepfamily life. In Disney animated films with stepfamilies, the stepfamilies are oversimplified, and only one family subsystem is shown.[7] This absence can reinforce children's fear that divorce will lead to a permanent loss of a parent.[7] Sitcoms tend to depict stepfamilies as new nuclear families, and the problems of family life portrayed in these fictional stepfamilies are similar to those of nuclear families.[2] These shows oversimplify the difficulties of merging multiple family subsystems to create new stepfamily traditions and routines. In the 1990s, the shows on ABCs Friday night prime time line up highlighted nontraditional family structures,[17] including the Foster-Lambert stepfamily on *Step by Step* (1991–98). This series begins after Frank and Carol meet while on vacation and immediately fall in love and marry. Upon their return home, they announce their marriage to their children and immediately all move in together. Although tensions created in merging two different families is a frequent theme, these conflicts are all resolved in under 30 min and issues related to Frank and Carol's former marriages are largely ignored. Instead, the dilemmas focus around how the Lamberts and the Fosters can become a new family, and the resolutions highlight the importance of love and connection within the stepfamily.[17]

Leon[6] looked at 26 films between 1990 and 2003 that prominently featured stepfamilies and found that film clips could illustrate common stepfamily dynamics, which include "issues related to the former marriage," conflict between the adults, and the loyalty binds that occur when children feel that allying with a stepparent is betraying the absent biological parent. Leon[6] also found that films can provide examples of the stepparent as supportive of the stepchild, which counteract the stereotypes of evil stepmothers, abusive stepfathers, and neglected, resentful stepchildren. Leon[6] found these film clips could be used in facilitating discussions in parent and stepparent groups. Psychoeducation around the process of becoming a stepfamily should emphasize the importance of teamwork between all the adults, as the additional support for children is commonly cited as a stepfamily strength.[6] Both biological and stepparents should recognize that the disruption of previous family routines is hard for children, even when the transition to stepfamily life is going well.[5,16] Parent guidance should also focus on helping stepparents build friendships with the stepchildren while the biological parent takes on the role of a disciplinarian.[18] In addition to highlighting these concepts for parent and stepparent education, film clips can be used to generate similar discussions with child psychiatry trainees who will inevitably be working with stepfamilies.

Single Parent Families

In television programming geared toward children, there is less representation of single parenting,[13] and parental absence is often a peripheral detail. For example, when Disney animated films feature single parents, mothers are frequently missing without much explanation.[7] This can be difficult for single parents who are looking for models of developmentally appropriate explanations of parental absence. However, children's television and film can still be used to facilitate these conversations because parents or therapists can engage children in "re-authoring" exercises where the adult asks the child for their perspective on the missing parent.[7] For example, after watching *The Little Mermaid* with a child, one could ask questions such as "Where do you think Ariel's mother is? What would be different if Ariel was raised by her mother instead of her father? Where do you think her father would be in this version of the story?" This can give insight into the child's thoughts about parental absence, as children are often more comfortable talking about big feelings in displacement. Reauthoring exercises can lead to adult-guided discussions about how parental absence is never the child's fault and does not mean that the parent does not love the child. A parent can love a child but be unable to care for them or be present in their life daily.

Sitcoms and dramas targeted at adults and teenagers may focus more on a parent's personal life and romantic interests. *Gilmore Girls* originally aired on the CW network from 2000 to 2007 and, due to the show's continued popularity, returned in 2016 for a four-episode mini-series on Netflix. This show focuses on the intergenerational relationships within the Gilmore family, especially the single mother, Lorelei, and her daughter, Rory. Lorelei experiences her own mother's attempts at affection as coercive and controlling, and there are many splits in their enmeshed relationship.

Although Lorelei's relationship with Rory is warmer, it also has permeable boundaries and is an idealized example of an enmeshed mother-daughter relationship. This show provides an unrealistic depiction of single parenting, including that teenagers are mini-grownups who are able to put a parent's desire for romantic love and happiness ahead of their own concerns and fears regarding major life transitions. The idea that single parents find their best friend in their child is valid only as a wish, and viewers may miss ways that parentification and enmeshment can be damaging to parent-child relationships.

Effective parenting requires significant emotional regulation, as parents must be calm in order to either hold to consistent limits or negotiate acceptable compromises. The more stressed and overwhelmed the parent, the more difficult it is to remain regulated in the face of everyday parenting challenges.[5,16] Limited parental support and the stress of providing for children on a single income can create toxic levels of stress for single parents. Single-parent-only child dyads can fall into patterns of enmeshment where there is a blurring of the boundaries between parent and child, and this enmeshment can exacerbate conflict during adolescence when it is developmentally normative for teenagers to be forming their own identities and separating from their parents. *Gilmore Girls* illustrates several "wishes" associated with single mothering and can be used to foster discussion on healthy boundaries that promote strong and secure attachments within mother-daughter relationships. Despite the challenges inherent in single parenting, single parents can balance nurturing and effective limit-setting to promote clear boundaries and secure relationships with their children.

Sexual Minority Parents

Gay and lesbian parents are becoming increasingly visible,[19] and parents in same-sex romantic relationships have begun to be depicted in the media, including television sitcoms and dramas.[12] Two popular examples of television shows featuring parents in same-sex relationships include *Modern Family* (2009–present) and *The Fosters* (2013–present). *Modern Family* focuses on several family subsystems within a large extended family, including a gay couple raising their internationally adopted daughter. *The Fosters* is an hour-long cable drama featuring an interracial lesbian couple raising five children: one is a biological child from a previous relationship, two are adopted twins, and two are foster children. These programs show same-sex parents successfully raising children and creating family cultures that emphasize love and connection. Research on gay and lesbian parenting has shown that children raised by same-sex partners are as psychologically well adjusted as their peers raised in heterosexual households, and it is the quality of the children's attachment relationships with their parents, not their parents' genders, that are the most important for healthy emotional development.[19]

The diversity of sexual minority family structures portrayed in the media has continued to evolve as television platforms have expanded to include Internet streaming services. Jill Solloway, the creator of *Transparent* (2014–present), identifies as gender nonbinary (and prefers they/their pronouns), and the show is loosely based on the life experiences of their father's transition. *Transparent* follows the Pfefferman family, including Maura (formerly Mort), a retired professor who identifies as transgender and begins transitioning in late life. The show also follows Maura's three grown children and highlights their difficulties in romantic relationships. This nontraditional family structure also has the least traditional values as the adult children are self-centered and struggle to maintain meaningful relationships. Perhaps Maura's suppression of identity until later in life can be viewed as an intergenerational trauma that was passed down to her children, who remain stuck and preoccupied with creating their own identities and fulfilling their own unmet emotional needs. Despite the imperfections of the characters, the show highlights that parents can embrace their true identity and still maintain relationships with their children.

When working with same-sex or transgender parents, it is important to assess the levels of psychosocial support available and the ways discrimination impact their family life.[5,19] Work with sexual minority parents might include helping them create developmentally appropriate explanations about a child's conception, as it is typical for children to wonder about their biological origins.[19] In addition to highlighting the unique challenges facing same-sex and transgender parents, a clinician should also highlight when universal parenting dilemmas are present and provide reassurance that such challenges are a normal part of family life.[5,16] For example, parents who are unprepared for the normal increase in parent-child tensions during adolescence may interpret this stage as deeply painful and respond in ways that exacerbate the conflict. The primary task for the clinician working with same-sex or transgender parents is to help promote warm, supportive parent-child relationships with clearly differentiated boundaries, as these characteristics are associated with a child's psychological well-being.

Families of Color

Racial and ethnic minority families come in all family structures, and additional stresses arise when there is conflict between the family system and external systems due to cultural differences or institutional racism.[16] Television series highlighting positive stories of families of color can provide counter examples to the negative stereotypes that perpetuate myths of racial inferiority.[20,21] *The Cosby Show* (1984–92) focused on the Huxtables, an upper-income black nuclear family living in Brooklyn, NY. This network sitcom focused on stories of love and connection within the nuclear family, and the Huxtables were presented as a close knit family. The show focused on stories of assimilation, in which the similarities between the Huxtables and other families were emphasized.[21] *The Cosby Show* has been criticized for ignoring topics that might make white audiences uncomfortable, including racism and discrimination.[21] Care must be taken not to use these stories of success to ignore or dismiss the impact of systematic injustices, institutional racism, and the legacy of slavery.[20] The legacy of *The Cosby Show* has been further complicated by the numerous allegations of sexual assault against creator and star Bill Cosby, and the show has been dropped from syndication by many networks.[22] The modern network sitcom *Blackish* (2014–present) depicts an upper-income black nuclear family and includes stories focusing directly on race, class, and the current political context.[21] *Blackish* focuses on themes of love and connection in family life and directly discusses systemic racism, including police brutality and the effect of slavery on the creation of the racial wealth gap.

The new revenue model of subscription streaming services has led to a creative renaissance in television that has increased diversity both behind and in front of the camera.[23] In addition to traditional sitcoms, depictions of black family life can be found in programs such as Donald Glover's groundbreaking *Atlanta*, which follows two cousins and their efforts to navigate the Atlanta hip hop scene, as well as Ava DuVernay's *Queen Sugar*, which explores intergenerational family dynamics as estranged siblings reunite to save their family's sugarcane farm.[23] The Netflix series *Master of None* (2015–present), created by Aziz Ansari and Alan Yang, features stories written by racial and/or sexual minorities and acted by a racially diverse cast complete with a token white friend. The episode "Thanksgiving" focused on Denise, an African-American lesbian, played by Lena Waithe, who also co-wrote the episode based loosely on her own experiences coming out. Set over a series of Thanksgivings,

Denise's family's understanding and acceptance of her sexuality occurs slowly and in stages. Denise's mother's reluctance to accept Denise's sexuality is rooted in a parental desire to protect Denise from additional experiences of discrimination. However, the episode ends on a hopeful note with Denise's mother and girlfriend bonding over mocking Denise's clothing choices. There is an increasing intersectionality in the stories depicted on television, but many marginalized groups still remain invisible and without a voice.

It is important for child psychiatrists and family therapists to understand the ways in which racism and privilege affect family life.[24] In clinical work with families, therapists have an important opportunity to facilitate discussions of the families' experience of race and culture. Therapists of all racial and ethnic backgrounds should seek to be aware of their own biases and take a nonjudgmental stance that allows the patient to explore their own identity.[16] Media gives therapists and patients opportunities to talk about race and culture in displacement. Facilitating discussions around characters to whom patients might relate and inquiring about the parts of their lived experiences that feel absent from media are techniques that therapists can use to allow patients to take the lead in discussing the way their life experience is shaped by race and ethnicity.

It is also important to validate a patient's experience of racist microaggressions as painful and due to a problem in society rather than a problem within the individual or family unit.[25] Microaggressions on the part of the therapist are painful empathic failures, and the therapeutic work lies in the repair of the relationship.[25] If a patient feels marginalized in the course of treatment, the therapist should avoid defensiveness and seek to repair the relationship by understanding the patient's point of view and incorporating this feedback into the therapeutic work.

CONCLUSIONS

The structure of the American family has been changing over the decades, and family depictions in television and film today are more inclusive of different family structures and are more racially and ethnically diverse compared to the past. The increase in the number of cable channels and subscription streaming services has led to an increase in viewer choices, including more opportunities to find stories of family life to compare or contrast to our own lived experiences. However, it is important to remain a critical viewer of media because television and film are embedded in a societal context and most are created for profit.[2]

Healthy families come in a variety of structures, and it is important for clinicians working with families to use a nonjudgmental stance and focus on supporting healthy relationships within the family. Divorce results in a period of conflict and painful transition, especially for children, and it is important for parents to put aside conflict in order to effectively co-parent. Becoming a stepfamily is a time-consuming process consisting of merging family subsystems to create a new family culture, and the painful difficulties associated with this process are often overlooked by television sitcoms. Single parents face all the same challenges as two-parent households but with less support. Providing developmentally appropriate explanations for young children about the other parent's absence can be a unique challenge of single parenting. It is important to help all parents, especially single parents and same-sex parents, to be prepared for the process of differentiation that occurs during adolescence and to view this as a normal part of growing up rather than a personal rejection. Racial, ethnic, and sexual minorities are increasingly represented on television, and these minority groups may have different relationships to the power structures in the dominant culture. Well-differentiated parent-child boundaries are essential to effective parenting. These boundaries support parents in exploring their children's unique perspective and encouraging them to find their own place in the world. This supportive stance is essential for all children, but it is especially important for children with any kind of disability or difference.

Although there has been increasing diversity on television and an increasing intersectionality in the stories depicted, many marginalized groups remain invisible and without a voice. It is important for clinicians to talk with patients about their experiences of identity, including their racial and ethnic background, sexual orientation, and gender identity. Although clinicians should feel comfortable talking about these topics directly, they may also find it helpful to explore with patients the way their family life compares with the depictions of family life on television and film.

REFERENCES

1. Levy E. The American dream of family in film: from decline to a comeback. *J Comp Fam Stud.* 1991:187–204.
2. Cantor MG. The American family on television: from Molly Goldberg to Bill Cosby. *J Comp Fam Stud.* 1991; 22(2):205–216.
3. Leavitt PA, Covarrubias R, Perez YA, Fryberg SA. "Frozen in time": the impact of Native American media representations on identity and self-understanding. *J Soc Issue.* 2015;71(1):39–53.

4. Tukachinsky R. Where we have been and where we can go from here: looking to the future in research on media, race, and ethnicity. *J Soc Issue*. 2015;71(1):186−199.

5. Sargent J. Variations in family composition. Implications for family therapy. *Child Adolesc Psychiatr Clin N Am*. 2001;10(3):577−599.

6. Leon K, Angst E. Portrayals of stepfamilies in film: using media images in remarriage education. *Fam Relat*. 2005; 54(1):3−23.

7. Tanner L, Haddock S, Zimmerman T, Lund L. Images of couples and families in disney feature-length animated films. *Am J Fam Ther*. 2003;31(5):355−373.

8. Skill T, Robinson JD. Trend: four decades of families on television: a demographic profile, 1950−1989. *J Broadcast Electron Media*. 1994;38(4):449−464. https://doi.org/10.1080/08838159409364278.

9. Moore ML. The family as portrayed on prime-time television, 1947−1990: structure and characteristics. *Sex Roles*. 1992;26:41−61. https://doi.org/10.1007/BF00290124.

10. Skill T, Robinson J, Wallace S. Portrayal of families on prime-time TV: structure, type, and frequency. *Journal Q*. 1987:360−398.

11. Tukachinsky R, Mastro D, Yarchi M. Documenting portrayals of race/ethnicity on primetime television over a 20-year span and their association with national-level racial/ethnic attitudes. *J Soc Issue*. 2015;71(1):17−38.

12. Wiscombe SA. *Family Ties: A Profile of Television Family Configurations, 2004−2013*. 2014.

13. Callister MA, Robinson T, Clark BR. Media portrayals of the family in children's television programming during the 2005−2006 season in the US. *J Child Media*. 2007;1(2): 142−161. https://doi.org/10.1080/17482790701339142.

14. Josephson A. From family therapy to family interventions. *Child Adolesc Psychiatr Clin N Am*. 2015;24:457−470.

15. Kramer D. History of family psychiatry: from the social reform era to the primate social organ system. *Child Adolesc Psychiatr Clin N Am*. 2015;24:439−456.

16. Sargent J, Sharma N. Family therapy. In: Sadock BJ, Sadock VA, Ruiz P, eds. *Kaplan & Sadock's Comprehensive Textbook of Psychiatry*. 10th ed. vol. 2. Philadelphia: Wolters Kluwer; 2017.

17. Smith KH. *TGIF: Thank Goodness It's Family: Family Messages in ABC's 1990s Friday Night Lineup*. 2015.

18. Papernow P. *Surviving and Thriving in Stepfamily Relationships: What Works and What Doesn't*. New York: Routledge; 2013.

19. Telingator CJ, Patterson C. Children and adolescents of lesbian and gay parents. *J Am Acad Child Adolesc Psychiatry*. 2008;47(12):1364−1368. https://doi.org/10.1097/CHI.0b013e31818960bc.

20. Scharrer E, Ramasubramanian S. Intervening in the media's influence on stereotypes of race and ethnicity: the role of media literacy education. *J Soc Issue*. 2015;71(1):171−185.

21. Stamps D. The social construction of the African American family on broadcast television: a comparative analysis of The Cosby Show and Blackish. *Howard J Commun*. 2017: 1−16.

22. Poniewozik J. So what do we do about *The Cosby Show*? *Time*; November 21, 2014. Entertainment. Available from: http://time.com/3599978/cosby-show-reruns-rape/.

23. Qureshi B. Elsewhere: the cultural consolation of Ava DuVernay's Queen Sugar. *Film Q*. 2017;70(3):63−68.

24. McDowell T, Fang SR, Gomez-Young C, Khanna A, Sherman B, Brownlee K. Making space for racial dialogue: our experience in a marriage and family therapy training program. *J Marital Fam Ther*. 2003;29(2):179−194.

25. Derald WS, Capodilup CM, Torino GC, et al. Racial microaggressions in everyday life implications for clinical practice. *Am Psychol*. 2007;62(4):271−286.

CHAPTER 16

Digital Media Use by Young Children: Learning, Effects, and Health Outcomes

ELLEN A. WARTELLA, PHD • SILVIA B. LOVATO, MA • SARAH PILA, MA • ALEXIS R. LAURICELLA, PHD, MPP • RUBEN ECHEVARRIA, MA • JABARI EVANS, MSW • BRIANNA HIGHTOWER, MA

Recent years have seen a steep growth in young children's access to media. In the United States, nearly all (98%) children aged 0–8 years live in a home with a tablet or smartphone.[1] Not only is there a wide proliferation of digital media devices such as tablet computers and smartphones, but touchscreen technology has led to significant improvements in the ease of use. Touchscreens are easier for children to manipulate and cheaper than traditional computers and television sets. In parallel with the proliferation of touchscreens in homes, the last decade has seen a steep increase in technology adoption by school systems. In 2013, Apple reported 4.5 million iPads in American schools, three times as many as there were only 1 year earlier.[1] Further, 58% of preschool and kindergarten teachers surveyed were using iPads or other tablets at least weekly.[2]

As with any new media technology, research has not kept pace with the growth of digital media devices, and an abundance of unanswered questions exist about the impact of digital device use on children and youth. This chapter covers the research findings from the past decade on how young children, aged 8 years and younger, are impacted by digital media use. Given the variety of media technology available and used by children today, some of the studies focus on television while others investigate characteristics that are unique to newer digital media, such as learning from interactive systems.

We have organized the findings into three main research areas: the first examines studies that focus on the impact of media on children's learning and cognitive development. Next, we review studies that cover social and emotional development, and finally, given that we expect this volume to be especially interesting to clinicians, we describe the findings from studies focused on health outcomes, including topics such as sleep, attention, exercise, and obesity.

LEARNING FROM MEDIA
Theoretical Background
Children employ several different cognitive faculties when they use and consume media. These capacities include the processes of attention, comprehension, memory, and perspective-taking, known in the cognitive literature as Theory of Mind.[3,4] The first of these processes, attention, is central to understanding cognition while using media because it can be seen as a prerequisite for the other, higher-order processes to take place.

There are two guiding hypotheses about how young children attend to screen media: the formal features[5] and comprehensibility hypotheses.[6] Singer[7] believed that it is the formal features of the screen media program that influence young children's attention to the screen. Formal features are the use of production techniques designed to drive attention toward the screen.[8] The flashing lights, movement, cuts, pans, and zooms have the ability to attract young children to the screen, orienting them to the program in such a way that maintains attention. Support for this claim is found in earlier studies like Hollenbeck and Slaby's[9] research with 6-month-olds and television stimuli, as well as Calvert et al.'s[10] study of attention attributed to the pacing of a show. According to this hypothesis, even newborns pay attention to screens because the visual stimuli are perceptually appealing.

On the other hand, Anderson and Lorch[6] claim that young children attend more to screen media when they are able to comprehend what they see. This hypothesis assumes that attention is driven by whether the content on the screen makes sense. Young children seem to sustain more attention toward a screen when what they are watching is comprehensible than when it is not; they do not simply attend to the salient visual and auditory cues. Recent support for this view comes from work with infants that shows 2-year-olds (and some 18-month-olds) pay more attention when screen stimuli are comprehensible than when they are incomprehensible (backward, violate expectations, etc.), but the 6- and 12-month-olds did not appear to notice such differences.[11] This hypothesis argues that very young children pay little attention to screens. Indeed, scholars who use comprehensibility framing make the case that perceptually salient features are meaningless in infants' attention toward screens unless they help with the comprehension of the program. In the same way, comprehensibility of the screen content drives infant attention toward it since it appears to make logical sense rather than merely a mess of lights, sounds, and flashes.

At first glance these ideas are seemingly dichotomous, but research has demonstrated that both hypotheses are important for understanding children's learning from a screen. However, research from Kirkorian et al.[12] posits that children's understanding and comprehension of the salient perceptual features of television (in this case, a cut in the scene) increases with age. In their study, the youngest children were unaware of such transition, but older children quickly understood.[12] Salient perceptual features may draw attention to the screen at some developmental time points while comprehensible, logical plotlines may foster attention at others. It makes sense that both are at play and fluctuate in their importance throughout development. These hypotheses help us consider how very young children attend to, and possibly learn from and engage with, media because comprehension and learning are not possible without first attending to the screen.

Learning From Educational Television
Evaluation studies done on educational content like *Sesame Street* have been able to demonstrate positive developmental outcomes for television viewing in the youngest set.[13–16] The summative research on the earliest years of *Sesame Street* found that children who watched the show were more likely to have learned the readiness skills that the program taught in its first years.[14,15] For children 3–6 years of age, *Sesame Street* appears to have significant effects on school-readiness and can be most helpful to those

from disadvantaged backgrounds.[14–18] A longitudinal project found that watching *Sesame Street* and other educational television programs by 2- and 3-year-olds predicted better scores on measures of math and language ability as well as school readiness at the age of 5 years.[19] Of course, these academic outcomes were most apparent when children were watching high-quality media with appropriate parental co-viewing support.[17,20,21] Researchers who followed up on these children years later also found that watching *Sesame Street* and other educational programming as a preschooler was positively related to academic achievement in terms of transcript grades in adolescence.[13] These findings provide support for the developmental benefits of early educational media use.

Video Deficit
One of the earliest beliefs on learning from screens is that children would simply imitate what they saw, and this imitation was a part of cognition in general.[22] In fact, even infants only hours old can imitate adult facial expressions like tongue protrusions,[23] and the earliest studies on imitation from television suggest children as young as 14 month can imitate what they see on a television screen, even days later.[24] For these reasons and more, it's not unreasonable to consider imitation from the screen as a cognitive process for young children.

Across the field, however, there is strong evidence that supports the idea that infants and young toddlers learn and imitate better from live actors and demonstrations than from screens. This phenomenon has been termed the "video deficit"[25] or the "transfer deficit."[26] Several experimental studies show that young children imitate and model demonstrations made by live researchers in the lab better than those they see on television. This difference continues until about 3 years of age, when the screen media becomes a more robust learning opportunity for young children.[12,27–31] In a landmark study by Troseth and DeLoache,[32] the researchers found that 2-year-olds who watched an experimenter hide a toy over closed circuit television performed worse at the object-retrieval task than another group who saw the experimenter hide the same toy through a window in real-time (a nonmediated demonstration). However, the researchers also found that 30-month-olds in the same experimental paradigm were successful in the object retrieval task in both circumstances, demonstrating that there is, in fact, a developmental difference between these age groups and that the video deficit is nonexistent by 2½ years of age. This research was also supported by Barr and Hayne,[27] who found that during five experiments with 12-, 15-, and 18-month-old infants, those who watched an experimenter live performed better on an imitation task than those who watched the experimenter on television. There were also age-related differences in that 18-month-olds were more likely to correctly imitate actions from television than the other age groups, although their ability to imitate from live actors was better in almost all conditions,[27] echoing findings from the Troseth and DeLoache[32] work.

However, research has also demonstrated that other factors can reduce or eliminate the video deficit. Barr and Hayne[27] found that when the task was easier, infants' ability to reproduce the actions from television was nearly equivalent to their ability to do the same from a live model. When the task is repeated, infants and toddlers can learn to imitate the behaviors.[33] Several repetitions of the video task may support young children's memory of the object retrieval or search or other imitation tasks (e.g., word learning) even after an extended period of time.[34,35] But while repeat exposure may help reduce the video deficit for very young children in other tasks, Krcmar[35] found that it only did so for older infants (17 month and older) in terms of learning words. Surely, repetition is one mechanism for reducing the video deficit, but perhaps it is more appropriate for some types of learning rather than others.

Another possible technique in reducing the video deficit is to use familiar and socially relevant stimuli. When the characters are socially meaningful to the child or the technology supports social interaction, young children can demonstrate learning from a screen.[36–39] Not only are familiar partners more likely to reduce the video deficit but contingency is also related to such reduction. Contingency here means that what appears on the screen next depends, or is *contingent*, on the child's actions. Repeating words or phrases back to the child demonstrates this. Troseth et al.[40] found that 2-year-olds exposed to an experimenter via closed circuit television explaining where an object was hidden (contingent condition) were more successful at finding the object than another group who watched these directions on a pretaped video (noncontingent condition). Surprisingly, participants in the closed circuit television condition were also as successful as a similar group of 2-year-olds who were told these instructions in person. These findings continue to hold with new technologies like video chatting. For example, Myers et al.[41] found that 12- to 25-month-olds learned more novel words and actions from a socially contingent partner over

video chat than another group who watched a prerecorded video of the same experimenter, but there was also an interaction of age by condition. Similarly, Roseberry and colleagues (2014) found that 24- to 30-month-olds in their study learned novel words from both socially contingent interactions (the video chat and live conditions), but not from a prerecorded video of the same information. In all, socially meaningful and contingent interactions available on new technologies seem to have the power to reduce the video deficit.

Finally, minimizing the disparity between tasks aids transfer. For example, children are better at imitating a task seen on a two-dimensional screen if they are tested on a similar two-dimensional screen.[26,42,43] In one study, Zack et al.[43] found that even though 15-month-olds can imitate target actions from either a two-dimensional or three-dimensional stimulus, those who saw the action in the same dimension as the task they were asked to do (within-dimension condition) performed significantly better than those who had to reproduce the task in another dimension (cross-dimension condition). The researchers suggested that nearer transfer (within-dimensions) can help improve imitation performance and eliminate the video deficit.

Taken together, using the same dimensional transfer, familiarity, repetition, and contingency might help reduce the video deficit effect before the age of 3 years.[44] As much as we can help very young children learn from screen media in order to minimize the video deficit, once children reach about 3 years of age, they have seemingly developed the natural skills to transfer tasks they have seen done on a screen to their three-dimensional world due to either increased experience with screen media or more elaborate cognitive skills (see Barr[45] for a review of the literature). After 3 years of age, the video deficit is largely overcome, and children seem to learn as well from television and interactive media as they do from live actors. This developmental change seems to support the dual representation hypothesis in that children eventually come to understand that video images can "stand in for," or be a symbol, for something else, which also allows children to learn from video content (see Strouse and Troseth[31] for a similar conclusion).

Word learning and television

Another area for potential cognitive and developmental outcomes is the research on word learning from television. Infant-directed programs (e.g., *Baby Einstein*) were designed with the idea that screens have the potential to teach even the youngest children. These programs are thought to negatively impact young children's language development by some scholars,[46,47] but other research suggests that while exposure to infant-directed television does not negatively affect word learning, it does not positively impact it either.[48,49] In fact, the most significant predictor of vocabulary after controlling for other demographic factors was how often children were read to.[49] Although these mixed findings are not encouraging for those who think children should be able to learn words from television, researchers have attributed the negative directionality to the fact that parents are less likely to talk to infants while the television is on.[49a] Indeed, research suggests that merely having the television on may negatively impact word learning because it limits the amount of language interaction between children and parents.[50,51] All this to say, media could be one mechanism for word learning as mentioned earlier, but if the socially relevant and contingent partner is elsewhere, it could negatively impact language learning.

Learning From Interactive Media

Though it is well-known that children can learn from educational television, the jury is still out on whether and how children might be able to learn from new interactive tablet applications designed to promote learning. So far, the research on this topic has focused primarily on literacy outcomes, usually comparing e-books to traditional print books.[52,53] Findings from these studies have been mixed. Krcmar and Cingel[52] found that children had better comprehension of a traditional storybook than the electronic copy of the same story. However, Lauricella et al.[53] saw no difference in children's comprehension from the two different types of books. New research on word learning from interactive e-books by Beschorner and Hutchison[54] points to the possible affordances of interactive screens, while other researchers find that the interactivity might be too distracting for the youngest users, limiting their comprehension of the content.[55,56] Based on a recent review of this literature, it is recommended that parents and other adults thoughtfully select e-books with limited distracting features, engage in reading these electronic books with children, and while they might use them with older children, to do so sparingly with infants younger than 2 years of age.[57]

Beyond research on e-books, we are seeing initial results regarding children's ability to learn from interactive tablets in other domains and contexts. Studies on imitation tasks from touchscreens are just starting to shed light on how young children might be able to use the interactivity of the touchscreen to learn. Huber et al.[58] found that 4- to 6-year-olds are able to transfer learning from a touchscreen fairly seamlessly to the physical version of a challenging cognitive task (Tower of Hanoi).[58] They found that regardless of the original modality children practiced the task on (2D or 3D), all children improved in the final problem-solving task. Similarly, preschoolers who played a tablet game that focused on teaching approximate measuring experienced smooth transfer of learning to near-transfer tasks, but those who viewed a prerecorded, noninteractive version of the game did better on far-transfer tasks.[58a] The researchers posit that although children can transfer approximate measuring skills from either watching or playing a game meant to teach that topic, the interactive nature of playing the game might only help in conditions closest to game play and distract from the overall conceptual learning.

Some studies have begun to examine toddlers' transfer of learning from touchscreen interactions.[30,59] The researchers found that the youngest children learned best with media that required the specific interaction—meaning the child had to touch the labeled object directly on the screen, while slightly older children learned best from the noninteractive video—in which they simply observed an actress labeling the object. In a similar experiment, toddlers were asked to watch an animated character hide using the same three conditions (no, general, or specific interaction).[59] Again, the youngest viewers were more likely to successfully find the character when exposed to the specific interaction condition, while the effect was reversed for older toddlers, who learned best in the noninteractive condition.

Science, Technology, Engineering and Mathematics Learning From Media

One element related to the potential of Science, Technology, Engineering and Mathematics (STEM) learning from media is the possibility of using screen media to influence children's spatial skills. It is well known that earlier spatial ability is related to later success in STEM occupations.[60] Edited television, for all intents and purposes, relies on at least some spatial capacity in that children have to understand that the same action can be shown from many different angles, and they may have to rotate these images in their minds to consider the different perspectives that they see. Interactive media are also believed to be inherently rich for spatial skills because many of the games on tablets, gaming consoles, and computers are created with the intention of developing these skills. Research with adolescents and adults, using both correlational and experimental designs, demonstrates that video game playing (even fairly brief exposure) is related to improvements in tests measuring spatial ability (see Grancic et al.[61] for a review). However, across both lines of research, it appears that television and interactive media designed to promote spatial skills are successful in doing so, but that television-like media in and of itself is not supportive enough.

COGNITIVE AND SOCIAL EMOTIONAL MEDIA EFFECTS

The social cognitive theory (SCT) explains how people acquire and maintain behavioral patterns through observation of others' behavior.[62] According to SCT, modeling is not simply a process of response mimicry; rather, observers extract the rules underlying the modeled style of thinking and behaving, and those rules enable them to generate new behaviors in that same style.[63] Research with youth and media have consistently demonstrated that the repeated observation of behavior from a screen can influence children's behaviors postviewing, both positively and negatively. We use SCT as a theoretical backdrop to consider the ways in which media affect the cognitive and social emotional development of young children.

Violence, Aggression, and Fear

Much of the empirical research about media effects on social cognition has centered on the effect of televised violence.[64,65] Exposure to televised violence has at least three distinct effects.[65a] It teaches aggressive styles of conduct, reduces restraints over aggressive conduct, and portrays violence as a preferred solution to conflict in a way that is often successful and relatively clean. Frequently in children's media, superheroes are doing most of the killing. When good triumphs over evil by violent means, such portrayals can legitimize and glamorize violence. In addition, heavy exposure to televised violence desensitizes and habituates people to human cruelty (Wilson, 2011). Historically, empirical findings from many scholars claimed that children who are exposed to media violence have increased probability of aggression[66–69] and that exposure to violent content during childhood years has lasting impacts on aggressive behavior into adulthood.[70,71,71a] However, more recent work has refuted the design of those prior studies on the effects of violent media.[70] These recent studies found consistent results that increased violent and aggressive behavior is overestimated and

largely dependent on the preexisting conditions of the child, the specific nature of the content, and the context with which the violent content is viewed.[71–74] Across this aggregate of research, both experimental and self-selected exposure to media violence have been shown to be only moderately associated with negative outcomes when controlling for individual factors: more aggressive behaviors, thoughts, and feelings, as well as reduced helping behavior.[71] Empirical research has also noted that although short-term effects (measured experimentally) were somewhat stronger for adults than for children, long-term relationships between self-selected exposure and subsequent aggression (in some studies, measured years later) were stronger for exposure during childhood than during adulthood.[75]

Most work has focused on the effect of media on physical aggression. However, social aggression is another important variable that has been influenced by antisocial programming. Social aggression is a type of aggression that damages a target's self-esteem or social standing.[76] Social aggression includes both indirect (e.g., spreading a rumor) and direct (e.g., ignoring another) acts of aggression. Social aggression may be delivered via verbal and nonverbal means, which distinguishes it from other conceptually related overlapping constructs such as indirect or relational aggression (for further review, see Archer and Coyne[77]). Research indicates that social aggression is more prevalent among girls. Research results revealed a significant relationship between exposure to televised social aggression and increased social aggression at school, but only for girls.[78]

Historically, the primary focus of concern about children's media use has been whether it makes them more hostile and aggressive, and increases their chances of becoming violent adults. Another important concern is the effect media have on children's feelings of safety, comfort, and fear. The results of numerous studies suggest that children aged 3–7 years tend to be scared or disturbed by visually grotesque images or scary sounds, such as those often found in fantasy content, even if the actual threat implied by the narrative is relatively minimal.[79] Additionally, material that does not contain visual or auditory distortions, such as scenes focusing on a character's anxiety or scenes in which abstract threats are conveyed via words, tend to disturb younger children relatively less.[75] Age differences in fear responses to news stories are consistent with this pattern; in several studies, kindergarten children were much more likely to be frightened by stories of natural disasters (typically shown with scenes of destruction) than by stories of stranger violence (which typically do not have disturbing visual images) (Wilson, 2011) [also see Chapter 5 in this volume]. At the age of 8 years, most children are no longer as focused on the perceptually striking characteristics of a situation, can understand more abstract threats, and respond empathically to the emotional displays of the characters.[79]

Prosocial Effects

While there is evidence of some negative, indirect effects of media, research has also indicated several positive effects of media on prosocial behavior and subsequent mental health. A smaller body of research has focused on whether, and under what conditions, there may be prosocial outcomes of media use. Studies have documented that exposure to prosocial content, such as *Mister Rogers' Neighborhood*, is associated with increased prosocial behaviors in preschool-age children.[80] More recent studies and meta-analyses have found that prosocial programming can positively enhance children's prosocial behavior, with the strongest effect on altruism, or helping others.[81–85,85a] Scholars also suggest that prosocial content has stronger effects on older children and those from middle- and upper-class families, but no gender differences emerged.[86–88] Surprisingly, Mares and Woodard's[83] meta-analysis on prosocial programming also asserted that the effect of prosocial content on altruism is higher than the effect of any other programming on any other behavior, including the effect of violent television on aggressive behavior.

In recent years, *Sesame Street* has incorporated emotions and emotional coping into its curricular goals. Storylines have incorporated childbirth, death, and marriage. Many early studies demonstrated that regular viewing of *Sesame Street* can help preschoolers develop a fuller understanding of emotions and difficult situations.[88a] In 2001, *Sesame Street* sought to help preschoolers cope with 9/11 by featuring a storyline which required brave firefighters to save people from injury in a grease fire.[89] That same year, a series of episodes also focused on a hurricane that hit New York City and destroyed a character's home.[90] However, to date, there is no wide body of scholarly work that explains whether there are long-term effects of watching this type of content on children's emotional development.

MEDIA USE AND HEALTH EFFECTS

The United States and other countries around the world have recently been facing new health concerns, with diseases and disorders that were largely associated with adults now observed in young children, including obesity.[90a] With increased access to media technology, both traditional media like television and new mobile media like smartphones and tablets, there is increased interest in the role that media have on children's health. Here, we examine how media and technology may influence sleep, obesity, attention, addiction, pain management, the physical body, and autism and social development in young children.

Sleep

Even though the majority of parents endorse the importance of sleep, an online survey conducted with 1103 parents of children aged 6–17 years found that 90% of children obtained less sleep than the recommended "at least 10 h a day."[91] Significant predictors of children sleeping a sufficient amount (conservatively estimated as ≥ 9 h/night for children aged 6–11 years by Buxton et al.[91]) of time included parents' education level, regular enforcement of rules about caffeine, and whether children had technology in their bedroom overnight. Significant predictors of excellent sleep quality of children as reported by parents included whether a family always enforced a bedtime and whether children did not have technology on overnight.

In addition to Buxton's findings, several studies indicate that the presence of screens, such as televisions, tablets, and smartphones, in a child's bedroom can lead to adverse sleep outcomes. Hale and Guan[92] conducted a systematic literature review of 67 youth sleep studies published between 1999 and 2014. Ninety percent of the reviewed studies indicated screen time negatively impacted sleep for school-aged children and adolescents by adversely influencing outcomes like sleep duration and onset of sleep. Despite these findings and recommendations to not allow screens and technology in children's bedrooms overnight,[93] the National Sleep Foundation found that 42.4% of children aged 6–10 years had a television in their bedrooms.[94] However, that percentage has recently declined; in 2017, 29% of children younger than 8 years of age were found to have a television in their bedroom (Rideout, 2017).

The presence of a television in the bedroom begins influencing sleep duration as early as infancy[95] and persists through adulthood. Adults also struggle with limiting screen exposure before bedtime, and this is related to adults perceiving their sleep as unrefreshing.[96] Parents' late night screen time may influence the dissonance for parents between knowing that technology negatively affects their child's sleep and permitting them to have access to screens immediately before onset of sleep. Despite the importance of establishing a consistent sleep pattern for children being emphasized to and believed by parents, media screens continue to pervade child bedrooms.

Obesity

The American Academy of Pediatrics reasserted the relationship between media use and obesity in their 2016 policy statement about media and young children, recommending the regulation of TV and Internet access for children. Their 2011 statement noted that "research has shown that the media contribute to the development of child and adolescent obesity, though the exact mechanism remains unclear" (p. 201)[97] and posits that late-night screen time may disrupt child sleep duration, which has a known correlation with childhood obesity.

An online survey of 1030 parents of children aged 4—18 years found that total media consumption predicted "ill-being" within the realms of physical problem symptomology, psychological symptom manifestation, attention problems, and home and classroom behaviors, even when controlling for daily exercise and eating habits.[98] Their findings suggest that managing a child's physical health goes beyond encouraging healthier food choices and promoting regular physical activity, to include limiting the use of technology and media. In a review of the extant literature assessing the relationship between children's patterns of media use and childhood obesity, Hingle and Kunkel[99] found that interventions that reduce screen media use, indicated through the decrease in the amount of time children spend with media, have been associated with improvement in child weight status. Additional studies found a link between children's exposure to unhealthy food marketing and children identifying unhealthy food items as healthy and nutritious.[99] Food advertising targeting children tends to market unhealthy products: one study found that 98% of all food advertising marketed to children featured foods that were high in fat, sugar, and sodium, like sugary cereals and salty potato chips.[99a]

Exercise

Children can physically interact with media and technology devices in ways that are both positive and negative for their bodies. Recommendations to combat negative effects include decreasing prolonged periods of uninterrupted sedentary time, encouraging proper postures and utilizing furniture that facilitates specific postures, and suggesting children respond to their own feelings of physical discomfort to combat irregular musculoskeletal development.[100] New technology that requires physical gestures to play could cause hand strain and accidental injury, but minimal data exist that captures how prevalent active videogame-related injuries.[100a] Active videogames and exergames, which are video games requiring the player to exert physical energy such as dancing or mimicking the motions of sport participation during video gameplay, have the potential to promote healthy activity and can even be successfully used as low-cost, home-based physical and psychological therapy interventions.[101] Despite active video games and exergames being a popular recreational activity for children,[102] existing research on the long-term physical effects, both positive and negative, that gameplay can have on typical body development outside of therapeutic settings is mixed.[103]

Pain Management

Technology devices and media can be used as a means of pain management for young children by distracting them from physical or anticipated pain or orienting them on a procedure before they undergo it to alleviate anxiety. A team of researchers reviewed 46 journal articles describing studies covering active and passive forms of distraction for children in medical settings.[104] Overall, the reviewed studies generally support distraction as a coping mechanism for young children receiving treatment. Given that there are so many distraction options available, selecting the best form for individual children is a difficult task for practitioners. [104]

Some disagreement exists on whether these distractors actually alleviate pain for young children or they simply ease parental anxiety. One intervention, which allowed child participants to select an age-appropriate distractor like music, video games, or viewing a cartoon video, found that the presence of distracting media alleviated parental perception of their young children's (6—10 years of age) pain distress, but that children did not report a difference in their own pain levels when they had access to distracting media.[105] Another study, which assessed parent perceptions of their child's anxiety while receiving immunizations, found that parents report that their child has less anxiety, need for being held, and amount of crying when they can be distracted from receiving an immunization using an iPad.[106] When capturing children's pain levels, practitioners and researchers should strive to use a multidimensional approach, including self-report, observational measures, and/or physiological indicators,[107] to indicate if there are differences in parental and practitioner perceptions of a child's pain and how a child reports feeling.

Another factor to consider when using new media as distraction devices is their cost. Novel distraction devices, like virtual reality helmets or robots, may be cost prohibitive in some settings, and it remains unclear if the additional costs are balanced by the efficacy of treatment and perceived pain alleviation.[107a] More easily available devices, like tablets that families may already own and bring with them to treatment settings, could be useful for both patients and practitioners in effectively distracting and treating young children. A group of child healthcare practitioners created a set of recommendations for using tablet applications, suggesting applications that are generic in nature, easy to use, require minimal user preparation, have visual and auditory components, allow many choices for players, and accommodate patient capabilities during procedures, such as requiring one hand, two hands, or no hands to participate in gameplay.[107b] Ultimately, practitioners should identify the best distractor to use, including media and technology options, based on individual patient preferences, child temperament, procedural situation, and cost to implement.

Attention and Executive Function

The recent increase in the prevalence of Attention Deficit Disorder and Attention Deficit and Hyperactivity Disorder (ADHD) has sparked a number of studies focusing on the relationship between attention disorders and media use, including whether exposure to media immediately influences children's executive function (e.g., self-regulation, attention span, and working memory). Lillard and Peterson[108] randomly assigned 60 four-year-olds to watch a fast-paced television cartoon or an educational cartoon or draw for 9 min. They were then given four tasks tapping executive function, including the classic delay-of-gratification and Tower of Hanoi tasks. Parents completed surveys regarding television viewing and children's attention. The authors of the study concluded that preschool-aged children were significantly impaired in executive function immediately after watching 9 min of a popular fast-paced television show compared to children watching educational television or drawing. Other correlational research suggests that more television viewing in the earlier years is related to later attention and executive function difficulties.[109,110] However, this relationship

is the strongest for children regularly exposed to adult-directed television in the background at home.[111] It is also possible that children who have poorer executive function skills or struggle with attention may be more likely to consume media rather than the reverse. Though research has suggested an association between entertainment television and later attention problems,[112] causation is difficult to demonstrate.

Besides television, research has also investigated the relationship between digital media use, including Internet, social media, and video games, and ADHD. While studies have shown that children diagnosed with ADHD tend to use digital media more, it is difficult to tease out whether the condition leads to heavier digital media use or the excessive use of digital media leads to ADHD symptoms[113,114] (see Ceranoglu[115] for a review). Video games might also be useful in treating ADHD in children; an initial clinical trial has found that children aged 8–12 years showed significant improvement in their ADHD symptoms after playing a tablet-based video game (*Project EVO*, by Akili Interactive Labs) designed for treatment when compared to a control group.[116]

Autism and social development

Children who are on the autism spectrum or identify as neuroatypical may engage with media and technology differently than children who are more typically developing. A recent study surveyed 210 caregivers of children aged 12–36 months about 10 of their daily routines (waking up, bath time, etc.) and how often media was used during their routines.[117] The researchers found that children at risk for social-emotional delay were 5.8 times more likely to have ≥5 routines occurring with a screen as compared to children not at risk for social-emotional delay.[117]

While this study included toddlers, most of the research on media and technology use and child social development involves older children. However, what we know about older children, while not directly transferable to younger children (aged 0–8 years), can inform our understanding of how media and technology may impact social development for young children.

One study found that children with Autism Spectrum Disorder (ASD) spent 62% more time watching television and playing video games than activities not centered around a screen.[118] Children with ASD also spent more time playing video games than their typically developing siblings but very little time using social media or playing socially interactive games.[118]

In contrast, another study found that preadolescents and early adolescents with autism were likely to engage with socially interactive games if certain parameters were directly stated and maintained by moderators.[119] *Autcraft*, a moderated world within Minecraft, specifically only permits members to join if they have autism or are an ally of a person with autism. The space is explicitly free of bullying and has forums where members can socialize with each other and ask others how to socialize with others in person.[119] Because members know that the space is "safe,"[120] this group may be more willing and comfortable engaging with socially interactive games than children sampled in other studies. Another study found that for children aged 8–11 years with autism, assistive technology can facilitate social relationships between pairs through supporting membership, partnership, and friendship.[121] However, social interactions in digital spaces can present some dangers during late childhood and early adolescence, such as cyberbullying, depressed feelings caused by social media, sexting, and exposure to inappropriate content.[122]

CONCLUSION

For the past half century, we have studied and learned how children use and are impacted by media, especially television. In just the last decade, we have seen a dramatic technological revolution that has shaken up the ways in which children access and use digital media, leading to the need for past research to be replicated on new technologies and a host of new research questions to be answered. Ubiquitous access to video and gaming content is still in its infancy, and the technology that supports this access continues to advance rapidly. Now children have access to voice agents on smartphones and through in-home devices such as Amazon's Echo and Google Home, and virtual reality headsets and content are rising in popularity. Additionally, mobile screens have been integrated into play activities that include physical objects (e.g., *Osmo* Kits, *Nintendo Switch* cardboard toys), essentially toys that mediate the screen experience. As a result, while much is known about children's media use and the effects of certain types of content or via specific platforms (e.g., television), much remains to be studied when it comes to digital media use by young children.

In this chapter, we present landmark studies and new research to provide evidence regarding the impact of media use on three main research areas: learning and cognitive development, social and emotional development, and child health. The effect that media may have on these crucial developmental areas is not only important for parents and educators but also for medical providers and clinicians to understand. Children today are growing up in a distinctive media-saturated world, and the role of media in young children's lives continues to be powerful in both its positive and negative impacts.

Children aged 8 years and younger spend on average over 2 h per day with electronic screen media—time spent with media increases with age, with children younger than 2 years spending an average of 42 min per day with screens while those aged 5–8 years spend close to 3 h (Rideout, 2017). Future research on young children's learning from digital media should pay close attention to the context in which they use such media. According to Vygotsky's sociocultural approach to development[123]; children's interactions with those around them play an important role in development, and so when we think about how children use digital media, we must recognize the influence the environment has on the child. By acknowledging the relationship between the child and the environment, researchers open a window for interpreting the child's motives for how and why they use digital media.[124] However, identifying the contexts where digital media is used is not always a straightforward task. Researchers argue that the mobility of digital media increases the complexity of defining a context[125] and others suggest that education research tends to oversimplify terms like "informal learning" and "formal learning" by connecting them to home or school, respectively.[126] Limiting environments to schools and homes can result in missed opportunities to study how children are using digital media in other surroundings, such as museums, community centers, and libraries.

It is imperative that the medical community recognize that screen media play a huge role in children's development. However, mental health physicians and media scholars alike must realize that the media's influence on youth depends far more on the type of content that children are engaging with rather than simply accounting for the average amount of screen time in a child's day. That said, we suggest that it is naïve to argue that media are solely detrimental or valuable to children's emotional states. It is the intermix of various media messages that can teach prosocial lessons as well as cultivate antisocial behavior. Thus, clinicians should be informed by research on the long-term consequences of repeated exposure to electronic media and emotional development. While we acknowledge that rapid changes in media technology and content genres make longitudinal studies challenging, such studies can explore issues of long-term exposure to underlying technologies (i.e., touchscreens) and clinicians will be able to utilize them to better inform their practice.

This review acknowledges that interactive digital media are now a part of most young children's lives; parents willingly provide their young children with digital media devices. Clinicians should consider this when addressing parents about digital media. This means fostering a discussion of the amount of children's exposure to digital media, the kind of content—whether or not it has a learning objective—they are using, and the expectation of the media's influence compared to other factors in the environment. Such a discussion may advance medical practice regarding young children and digital media.

REFERENCES

1. Rideout VJ. *The Common Sense census: Media use by kids age zero to eight.* San Francisco, CA: Common Sense Media; 2017;
1a. Paczkowski J. *Apple's ITunes U Hits One Billion Downloads;* February 28, 2013. Retrieved from: http://allthingsd.com/20130228/apples-itunes-u-hits-1-billion-downloads/.
2. Blackwell CK, Wartella E, Lauricella AR, Robb M. *Technology in the Lives of Educators and Early Childhood Programs: Trends in Access, Use, and Professional Development from 2012 to 2014.* Evanston, IL: Center on Media and Human Development at Northwestern University; 2015.
3. Gopnik A, Wellman HM. Why the child's theory of mind really is a theory. *Mind Lang.* 1992;7(1–2):145–171.
4. Meltzoff AN. Origins of theory of mind, cognition and communication. *J Commun Disord.* 1999;32(4):251–269.
5. Huston AC, Wright JC. *Children's Processing of Television: The Informative Functions of Formal Features.* New York, NY: Academic Press; 1983.
6. Anderson DR, Lorch EP. *Looking at Television: Action or Reaction?* New York, NY: Academic Press; 1983.
7. Singer JL. *The Power and Limitations of Television: A Cognitive-Affective Analysis.* Hillsdale, NJ: Erlbaum; 1980.
8. Bickham DS, Wright JC, Huston AC. *Attention, Comprehension, and the Educational Influences of Television and Other Electronic Media.* Los Angeles, CA: SAGE; 2012.
9. Hollenbeck AR, Slaby RG. Infant visual and vocal responses to television. *Child Dev.* 1979;50(1):41–45.
10. Calvert SL, Huston AC, Watkins BA, Wright JC. The relation between selective attention to television forms and children's comprehension of content. *Child Dev.* 1982;53(3):601–610.

11. Pempek TA, Kirkorian HL, Richards JE, Anderson DR, Lund AF, Stevens M. Video comprehensibility and attention in very young children. *Dev Psychol.* 2010;46(5):1283–1293.
12. Kirkorian HL, Anderson DR, Keen R. Age differences in online processing of video: an eye movement study. *Child Dev.* 2012;83(2):497–507.
13. Anderson DR, Huston A, Schmitt K, Linebarger D, Wright J. Adolescent outcomes associated with early childhood television viewing: the recontact study. *Monogr Soc Res Child Dev.* 2001;66(1):1–147.
14. Ball S, Bogatz GA. *The First Year of Sesame Street: An Evaluation: A Report to the Children's Television Workshop.* 1970. Retrieved from: Princeton, NJ.
15. Bogatz GA, Ball S. *The Second Year of Sesame Street: A Continuing Evaluation: A Report to the Children's Television Workshop.* Princeton, NJ: Educational Testing Service; 1971.
16. Zill N, Davies E, Daly M. *Viewing of "Sesame Street" by Preschool Children in the United States and its Relationship to School Readiness.* Rockville, MD: Westat; 1994.
17. Fisch SM, Truglio RT, Cole CF. The impact of Sesame Street on preschool children: a review and synthesis of 30 years' research. *Media Psychol.* 1999;1(2):165–190.
18. Mares ML, Pan Z. Effects of Sesame Street: a meta-analysis of learning in 15 countries. *J Appl Dev Psychol.* 2013;34(2013):140–151.
19. Wright JC, Huston AC. *Effects of Educational TV Viewing of Lower Income Preschoolers on Academic Skills, School Readiness, and School Adjustment One to Three Years Later: A Report to Children's Television Workshop.* University of Kansas, Center for Research on the Influences of Television on Children; 1995.
20. Baydar N, Kağitçibaşi Ç, Küntay AC, Gökşen F. Effects of an educational television program on preschoolers: variability in benefits. *J Appl Dev Psychol.* 2008;29(5):349–360.
21. Linebarger DL, Vaala SE. Screen media and language development in infants and toddlers: an ecological perspective. *Dev Rev.* 2010;30(2):176–202.
22. Bandura A. Self-efficacy: toward a unifying theory of behavioral change. *Psychol Rev.* 1977;84(2):191.
23. Meltzoff AN, Moore MK. Newborn infants imitate adult facial gestures. *Child Dev.* 1983;54:702–709.
24. Meltzoff AN. Imitation of televised models by infants. *Child Dev.* 1988;59(5):1221.
25. Anderson DR, Pempek TA. Television and very young children. *Am Behav Sci.* 2005;48(5):505–522.
26. Barr R. Transfer of learning between 2D and 3D sources during infancy: informing theory and practice. *Dev Rev.* 2010;30(2):128–154.
27. Barr R, Hayne H. Developmental changes in imitation from television during infancy. *Child Dev.* 1999;70(5):1067–1081.
28. Barr R, Zack E, Garcia A, Muentener P. Infants' attention and responsiveness to television increases with prior exposure and parental interaction. *Infancy.* 2008;13(1):30–56.

29. Kirkorian HL, Lavigne HJ, Hanson KG, Troseth GL, Demers LB, Anderson DR. Video deficit in toddlers' object retrieval: what eye movements reveal about online cognition. *Infancy.* 2016;21(1):37−64.

30. Kirkorian HL, Choi K, Pempek TA. Toddlers' word learning from contingent and noncontingent video on touch screens. *Child Dev.* 2016;87(2):405−413.

31. Strouse GA, Troseth GL. "Don't try this at home": toddlers' imitation of new skills from people on video. *J Exp Child Psychol.* 2008;101(4):262−280.

32. Troseth GL, DeLoache JS. The medium can obscure the message: young children's understanding of video. *Child Dev.* 1998;69(4):950−965.

33. Barr R, Muentener P, Garcia A, Fujimoto M, Chavez V. The effect of repetition on imitation from television during infancy. *Dev Psychobiol.* 2007;49(2):196−207. https://doi.org/10.1002/dev.20208.

34. Brito N, Barr R, McIntyre P, Simcock G. Long-term transfer of learning from books and video during toddlerhood. *J Exp Child Psychol.* 2012;111(1):108−119.

35. Krcmar M. Can infants and toddlers learn words from repeat exposure to an infant directed DVD? *J Broadcast Electron Media.* 2014;58(2):196−214.

36. Howard Gola AA, Richards MN, Lauricella AR, Calvert SL. Building meaningful parasocial relationships between toddlers and media characters to teach early mathematical skills. *Media Psychol.* 2013;16(4):390−411.

37. Krcmar M. Can social meaningfulness and repeat exposure help infants and toddlers overcome the video deficit? *Media Psychol.* 2010;13(1):31−53. https://doi.org/10.1080/15213260903562917.

38. Lauricella AR, Gola AAH, Calvert SL. Toddlers' learning from socially meaningful video characters. *Media Psychol.* 2011;14(2):216−232.

39. Roseberry S, Hirsh-Pasek K, Golinkoff RM. Skype me! Socially contingent interactions help toddlers learn language. *Child Dev.* 2014;85(3):956−970.

40. Troseth GL, Saylor MM, Archer AH. Young Children's use of video as a source of socially relevant information. *Child Dev.* 2006;77(3):786−799.

41. Myers LJ, LeWitt RB, Gallo RE, Maselli NM. Baby FaceTime: can toddlers learn from online video chat? *Dev Sci.* 2016. https://doi.org/10.1111/desc.12430.

42. Moser A, Zimmermann L, Dickerson K, Grenell A, Barr R, Gerhardstein P. They can interact, but can they learn? Toddlers' transfer learning from touchscreens and television. *J Exp Child Psychol.* 2015;137:137−155.

43. Zack E, Barr R, Gerhardstein P, Dickerson K, Meltzoff AN. Infant imitation from television using novel touch screen technology. *Br J Dev Psychol.* 2009;27(1):13−26.

44. Anderson DR, Kirkorian HL. Media and cognitive development. In: Liben LS, Muller U, eds. *Handbook of Child Psychology and Developmental Science.* 7th ed. Vol. 2. Hoboken, NJ: John Wiley & Sons, Inc; 2015.

45. Barr R. Memory constraints on infant learning from picture books, television, and touchscreens. *Child Dev Perspect.* 2013;7(4):205−210.

46. Krcmar M, Grela B, Lin K. Can toddlers learn vocabulary from Television? An experimental approach. *Media Psychol.* 2007;10(1):41−63.

47. Zimmerman FJ, Christakis DA, Meltzoff AN. Associations between media viewing and language development in children under age 2 years. *J Pediatr.* 2007;151(4):364−368.

48. Richert RA, Robb MB, Fender JG, Wartella EA. Word learning from baby videos. *Arch Pediatr Adolesc Med.* 2010;164(5):432−437.

49. Robb MB, Richert RA, Wartella EA. Just a talking book? Word learning from watching baby videos. *Br J Dev Psychol.* 2009;27(1):27−45;

49a. Vandewater EA, Bickham DS, Lee JH, Cummings HM, Wartella EA, Rideout VJ. When the television is always on: heavy television exposure and young children's development. *Am Behav Sci.* 2005;48(5):562−577.

50. Kirkorian HL, Pempek TA, Murphy LA, Schmidt ME, Anderson DR. The impact of background television on parent: child interaction. *Child Dev.* 2009;80(5):1350−1359.

51. Zimmerman FJ, Gilkerson J, Richards JA, et al. Teaching by listening: the importance of adult-child conversations to language development. *Pediatrics.* 2009;124(1):342−349. https://doi.org/10.1542/peds.2008-2267.

52. Krcmar M, Cingel DP. Parent−child joint reading in traditional and electronic formats. *Media Psychol.* 2014;17(3):262−281.

53. Lauricella AR, Barr R, Calvert SL. Parent−child interactions during traditional and computer storybook reading for children's comprehension: implications for electronic storybook design. *Int J Child-Computer Interact.* 2014;2(1):17−25.

54. Beschorner B, Hutchison A. iPads as a literacy teaching tool in early childhood. *Int J Educ Math Sci Technol.* 2013;1(1):16−24.

55. Chiong C, Ree J, Takeuchi L, Erickson I. *Print Books vs. E-books: Comparing Parent-child co-reading on Print, Basic, and Enhanced E-book Platforms.* New York, NY: The Joan Ganz Cooney Center; 2012.

56. de Jong MT, Bus AG. How well suited are electronic books to supporting literacy? *J Early Child Lit.* 2003;3(2):147−164.

57. Reich SM, Yau JC, Warschauer M. Tablet-based eBooks for young children: what does the research say? *J Dev Behav Pediatr.* 2016;37(7):585−591.

58. Huber B, Tarasuik J, Antoniou MN, Garrett C, Bowe SJ, Kaufman J. Young children's transfer of learning from a touchscreen device. *Comput Hum Behav.* 2016;56:56−64;

58a. Aladé F, Lauricella AR, Beaudoin-Ryan L, Wartella E. Measuring with murray: touchscreen technology and preschoolers' STEM learning. *Comput in Hum Behav.* 2016;62:433−441.

59. Choi K, Kirkorian HL. Touch or watch to learn? Toddlers' object retrieval using contingent and noncontingent video. *Psychol Sci.* 2016;27(5):726−736.

60. Wai J, Lubinski D, Benbow CP. Spatial ability for STEM domains: aligning over 50 years of cumulative psychological knowledge solidifies its importance. *J Educ Psychol.* 2009;101(4):817–835.

61. Grancic I, Lobel A, Engels RC. The benefits of playing video games. *Am Psychol.* 2014;69(1):66–78.

62. Bandura A. *Self-efficacy: The Exercise of Control.* Macmillan; 1997.

63. Bandura A. Human agency in social cognitive theory. *Am Psychol.* 1989;44(9):1175.

64. Atkin C. Effects of realistic TV violence vs. fictional violence on aggression. *Journal Q.* 1983;60(4):615–621.

65. Paik H, Comstock G. The effects of television violence on antisocial behavior: a meta-analysis. *Commun Res.* 1994; 21(4):516–546;

65a. Martins N, Wilson BJ. Mean on the screen: social aggression in programs popular with children. *J Commun.* 2012; 62(6):991–1009.

66. Anderson CA, Bushman BJ. The general aggression model: an integrated social-cognitive model of human aggression. *Annu Rev Psychol.* 2002;53(l):27–51.

67. Anderson CA, Berkowitz L, Donnerstein E, et al. The influence of media violence on youth. *Psychol Sci Public Interest.* 2003;4(3):81–110.

68. Bushman BJ, Huesmann LR. Effects of televised violence on aggression. In: *Handbook of Children and the Media.* 2001:223–254.

69. Frost JL, Wortham SC, Reifel RS. *Play and Child Development.* Merrill: Prentice Hall; 2001.

70. Adachi PJ, Willoughby T. Demolishing the competition: the longitudinal link between competitive video games, competitive gambling, and aggression. *J Youth Adolesc.* 2013;42(7):1090–1104.

71. Ferguson CJ. Does media violence predict societal violence? It depends on what you look at and when. *J Commun.* 2015;65(1);

71a. Carnagey NL, Anderson CA, Bushman BJ. The effect of video game violence on physiological desensitization to real-life violence. *J Exp Soc Psychol.* 2007;43(3):489–496.

72. Anderson CA, Bushman BJ. Effects of violent video games on aggressive behavior, aggressive cognition, aggressive affect, physiological arousal, and prosocial behavior: a meta-analytic review of the scientific literature. *Psychol Sci.* 2001;12(5):353–359.

73. Ferguson CJ, Kilburn J. Much ado about nothing: the misestimation and overinterpretation of violent video game effects in Eastern and Western nations: comment on Anderson et al. (2010). *Psychol Bull.* 2010;136(2):174–178.

74. Gentile DA, Anderson CA, Yukawa S, et al. The effects of prosocial video games on prosocial behaviors: international evidence from correlational, longitudinal, and experimental studies. *Pers Soc Psychol Bull.* 2009;35(6):752–763.

75. Bushman B, Huesmann LR. Short-term and long-term effects of violent media on aggression in children and adults. *Arch Pediatr Adolesc Med Res.* 2006;160(2006): 340–352.

76. Galen BR, Underwood MK. A developmental investigation of social aggression among children. *Dev Psychol.* 1997;33(4):589.

77. Archer J, Coyne SM. An integrated review of indirect, relational, and social aggression. *Pers Soc Psychol Rev.* 2005; 9(3):212–230.

78. Martins N, Wilson BJ. Social aggression on television and its relationship to children's aggression in the classroom. *Hum Commun Res.* 2012;38(1):48–71.

79. Cantor J. The media and children's fears, anxieties, and perceptions of danger. In: *Handbook of Children and the Media.* 2001:207–221.

80. Friedrich LK, Stein AH. Aggressive and prosocial television programs and the natural behavior of preschool children. *Monogr Soc Res Child Dev.* 1973;38(4):1–64.

81. Cingel DP, Krcmar M. Prosocial television, preschool children's moral judgments, and moral reasoning: the role of social moral intuitions and perspective-taking. *Commun Res.* 2017. https://doi.org/10.1177/0093650217733846.

82. Fisch SM. *Children's learning from educational television: Sesame Street and beyond.* Routledge; 2014.

83. Mares ML, Woodard E. Positive effects of television on children's social interactions: a meta-analysis. *Media Psychol.* 2005;7(3):301–322.

84. Wartella E, Beaudoin-Ryan L, Blackwell CK, Cingel DP, Hurwitz LB, Lauricella AR. What kind of adults will our children become? The impact of growing up in a media-saturated world. *J Child Media.* 2016;10(1):13–20.

85. Wilson BJ. Media and children's aggression, fear, and altruism. *Future Child.* 2008;18(1):87–118;

85a. Mares ML, Acosta EE. Teaching inclusiveness via TV narratives in the US: young viewers need help with the message. *J Child Media.* 2010;4(3):231–247.

86. Mares ML, Acosta EE. Be kind to three-legged dogs: children's literal interpretations of TV's moral lessons. *Media Psychol.* 2008;11:377–399.

87. Richert RA, Shawber A, Hoffman R, Taylor M. Learning from fantasy and real characters in preschool and kindergarten. *J Cogn Dev.* 2009;10:1–26.

88. Strasburger VC, Hogan MJ, Mulligan DA, et al. Children, adolescents, and the media. *Pediatrics.* 2013;132(5):958–961;

88a. Fisch S, Truglio R. *G is for "growing": Thirty years of research on children and Sesame Street.* Mahweh, NJ: Lawrence Elbaum; 2001.

89. Shuler C. *Sesame Workshop and 9/11. The Joan Ganz Cooney Center Blog;* 2011. Retrieved from: http://www.joanganzcooneycenter.org/2011/09/12/sesame-workshop-and-911/.

90. Busis H. 'Sesame Street' to air hurricane special. *Entertain Wkly;* November 7, 2012. Retrieved from: http://ew.com/article/2012/11/07/sesame-street-hurricane-special/;

90a. Lobstein T, Jackson-Leach R, Moodie ML, Hall KD, Gortmaker SL, Swinburn BA, McPherson K. Child and adolescent obesity: part of a bigger picture. *The Lancet.* 2015;385(9986):2510–2520.

91. Buxton OM, Chang AM, Spilsbury JC, Bos T, Emsellem H, Knutson KL. Sleep in the modern family: protective family routines for child and adolescent sleep. *Sleep Health.* 2015;1(1):15–27.

92. Hale L, Guan S. Screen time and sleep among school-aged children and adolescents: a systematic literature review. *Sleep Med Rev.* 2015;21:50–58.

93. American Academy of Pediatrics Council on Communications and Media. Media and young minds. *Pediatrics*. 2016;138(5).

94. Calamaro CJ, Yang K, Ratcliffe S, Chasens ER. Wired at a young age: the effect of caffeine and technology on sleep duration and body mass index in school-aged children. *J Pediatr Health Care*. 2012;26(4):276–282.

95. Cespedes EM, Gillman MW, Kleinman K, Rifas-Shiman SL, Redline S, Taveras EM. Television viewing, bedroom television, and sleep duration from infancy to mid-childhood. *Pediatrics*. 2014;133(5):1163–1171.

96. Gradisar M, Wolfson AR, Harvey AG, Hale L, Rosenberg R, Czeisler CA. The sleep and technology use of Americans: findings from the National Sleep Foundation's 2011 Sleep in America poll. *J Clin Sleep Med*. 2013;9(12):1291–1299.

97. Strasburger VC. Children, adolescents, obesity, and the media. *Pediatrics*. 2011;128(1):201–208.

98. Rosen LD, Lim AF, Felt J, et al. Media and technology use predicts ill-being among children, preteens and teenagers independent of the negative health impacts of exercise and eating habits. *Comput Hum Behav*. 2014; 35:364–375.

99. Hingle M, Kunkel D. Childhood obesity and the media. *Pediatr Clin N Am*. 2012;59(3):677–692;

99a. Powell LM, Schermbeck RM, Szczypka G, Chaloupka FJ, Braunschweig CL. Trends in the nutritional content of television food advertisements seen by children in the United States: analyses by age, food categories, and companies. *Arch Pediatr Adolesc Med*. 2011;165(12): 1078–1086.

100. Straker L, Abbott R, Collins R, Campbell A. Evidence-based guidelines for wise use of electronic games by children. *Ergonomics*. 2014;57(4):471–489;

100a. Biddiss E, Irwin J. Active video games to promote physical activity in children and youth: a systematic review. *Arch Pediatr Adolesc Med*. 2010;164(7):664–672.

101. Staiano AE, Flynn R. Therapeutic uses of active videogames: a systematic review. *Games Health J*. 2014;3(6): 351–365.

102. Rideout V, Foehr U, Roberts D. *Generation M2: Media in the Lives of 8- to 18-year-olds*. Menlo Park, CA: Kaiser Family Foundation; 2010.

103. Olson CK. Sports videogames and real-world exercise. In: *Sports Videogames*. New York: Routledge; 2013:278–294.

104. Koller D, Goldman RD. Distraction techniques for children undergoing procedures: a critical review of pediatric research. *J Pediatr Nurs*. 2012;27(6):652–681.

105. Sinha M, Christopher NC, Fenn R, Reeves L. Evaluation of nonpharmacologic methods of pain and anxiety management for laceration repair in the pediatric emergency department. *Pediatrics*. 2006;117(4):1162–1168.

106. Shahid R, Benedict C, Mishra S, Mulye M, Guo R. Using iPads for distraction to reduce pain during immunizations. *Clin Pediatr*. 2015;54(2):145–148.

107. Whitehead-Pleaux AM, Baryza MJ, Sheridan RL. The effects of music therapy on pediatric patients' pain and anxiety during donor site dressing change. *J Music Ther*. 2006;43(2):136–153;

107a. Birnie KA, Noel M, Parker JA, Chambers CT, Uman LS, Kisely SR, McGrath PJ. Systematic review and meta-analysis of distraction and hypnosis for needle-related pain and distress in children and adolescents. *J Pediatr Psychol*. 2014;39(8):783–808;

107b. McQueen A, Cress C, Tothy A. Using a tablet computer during pediatric procedures: a case series and review of the "apps". *Pediatr emerg care*. 2012;28(7):712–714.

108. Lillard AS, Peterson J. The immediate impact of different types of television on young children's executive function. *Pediatrics*. 2011;128(4):644–649.

109. Nathanson AI, Alade F, Sharp ML, Rasmussen EE, Christy K. The relation between television exposure and executive function among preschoolers. *Dev Psychol*. 2014;50(5):1497–1506. https://doi.org/10.1037/a0035714.

110. Zimmerman FJ, Christakis DA. Associations between content types of early media exposure and subsequent attentional problems. *Pediatrics*. 2007;120(5):986–992.

111. Barr R, Lauricella AR, Zack E, Calvert SL. Infant and early childhood exposure to adult-directed and child-directed television programming: relations with cognitive skills at age four. *Merrill-Palmer Q*. 2010;56(1):21–48.

112. Christakis DA, Zimmerman FJ, DiGiuseppe DL, McCarty CA. Early television exposure and subsequent attentional problems in children. *Pediatrics*. 2004; 113(4):708–713.

113. Bioulac S, Arfi L, Bouvard MP. Attention deficit/hyperactivity disorder and video games: a comparative study of hyperactive and control children. *Eur Psychiatry*. 2008; 23(2):134–141.

114. Ferguson CJ, Ceranoglu TA. Attention problems and pathological gaming: resolving the 'chicken and egg' in a prospective analysis. *Psychiatr Q*. 2014;85(1): 103–110.

115. Ceranoglu TA. Inattention to problematic media use habits: interaction between digital media use and attention-deficit/hyperactivity disorder. *Child Adolesc Psychiatr Clin N Am*. 2018;27(2):183–191.

116. Robbins R. Could this be the first prescriptive video game? New data show it helps kids with ADHD. *Stat News*; December 4, 2017. Retrieved from: https://www.statnews.com/2017/12/04/adhd-video-game-akili/.

117. Raman S, Guerrero-Duby S, McCullough JL, et al. Screen exposure during daily routines and a young Child's risk for having social-emotional delay. *Clin Pediatr*. 2017. https://doi.org/10.1177/0009922816684600.

118. Mazurek MO, Wenstrup C. Television, video game and social media use among children with ASD and typically developing siblings. *J Autism Dev Disord*. 2013;43(6): 1258–1271.

119. Ringland KE, Wolf CT, Faucett H, Dombrowski L, Hayes GR. Will I always be not social?: re-conceptualizing sociality in the context of a minecraft community for autism. In: *Proceedings of the 2016 CHI Conference on Human Factors in Computing Systems*. ACM; 2016:1256–1269.

120. Ringland KE, Wolf CT, Dombrowski L, Hayes GR. Making Safe: community-centered practices in a virtual world dedicated to children with autism. In: *Proceedings of the 18th ACM Conference on Computer Supported Cooperative Work & Social Computing*. ACM; 2015:1788–1800.

121. Boyd LE, Ringland KE, Haimson OL, Fernandez H, Bistarkey M, Hayes GR. Evaluating a collaborative iPad game's impact on social relationships for children with autism spectrum disorder. *ACM Trans Access Comput (TACCESS)*. 2015;7(1):3.

122. O'Keeffe GS, Clarke-Pearson K. The impact of social media on children, adolescents, and families. *Pediatrics*. 2011;127(4):800–804.

123. Vygotsky LS. The problem of the environment. In: *The Vygotsky Reader*. 1994:338–354.

124. Fleer M. Digital role-play: the changing conditions of Children's play in preschool settings. *Mind Cult Activity*. 2017;24(1):3–17.

125. Lauricella AR, Blackwell CK, Wartella E. The "New" technology environment: the role of content and context on learning and development from mobile media. In: *Media Exposure During Infancy and Early Childhood*. Springer International Publishing; 2017:1–23.

126. Furlong J, Davies C. Young people, new technologies and learning at home: taking context seriously. *Oxf Rev Educ*. 2012;38(1):45–62.

2. Chahal H, Fung C, Kuhle S, Veugelers PJ. Availability and night-time use of electronic entertainment and communication devices are associated with short sleep duration and obesity among Canadian children. *Pediatr Obesity*. 2013; 8(1):42–51.

3. Fisch SM, Truglio RT, eds. *G Is for Growing: Thirty Years of Research on Children and Sesame Street*. Routledge; 2014.

4. Garrison MM, Liekweg K, Christakis DA. Media use and child sleep: the impact of content, timing, and environment. *Pediatrics*. 2011;128(1):29–35.

5. Huesmann LR, Moise-Titus J, Podolski CL, Eron LD. Longitudinal relations between children's exposure to TV violence and their aggressive and violent behavior in young adulthood: 1977–1992. *Dev Psychol*. 2003;39(2):201.

6. Mares ML, Acosta EE. Teaching inclusiveness via TV narratives in the US: Young viewers need help with the message. *J Child Media*. 2010;4(3):231–247.

7. Rideout V. The common sense census: media use by tweens and teens. *Common Sense Media*; November 3, 2015. Retrieved from: https://www.commonsensemedia.org/research.

8. Squires J, Bricker D, Twombly E. *The ASQ: SE user's guide: for the ages & stages questionnaires: social-emotional*. Paul H Brookes Publishing; 2002.

9. Takeuchi L, Stevens R. *The New Coviewing: Designing for Learning through Joint Media Engagement*. New York, NY: The Joan Ganz Cooney Center at Sesame Workshop; 2011.

10. Vandewater EA, Bickham DS, Lee JH, Cummings HM, Wartella EA, Rideout VJ. When the television is always on: heavy television exposure and young children's development. *Am Behav Sci*. 2005;48(5):562–577.

FURTHER READING

1. Anderson JA. The production of media violence and aggression research: a cultural analysis. *Am Behav Sci*. 2008;51(8): 1260–1279.

CHAPTER 17

Use of Digital Media for Self-Expression in Children and Adolescents

ELVIRA PEREZ VALLEJOS, PHD

INTRODUCTION

The Internet is frequently held to transform social relationships, the economy, vast areas of public and private life across all ages, and, probably very soon, across all cultures. Such arguments are often recycled in popular debates, sensational tabloid news materials, and indeed in academic contexts as well. Research discussions on the topic of the Internet oscillate between celebration and fear, where on the one hand, technology is seen to create new forms of community and civic life and to offer immense resources for personal liberation and participation, while on the other, it poses dangers to privacy, creates new forms of inequality and commercial exploitation, in addition to increasing individual exposure to addiction triggers, abuse, and other forms of harm.

These kinds of ideas about the impact of technology tend to take on an even greater force when they are combined with ideas of childhood, youth, and well-being. The debate about the impact of media and technology on children has always served as a focus for much broader hopes and fears about social change. On the one hand, there is a powerful discourse about the ways in which digital technology is threatening or even destroying childhood. Young people are seen to be at risk, not only from more obvious dangers such as pornography and online pedophiles but also from a wide range of negative physical and psychological consequences that derive from their engagement with technology. Like television, digital media are seen to be responsible for a whole range of social ills— addiction, antisocial behavior, eating disorders, educational underperformance, commercial exploitation, depression, envy, and so on.

In recent years, however, the debate has come to be dominated by a very different argument. Unlike those who express regret about the media's destruction of childhood innocence, advocates of the new "digital generation" regard technology as a force of liberation and self-expression for young people—a means for them to reach past the constraining influence of previous generations and to create new, autonomous forms of communication and community. Far from corrupting the young, technology is seen to be creating a generation that is more open, more democratic, more creative, and more innovative than that of their parents.

Taking into account both the risks and opportunities associated with the Internet and digital technologies, this chapter considers the unavoidable dialectical in which the Internet is both socially shaped and socially shaping. In other words, by studying the way in which the Internet is utilized, we gain insights into its overall role and impact, but we also uncover its inherent constraints and limitations which are in turn largely shaped by the social and economic interests of those who control its production, circulation, and distribution. Understanding the values and ideas that are encoded in and promoted through the structure and use of the Internet is essential for successfully managing the social, economic, psychological, and cultural effects that it generates.

INTERNET SAFETY

At present, there appears to be little robust research evidence that compares the success of available Internet safety programs, or examines what materials or educational approaches are cost-effective, and how programs are being implemented in the community. Outcome evaluations have been limited in sophistication, and so far current results show little evidence that Internet safety programs reduce risky online behaviors or prevent negative experiences. On the contrary, studies have indicated that while children within test groups are able to retain the extra knowledge presented to them, the learning has been found to have little impact on children's online behavior.[1]

In response to increasing concerns about the extent to which Internet activities put children and young people at risk from sexual and psychological abuse, numerous Internet safety educational materials including online guidelines, tools, and advice for parents and teachers have been developed with the intention of minimizing such risks. Internet safety, however, appears to have more in common with risk prevention programs than programs aiming to promote digital rights among children and young people. For example, Internet victimisation risk factors, such as rule-breaking behavior, mental health issues, and social isolation, are very similar to the risk factors for so many other youth behavioral problems.[2–6]

Therefore, interventions aiming to promote digital literacy among children and young people may consider backing activities that have already been shown to reduce related risk factors.[1] While prevention and promotion interventions may have similar goals such as reducing cyberbullying or sexual exploitation, some important differences arise when focusing on the risks rather than on the opportunities that Internet can bring. Using the Internet can be a very healthy and rewarding activity as well as a potentially dangerous and unhealthy experience; it all depends on the user's awareness, knowledge, and intentions.

Livingstone[7] suggests that risk, harm, and vulnerability in children online can be researched by building on the literature for offline risk in children. Assessing risk and harm on the Internet, however, is particularly challenging because calculating the incidence rates of, for example, children being exposed to abuse online and the actual harm resulting from these hostile online encounters can be difficult. Indeed, there are no objectively verified and accurate statistics about how many children are exposed to inappropriate content, and therefore what is usually being reported is the "risk of the risk" that might result in harm, which may be completely disproportionate as not all risk results in harm.

At present, the literature regarding online harm is sparse, making it difficult to understand whether a risk results in harm or how the Internet plays a role in known harm. Clearly, the situation regarding online risk is quite different from offline risk, however, it has been documented that children who are vulnerable offline are also more likely to be at risk online.[8,9] Further understanding of the risk and protective factors that mediate the relationship between online and offline risk and harm seems mandatory, especially when considering a sociotechnological context that is in constant change where the use of the Internet is widely spread among children and young people, creating new interactions between risk and protective factors.

For example, a recent systematic review of the effect of online communication and social media on young people's well-being[10] has showed contradictory evidence, indicating that the Internet acts merely as a facilitator of human interaction and is itself value-free, neither promoting the good nor the bad. The findings from this review showed that online communication that allows young people to increase the size and composition of their social networks can be either beneficial, because it can increase social support and social capital, or harmful through increased likelihood of exposure to abuse content or promotion of maladaptive coping strategies, such as self-harm.[11] Taking these findings into consideration, strategies to support the well-being of young people may wish to focus on the particular application being used, the communicative and noncommunicative activities taking place, and the social support available offline to that individual to manage potential harm.

Due to the inevitable relation between humans and the digital world, it is more important than ever before that children and young people are familiar and confident with computers and technologies, not only because technology-related skills will optimize their future job opportunities but also because it promotes digital equalities and participation in society.[12] Therefore, it is vital that children are taught the benefits of new technologies and the associated risks but without frightening them or focusing too much on the risks associated with modern-day issues such as pornography, "trolling," "sexting," cyberbullying, and so on. For example, if we look back at previous research on youth prevention of substance misuse, we will find evidence showing that frightening messages do little to modify young people's risky or undesirable behavior.[13]

Recent evaluations and systematic reviews of Internet safety programs showed that while participants can retain messages as indicated in follow-up questionnaires, there is little apparent impact on participants' behavior.[14–18] There are several critical lessons to be learnt from previous research on prevention science that could guide new Internet safety educational materials. Recommendations include the development of interventions around strategies that are evidence-based and grounded in theory, meaning that the intervention explicitly defines why and how it is effective, indicating the social, behavioral, and communication theories from which such strategies have been developed.

According to the literature,[19,20] effective prevention programs target actual versus perceived risks factors.

For example, there is evidence to support that most young online sex crime victims are aware of the age difference of their perpetrator before meeting them face to face,[21] therefore educating young people about age deception is not as relevant as to provide education about judgment on sexual correspondence. Similarly, understanding risks and protective factors may help us understand who is actually vulnerable and avoid alarmist public perceptions that all children are "at risk," consequently increasing the media panic that results in demands to restrict children's Internet access, increase surveillance, or violate data protection and online freedom.

Prevention programs are most effective when they are integrated into school curricula, implemented consistently, and delivered by trained educators.[22,23] Extracurricular activities, however, are often perceived as more flexible and dynamic than activities within the national curriculum, which could prevent innovative activities from becoming a "program" ending up being bureaucratized and eventually fossilized. Understanding the relationship between young people and the Internet is crucial for designing effective interventions that promote not only the technical knowledge and skills necessary to successfully operate digital devices but also a number of other aspects.

For instance, interventions could be designed to cover the cognitive and social skills necessary to recognize and integrate new models of social interaction (e.g., Facebook) and develop emotional intelligence to deal with the affective feedback from online interaction (e.g., Twitter). Interventions should also acknowledge alternative views and cultures and adapting to them (e.g., online forums), adjust self-control and self-awareness to manage time spent online (e.g., online gaming), recognize and address new types of malign intention (e.g., online grooming), adapt from a close, individual-based model of learning and creation to one based on collectively sourced collaboration (e.g., crowdsourcing), and so on. In this chapter, the concept of *digital literacy for self-expression* takes the humanities approach to consider the social skills and cultural competencies required to enabling participation within the new media culture.

According to Jenkins et al.,[24] there are three main problems that any digital literacy program should address: the first issue tackles the inequalities in young people's access not only to new media technology and the Internet but also to skills and content that is most beneficial (i.e., what they call the participatory gap). The second issue focuses on the transparency problem or the potential commercial interests that may influence online decisions. This problem becomes apparent when analyzing the advertising practices displayed on online gaming or the dangers of blending false or inaccurate information from facts. This is especially relevant when taking into consideration results from a systematic review on how children make sense of online resources, showing a lack of both knowledge and interest in assessing how information was produced.[25] The third challenge focuses on the ethics or how to encourage young people to become more reflective about the ethical choices that they make online, and the potential impact on others. The ethics challenge is linked to digital citizenship and relates to the content young people post online, the content they access to (e.g., adult content), and compliance with implicit/explicit online community rules. These three issues (i.e., participatory gap, transparency, and ethics) are central themes developed and dramatized in the Youth Juries. These three problems related to the Right to Agency, the Right to Know, and the Right to Digital Literacy are described further below.

Finally, experts on prevention science[1] have also pointed out that creative and multifaceted approaches involving peers, parents, teachers, and the general public on either generic awareness campaigns or more specific/targeted training is also desirable.

YOUTH JURIES

This section briefly describes the Youth Juries, a new methodological approach for the promotion of well-being through self-expression among children and young people. These juries take into consideration all the cumulative evidence and recommendations on online risk and protective factors, including the fuzzy links between risk, harm, and vulnerability, the need for a theoretical context, known predictors for successful prevention programs such as implementation and delivery, the issues that literacy programs should address, and who to involve in such programs.

Juries

This section presents an innovative methodology to bring people together and facilitate reflection upon the issue of online self-expression. What we are calling juries are similar to focus groups, but unlike many focus groups, juries have an explicit objective of arriving at clear recommendations regarding digital rights. Using the terminology "juries" is an important decision, as it is to be hoped that participants will subsequently feel a sense of responsibility as decision makers and facilitate participation and discussion.

How the jury is delivered and implemented is also extremely important, not only because the juries should be replicable and participants' outputs should not depend on the personal attributes of the facilitator or educator but also because explicit training, guidelines, and processes are in place and a sense of ownership, responsibility, and care are also part of the training. For example, understanding the current evidence on online risks and protective factors is important to ensuring that accurate information and facts are discussed during the deliberation process.

It has been consistently shown that interactive programs with skills training offered over multiple sessions outperform noninteractive, lecture-based, one-shot programs.[19,26] Currently, our juries are highly interactive and the scripts developed to dramatize the scenarios have been co-produced with young people to explore their personal concerns and online experiences. When co-producing scenarios with young people, we are enhancing engagement opportunities, making these more real, easier to relate to, and, consequently, maximizing youth involvement in discussions.

The aim of our juries is not only to find out what participants (i.e., the "jurors") think and feel about the experiences of the digital world and how these may affect their sense of well-being but also to discover what shapes their thinking and whether they are open to changing their minds in the light of discussion with peers or exposure to new information. In order to explore such questions, we are interested in discussing (1) the reasons that jury members give for adopting particular perspectives and positions and (2) the extent to which participants' perspectives and positions change, individually and collectively, between their arrival on the jury session and their departure. The jury session is typically lead by a trained facilitator, whose task is to provide a safe space for participants to express themselves freely and critically while demystifying issues around technology and well-being, data privacy, informed consent, and so on.

Vignettes

The use of dramatic scenarios builds upon the methodological research tradition of using *vignettes* as prompts to elicit reflective responses from participants. Vignettes are more frequently used in applied drama within educational settings, which has a long tradition and for which there is extensive evidence on the underlying social, cognitive, and emotional processes associated to applied drama for facilitating learning and development.[27–29]

Bloor and Wood[30] define vignettes as: "A technique used in structured and in-depth interviews as well as focus groups, providing sketches of fictional (or fictionalized) scenarios. The respondent is then invited to imagine, drawing on her own experience, how the central character in the scenario will behave. Vignettes thus elicit situated data on individual or group values, beliefs and norms of behaviour. While in structured interviews respondents must choose from a multiple-choice menu of possible answers to a vignette, as used in in-depth interviews and focus groups, vignettes act as a stimulus to extended discussion of the scenario in question."(pp. 183).

While the format of vignette presentation can vary including short video clip presentation and live acting, its aims and objectives are usually the same: to facilitate discussion, reflection, and deliberation amongst a group of young people (e.g., in this case, the jury) that may develop new attitudes, opinions, and interpretations about their digital rights and therefore the potential benefit and harm associated with specific online activities. Vignettes can take several forms, and their development and administration should always protect the research participants, especially when sensitive issues are being presented.[31] Usually vignettes are short stories that are read out loud to participants. Some researchers have used film and music, while others have used interactive Web content or live acting, with its value deriving from combining the stimulus of the vignette method with the liveness and indeterminacy of the applied drama/theatre-in-education tradition.

The interpretation of responses to the scenarios entails complex analysis, involving the need to be clear about what we think responses represent, the extent to which there is a relationship between expressed beliefs and actions, the possibility that some participants might have felt under pressure to "give the right answer," and the degree of consistency between post-scenario comments and broader findings from the group session tapes and transcripts.[32,33]

Vignettes have been used by researchers from a range of disciplines, including scholars studying public acceptance of mentally ill residents within a community,[34] multicultural integration in neighborhoods,[35] the neglect and abuse of elderly people,[36] and early onset dementia.[37] Vignettes have proved to be particularly useful in eliciting reflective responses from groups of young people: Barter and Renold[38] used them very successfully in their research with young people exploring violence in residential children's homes; Conrad[39] used vignettes as a way of talking to young rural Canadians about what they considered to be "risky activity"; Yungblut et al.[40] used them in their work with adolescent girls to explore their lived experiences of physical exercise; and Bradbury-Jones et al.[41] employed vignettes to explore children's experiences of domestic abuse. To date we are not aware of any published research using vignettes to promote digital literacy.

Youth Juries

This chapter follows a series of Youth Juries held in three United Kingdom cities including 12 young people per session aged 12–17 years and from diverse socioeconomic backgrounds. Participant as well as parental consent was obtained prior to participation. These juries illustrate the "improvised drama" element of a piece of research lead by iRights,[42] a new civil society initiative that is working to create a future where all young people have the fundamental right to access the digital world "creatively, knowledgeably and fearlessly." The juries were developed and co-produced with young people in collaboration with the SHM Foundation, the University of Leeds, and the University of Nottingham to explore five predefined digital rights and their implications with juries of young people. There was no restriction on the content used for the juries. The following are the five digital rights covered:

1. The Right to Remove: "Every child and young person under 18 should have the right to easily edit or delete any and all content they themselves have created. It must be right for under 18s to own content they have created, and to have an easy and clearly signposted way to retract, correct and dispute online data that refers to them."

2. The Right to Know: "Children and young people have the right to know who is holding or profiting from their information, what their information is being used for and whether it is being copied, sold or traded. It must be right that children and young people are only asked to hand over personal data when they have the capacity to understand they are doing so and what their decision means. It must also be right that terms and conditions aimed at young people are written so that typical minors can easily understand them."

3. The Right to Safety and Support: "Children and young people should be confident that they will be protected from illegal practices and supported if confronted by troubling or upsetting scenarios online. It must be right that children and young people receive an age-appropriate, comparable level of adult protection, care and guidance in the online space as in the offline. And that all parties contribute to common safety and support frameworks easily accessible and understandable by young people."

4. The Right to Make Informed and Conscious Decisions (The Right to Agency): "Children and young people should be free to reach into creative and participatory places online, using digital technologies as tools, but at the same time have the capacity to disengage at will. It must be right that the commercial considerations used in designing software should be balanced against the needs and requirements of children and young people to engage and disengage during a developmentally sensitive period of their lives. It must also be right that safety software does not needlessly restrict access to the Internet's creative potential."

5. The Right to Digital Literacy: "To access the knowledge that the Internet can deliver, children and young people need to be taught the skills to use and critique digital technologies, and given the tools to negotiate changing social norms. Children and young people should have the right to learn how to be digital makers as well as intelligent consumers, to critically understand the structures and syntax of the digital world, and to be confident in managing new social norms. To be a 21st century citizen, children and young people need digital capital."

During these Youth Juries, participants put the Internet on trial by deliberating on a series of real-life digital scenarios, previously produced in partnership with young people and brought to life by live actors. To work in equal partnership with children and young people is relevant to further develop the Youth Juries and ensure vignettes present real issues and experiences to which young people can relate to and maximize their ecological validity. Working with young people as equal partners is also important to guarantee that the language used to dramatize the scenarios resonates with their vocabulary and expressions. Because scenarios have to be co-produced with local young people, vignettes are idiosyncratic and sensitive to cultural differences as they should represent a specific and distinct point in time, avoiding universalistic terms. In this way, the scenarios developed for this first wave of Youth Juries will differ from those developed in the near future as smartphone applications, computer games, and lexicon around technologies rapidly evolve with time.

In relation to the three main problems outlined by Jenkins et al. (i.e., participatory gap, transparency, and ethics), our juries have been designed to promote social skills and cultural competencies through dialog, collaboration, and discussion. The juries offer objective information about data privacy issues and a space for reflection to develop critical-analysis skills on how media shapes perceptions of the word. The dilemmas or conflicts that the scenarios bring to life include an element of reflection on the negative as well as the positives exhibited on the Internet. These dilemmas also encourage young people to pull knowledge and reconcile conflicting information to form a coherent picture. This is a form of problem solving valuable in shaping all kinds of relationships (e.g., knowledge, community, tools, etc.).

The presence of live actors added a realistic dimension to the deliberation process and served to highlight key themes and issues by bringing them to life and stimulating discussions. This could be considered a form of simulation, encouraging young people to interpret and construct models of real-world processes. As the dramatized scenarios are highly dynamic, allowing space for improvisation and interaction between actors and participants, young people can formulate hypotheses of "what is going to happen next," test different variables in real time, and modify or refine their interpretation of the "real world" while engaging them in a process of modeling (i.e., learning that takes place in a social context through observation). It is well known[43] that students learn more through direct observation and experimentation than simply by reading text books, or listening in the classroom setting. Simulations not only broaden the kinds of experiences students may have but also bring capacities to understand problems from multiple perspectives, to assimilate and respond to new information.

These juries are embedded in a research process designed to explore online self-expression and their implications with juries of young people. Specifically, the research project has been designed to capture reflections on (1) their experiences of anxiety, uncertainty, frustration, and aspiration in using digital technologies, (2) their understanding of who "runs" the Internet, who polices it, what "it" is, and how far they feel they can control their digital experiences, (3) their sense of their own digital literacy and its limitations, (4) their responses to new information about the Internet and digital technologies, (5) the relevance and effectiveness of specific digital rights (see below) in relation to such experience, (6) appropriate language and techniques for sharing and disseminating digital rights, and (7) ways of further engaging young people in thinking about the use of digital media for self-expression.

Future Youth Jury developments should incorporate skills training over multiple sessions. For example, if a scenario focuses on the "right to know," a more hands-on session or workshop could focus on how to avoid third-party tracking cookies designed to compile long-term records of individuals' browsing histories. Skills training could complement the deliberation process on potential privacy concerns that cookies represent when storing passwords and sensitive information, such as credit card numbers and addresses. Ideally, juries should be offered on more than one session and present a repertoire of scenarios that have been co-produced with a local representative sample of children and young people to illustrate up-to-date and culturally relevant online youth concerns and celebrations. The core measures used within the current study included semi-structured interviews and questionnaires completed before and after the jury, designed to assess attitudinal changes.

OPEN EDUCATIONAL RESOURCE

In addition to helping researchers interested in how young people consider their online lives, the Youth Juries are a valuable tool for engagement, increasing awareness and giving young people agency to influence their online lives. As such, it is valuable for others, for example, teachers and youth workers, to be able to use this method to run Youth Juries with their own groups. To this end, an online open educational resource has been developed, detailing the method and providing downloadable versions of suggested jury scenarios. This resource can be found at https://oer.horizon.ac.uk/.

This method of deliberation—space for participants to express, compare, and make sense of their views and experiences—is expected to generate thoughts among the jurors for critical and reflective thinking about digital rights with the view to modify undesirable behavior and promote well-being.

To conclude, this method of deliberation fosters self-expression in adolescents, allowing and promoting young people to reflectively present themselves. This act can be beneficial in revealing insights and new perspectives into the self-concept of young people and positively influence psychological processes and development.

ACKNOWLEDGMENTS

This work forms part of the Citizen-centric Approaches to Social Media Analysis (CaSMa) project, supported by Economic and Social Research Council (ESRC) grant ES/M00161X/1 and based at the Horizon Digital Economy Research Institute, University of Nottingham. For more information about the CaSMa project, please see http://casma.wp.horizon.ac.uk/. Elvira Perez Vallejos acknowledges the financial support of the Nottingham Biomedical Research Centre (NIHR).

REFERENCES

1. Jones LM. The future of Internet safety education: critical lessons from four decades of youth drug abuse prevention. *Pubios Proj*; 2010. http://publius.cc/printpdf/future_internet_safety_education_critical-lessons_four_decades_youth_drug_abuse_prevention (page-1). Accessed 11.06.2018.

2. Stice E, Shaw H, Bohon C, Marti CN, Rohde P. A meta-analytic review of depression prevention programs for children and adolescents: factors that predict magnitude of intervention effects. *J Consult Clin Psychol*. 2009;77(3): 486−503. https://doi.org/10.1037/A0015168.

3. Skiba D, Monroe J, Wodarski JS. Adolescent substance use: reviewing the effectiveness of prevention strategies. *Soc Work*. 2004;49(3):343−353.

4. Durlak JA, Wells AM. Primary prevention mental health programs: the future is exciting. *Am J Community Psychol*. 1997;25(2):233−243. https://doi.org/10.1023/A:10246 74631189.

5. Wells M, Mitchell KJ. How do high-risk youth use the Internet? Characteristics and implications for prevention. *Child Maltreat*. 2008;13(3):227−234. https://doi.org/10.117 7/1077559507312962.

6. Durlak JA. Common risk and protective factors in successful prevention programs. *Am J Orthopsychiatry*. 1998; 68(4):512−520. https://doi.org/10.1037/H0080360.

7. Livingstone S. E-Youth:(future) policy implications: reflections on online risk, harm and vulnerability. In: *Proceedings at the e-Youth: balancing between opportunities and risk (Antwerp, Belgium 27-28 May 2010)*. UCSIA & MIOS; 2010. http://eprints.lse.ac.uk/27849.

8. Livingstone S, Haddon L, Görzig A, eds. *Children, Risk and Safety Online: Research and Policy Challenges in Comparative Perspective*. Bristol: The Policy Press; 2012.

9. Bradbrook G, Alvi I, Fisher J, et al. *Meeting Their Potential: The Role of Education and Technology in Overcoming Disadvantage and Disaffection in Young People*. Coventry: Becta; 2008.

10. Best P, Manktelow R, Taylor B. Online communication, social media and adolescent wellbeing: a systematic narrative review. *Child Youth Serv Rev*. 2014;41:27−36. https://doi.org/10.1016/j.childyouth.2014.03.001.

11. Duggan M, Brenner J. *The Demographics of Social Media Users*. Pew Internet Research Centre's Internet and American Life Project; 2013. http://pewInternet.org/Reports/2013/Social-media-users.aspx.

12. Mossberger K, Tolbert C, McNeal R. *Digital Citizenship*. MIT Press; 2007.

13. Lynam DR, Milich R, Zimmerman R, et al. Project DARE: No effects at 10-year follow-up. *J Consult Clin Psychol*. 1999;67(4):590−593.

14. Dresler-Hawke E, Whitehead D. The behavioral ecological model as a framework for school-based anti-bullying health promotion interventions. *J Sch Nurs*. 2009;25(3):105−204. https://doi.org/10.1177/1059840509334364.

15. Chibnall S, Wallace M, Leicht C, Lunghofer L. *I-SAFE Evaluation: Final Report*. Fairfax, Virginia: Caliber; 2006.

16. Brookshire M, Maulhardt C. *Evaluation of the Effectiveness of the NetSmartz Program: A Study of Maine Public Schools*. Washington, DC: The George Washington University; 2005.

17. Crombie G, Trinneer A. *Children and Internet Safety: An Evaluation of the Missing Program. A Report to the Research and Evaluation Section of the National Crime Preventure Centre of Justice Canada*. Ottawa: University of Ottawa; 2003.

18. Shillair R, Cotten SR, Tsai HYS, Alhabash S, LaRose R, Rifon NJ. Online safety begins with you and me: convincing Internet users to protect, themselves. *Comput Hum Behav*. 2015;48:199−207. https://doi.org/10.1016/j.chb.2015.01.046.

19. Bond LA, Carmola Hauf AM. Taking stock and putting stock in primary prevention: characteristics of effective programs. *J Prim Prev*. 2004;24(3):199−221.

20. Winters KC, Fawkes T, Fahnhorst T, Botzet A, Augsut G. A synthesis review of exemplary drug abuse prevention programs in the United States. *J Subst Abuse Treat*. 2007; 32:371−380. https://doi.org/10.1016/j.jsat.2006.10.002.

21. Wolak J, Finkelhor D, Mitchell KJ, Ybarra ML. Online "Predators" and their victims - myths, realities, and implications for prevention and treatment. *Am Psychol*. 2008;63(2): 111−128. https://doi.org/10.1037/0003-066x.63.2.111.

22. Durlak JA, DuPre EP. Implementation matters: a review of research on the influence of implementation on program outcomes and the factors affecting implementation. *Am J Community Psychol*. 2008;41(3−4):327−350. https://doi.org/10.1007/s10464-008-9165-0.

23. Payne AA, Eckert R. The relative importance of provider, program, school, and community predictors of the implementation of quality of school-based prevention programs. *Soc Prev Res*. 2009:1−16.

24. Jenkins H, Purushotma R, Weigel M, Clinton K, Robison. *A Confronting the Challenges of Participatory Culture. Media Education for the 21st Century*. MIT Press; 2009.

25. Buckingham D. *The Media Literacy of Children and Young People: A Review of the Literature*. Centre for the Study of Children, Youth and Media, Institute of Education, University of London; 2005. http://www.ofcom.org.uk/advice/media_literacy/medlitpub/medlitpubrss/ml_children.pdf.

26. Ennett ST, Tobler NS, Ringwalt CL, Flewelling RL. How effective is drug abuse resistance education? A metaanalysis of project DARE outcome evaluations. *Am J Public Health*. 1994;84(9):1394−1401.

27. Tombak A. Importance of drama in pre-school education. In: *3rd Cyprus International Conference on Educational Research (Cy-Icer 2014)*. Vol. 143. 2014:372−378. https://doi.org/10.1016/j.sbspro.2014.07.497.

28. Winston J. Imagining the real: towards a new theory of drama in education. *Br J Educ Stud*. 2015;63(2):252−254. https://doi.org/10.1080/00071005.2015.1035913.

29. Burn A. Drama education with digital technology. *Engl Educ*. 2011;45(1):104−106. https://doi.org/10.1111/j.1754-8845.2010.01086.x.

30. Bloor M, Wood F. *Keywords in Qualitative Methods: A Vocabulary of Research Concept*. London: Sage Publications Ltd; 2006.

31. Bradbury-Jones C, Taylor J, Herber OR. Vignette development and administration: a framework for protecting research participants. *Int J Soc Res Methodol*. 2014;17(4):427−440. https://doi.org/10.1080/13645579.2012.750833.

32. Barter C, Renold R. The use of vignettes in qualitative research. *Soc Res Update*. 1999;25. http://sru.soc.surrey.ac.uk/SRU25.html.

33. Finch J. The vignette technique in survey research. *Sociology*. 1987;21(2):105–114.

34. Aubry TD, Tefft B, Currie RF. Public-attitudes and intentions regarding tenants of community mental-health residences who are neighbours. *Community Ment Health J*. 1995; 31(1):39–52. https://doi.org/10.1007/Bf02188979.

35. Schuman H, Bobo L. Survey-based experiments on white racial-attitudes toward residential integration. *Am J Sociol*. 1998;94(2):273–299. https://doi.org/10.1086/228992.

36. Rahman N. Caregivers' sensitivity to conflict: the use of the vignette methodology. *J Elder Abuse Negl*. 1996;8(1): 35–47. https://doi.org/10.1300/J084v08n01_02.

37. Smythe A, Bentham P, Jenkins C, Oyebode JR. The experiences of staff in a specialist mental health service in relation to development of skills for the provision of person centred care for people with dementia. *Dementia-Int J Soc Res Pract*. 2015;14(2):184–198. https://doi.org/10.1177/1471301213494517.

38. Barter C, Renold E. 'I wanna tell you a story': exploring the application of vignettes in qualitative research with children and young people. *Int J Soc Res Methodol*. 2000; 3(4):307–323.

39. Conrad M. Family life and sociability in upper and lower Canada, 1780–1870. A view from diaries and family correspondence. *Rev Hist Am Fr*. 2004;58(1):124–126.

40. Yungblut HE, Schinke RJ, McGannon KR. Views of adolescent female youth on physical activity during early adolescence. *J Sports Sci Med*. 2012;11(1):39–50.

41. Bradbury-Jones C, Taylor J, Kroll T, Duncan F. Domestic abuse awareness and recognition among primary healthcare professionals and abused women: a qualitative investigation. *J Clin Nurs*. 2014;23(21–22):3057–3068. https://doi.org/10.1111/Jocn.12534.

42. www.iRights.uk.

43. Gaba D. Human work environment and simulators. In: Miller RD, ed. *In Anaesthesia*. 5th ed. Churchill Livingstone; 1999:18–26.

Index

Note: Page numbers followed by "f" indicate figures and "t" indicate tables.

Printed in the United States
By Bookmasters